FRONT END, OR BACK?

Published by

Librario Publishing Ltd

ISBN: 1-904440-59-2

Copies can be ordered via the Internet
www.librario.com

or from:

Brough House, Milton Brodie, Kinloss
Moray IV36 2UA
Tel /Fax No 00 44 (0)1343 850 617

Printed and bound by Digisource GB Ltd

Front End, Or Back?

A Year in the Life of a Small Animal Vet

Claire Poole

Librario

Chapter 1

The first day of the new century – indeed of the new millennium – dawns reassuringly normally. Power and telephones are still functioning, and the only millennium bugs so far seem to be those bothering our dogs. For the last hour there has been much scratching and nibbling, but this may just be disgruntlement at our attempts to have a slightly long lie. Giving up, I let them out and dole out their breakfast. The cattle at the farm are also shouting for their food. Animals do not know that it is the day after Hogmanay, and all of Scotland is deep in slumber. I could have cheerfully slept longer, but have to get up anyway, as there is a patient in the surgery to be checked.

I should at this point explain who I am. My name is Claire Poole and I am a single-handed vet based in the village of Clayfern on the border of the Scottish Highlands. I only deal with small animals, that is – household pets such as dogs, cats, rabbits and other small furries. Every morning and evening during the week, and on Saturday mornings, I drive to Clayfern where I hold an hour's surgery. The rest of my working day is spent in the surgery attached to my home – a cottage on Fern Farm, four miles from Clayfern. I live here with my partner Jay, and our two dogs, Kippen, an old hairy boy of indeterminate ancestry, and Fintry, the youngster, a sleek but wimpy black Labrador bitch. The festive season this year has been refreshingly peaceful, and Jay and I have enjoyed a relaxing interlude with our families – unlike last year, when seasonal revelling had to be fitted in between a flurry of epidemics and emergencies. However, into every life a little rain must fall, and I should have realised that we would be unlikely to get through an entire holiday period without *some* timely interruption from the surgery. The little cat in the surgery proves my point.

Jay's brother and family were due to arrive here yesterday to join in our New Millennium celebrations, and I was hurriedly doing last minute shopping after morning surgery in Clayfern when my pager went off, shaking me rudely out of holiday mode.

Ten minutes later, a twitching, jerking cat was on the consulting table at Clayfern surgery, barely restrained by her distraught owner. There was no clue as to what had befallen her – when she had asked out at 1 a.m., she had been perfectly normal, but had just been found under a bush by her owner. With some difficulty, I carried out an examination, mentally running through the various possibilities. In the absence of any sign of injury or trauma, poisoning seemed a possibility, but which poison? There was no increased salivation, which tended to rule out organophosphorus poisoning, and her temperature was below normal.

My brain gradually compared the cat's symptoms with the knowledge of common poisonous materials stored in its data banks and came up with the most probable diagnosis – *Alphachloralose poisoning*. *Alphachloralose* is a rodenticide, and Rosie could have been poisoned either by eating the bait directly or in a poisoned mouse. Her tearful owner confirmed that Rosie was indeed a hunter.

Confirmation of a suspicion is seldom achieved in veterinary poisonings – for this, analysis of either blood or stomach contents is required, and by the time the results return, the victim is either better or dead. Luckily, vets are familiar with the symptoms of the more common poisons, and can usually treat as necessary. There are seldom exact antidotes to animal substance abuse, and this is the case with *alphachloralose*, so my only course of action was to treat the symptoms and hope for the best. I administered a sedative, swathed Rosie in bubble wrap to conserve body heat, and put her in a basket with a hot water bottle for the trip to the farm surgery. Jay and I live four miles from Clayfern on Fern Farm, and the surgery is attached to the side of the house. While most consultations are carried out in Clayfern, all surgical cases and in-patients are brought to Fern.

Our visitors had arrived early – before Jay returned from work – and greeted me as I drew up outside our cottage. Oh, the opposing demands of family and work. There were hurried greetings and explanations with the newcomers before I vanished into the surgery with Rosie. Luckily, our friends and relatives are used to our oddball veterinary lifestyle, and this lot were not disconcerted in the least. They took in their own luggage and made their own cups of tea.

Meanwhile, I increased the heating in the surgery, and prepared equipment for an intravenous drip.

Normally, it would not be possible to single-handedly insert a canula into a cat's vein, and I would need to call out Julie, my faithful nurse, but this one was refreshingly easy – having a flat-out patient had its advantages. My plan was to maintain Rosie on a drip to aid elimination of the poison from the body, keep her warm to counteract the hypothermia associated with alphachloralose and keep her sedated to prevent the tremors. Time just flies by while attending to such an emergency, so it was lucky the visitors were there to prepare lunch! Some holiday for them.

The cat was stable after a while, and could be left for short spells. This was fortunate, as I had a vital mission for the afternoon – the placing of the clues for a New Year's Day treasure hunt. This was to be the high spot of the kids' visit, so it had to be done. Trudging through the woods with assorted signs and props, I felt slightly disgruntled – it should have been a pleasure, not a chore to be rushed through in between cat checks. However I relaxed as it took shape and began to enjoy myself. The treasure was to be found in 'The Beast of Fern's Lair.' Jay and I had been working on the lair for a while, and the end result looked suitably intimidating. To get there, the dogs and I followed our usual route. We rambled slowly through the woods securing clues to trees and investigating interesting landmarks – the fox's den, the old tree trunk with the woodpecker's hole, the squirrel's drey. All the undergrowth dies back in winter, allowing us to venture into areas which are impenetrable in summer.

Reaching the Beast of Fern's Lair, the dogs disappeared into the trees, leaving me to stash the treasure and add the finishing touches to the site. With some difficulty, I resisted the impulse to drag more fallen boughs to add to the den. It looked quite cosy and dry inside, a useful shelter if ever caught out in rain or snow. Two roe deer silently bounded away as I worked, noticed only when I caught a glimpse of their heart-shaped rear ends. After fleeing to a safe distance, they stood stock still and observed the dogs and me with interest.

The dull 'craik' of a pheasant sent Fintry crashing into the woods, causing the 'craiking' to increase in pitch and agitation before the bird burst into flight directly in front of me. Another near-miss. There are dozens of pheasants around this winter. The estate over the hill rears them for 'sport,' but much to the locals' delight, they appear to have merely walked down the hill and found safe haven in our woods. I wonder if our beautiful bottle-green pheasant from last year – dubbed Farquhar – has survived the winter. In view of his low mental capacity it is probably unlikely.

The rest of Hogmanay passed in a blur – a surprisingly brisk evening surgery, then home to check the cat and top up her sedative again before returning en masse to Clayfern to watch the traditional annual procession. All the inhabitants turn out to watch burly locals carry flaming torches from one end of the town to the other, accompanied by a band and yet more locals in fancy dress who badger the crowd unmercifully for money to fill their buckets. The booty is used for local charities, hence the oft-heard plea 'Money for the old folk', and the jocular reply 'But I don't want one!' Stops at each of the local hostelries for 'refreshment' allowed the entire proceedings to become more disorganised and discordant as the evening progressed.

Clayfern is a friendly village, and the attraction of the procession for Jay and I is to see all our friends and customers out on the street, waving or stopping for a chat. After a quick trip home to check the cat, we then joined a group of friends and relatives for supper in a local restaurant.

A peculiarity of life as a single-handed vet is that on social occasions, I need to take my own car in case of emergency calls. This is less stressful than going in one car and either having to take the whole party along with me to an emergency call – which can be disconcerting when the meal has just been served – or going alone thus stranding them at the restaurant without transport home. Luckily, our meal was uninterrupted and was a great success. The surgery nurses Alice and Cath were both there with their families, but unfortunately, nurse Julie and her partner Bill were laid up with bad colds. Another trip home (alone) to check Rosie, then on to rejoin everyone at a millennium firework display in Stramar, the nearby market town. Rosie had her final check before I fell into bed at 3 a.m. Thank goodness! New Year – and the new millennium – successfully celebrated without too much interference from work.

In compensation for my earlier-than-desired rise, Rosie is looking much better today. She had a further low dose of sedative at 3 a.m., and has not resumed the jerking. She looks a little 'spaced out' but is otherwise normal, and hungrily demolishes a plate of food. A weight lifts off my shoulders – we can enjoy the day as planned without worrying about our in-patient.

Even more than Christmas day, New Year's Day can generally be relied on to be quiet. Only the direst emergencies will disturb us today.

After a relaxed breakfast, the excited family cram into our trusty Tundra, dogs leap in the back, and we set off on the treasure hunt up the hill behind the house. Bright sunlight greets us at the top, yet we have left the cottage still deep in shadow. For two months in winter, we lose the sun as it fails to rise above the hill. At midday at this time of year, it floods the field in front of the house, but stops at least one hundred yards short of our garden – so near and yet so far. Pulling off the track, we give the boys their first clue –

'Once the car is locked up tight,
Follow the track round to the right,
Look for a ribbon round a tree,
Further instructions there you'll see.'

Rod and Pete streak ahead, solving clues effortlessly, even the more subtle ones which we thought might fox them. The adults follow at a more sedate pace. Jay and I had great fun composing the clues, and are thrilled to see the hunt progressing so well. After last night's high winds, I offer a silent prayer of thanks that the clues are still in place. Mindful of our winter weather, they are well-wrapped in waterproof envelopes and tied securely in place. 'They look like parking-ticket envelopes,' says Rod who should know – his dad is a policeman. 'They're our old ones,' retorts Jay, quick as a flash. Round the hill the boys go, past the deer pen and into the woods. The trail gets more difficult now, and a compass appears with the next clue -

'Due South now pace steps 4 x 10,
Find where the rabbit has his den.'

This holds them up long enough for us to catch up, and the final section is completed together. The penultimate clue retrieved from the rabbit burrow reveals more of the sad tale of the Beast of Fern, and also contains a whistle, stopwatch and plastic glove which causes much hilarity -

'Three years ago, the Beast lost an ear,
To a hunter with a whistle like this one here,
Blow hard twice, then rush – don't tarry,
He'll run off panicking in a paddy,
You've got ten minutes till he gets suspicious,
And returns to find you taste delicious!'
'Follow the bones up through the firs,
Keep quiet in case his sidekicks stirs,

Soon you'll come to a stone grave,
That's Auntie Mary who we couldn't save.
Slowly turn your eyes to the right,
Behold the lair – a dreadful sight.

The 'bone trail' uses the bones from a roe deer, excavated last year by the boys' cousin Tom. Diverting him with difficulty from taking the bones back to the city, we have plans to 'rebuild' the deer when he next visits. As anticipated, the bones cause a great deal of excitement – in the dogs as well as the humans. Our old dog Kippen shambles along behind, staunchly clutching a femur in his mouth. He seldom chews bones these days, but does like to have something to carry. Fintry, the youngster, dashes around in ecstasy, discarding one bone for another, and even trying to cram two into her mouth at once.

Jay and I are rather proud of the lair – set in a clearing amongst the sombre firs, it comprises a den of fir branches enclosing a large hole in a fallen tree stump. The hole is large enough to swallow an entire shoebox full of treasure. Jay and I have 'decorated' the clearing to add to the fun. On one side are pine needle-covered mounds, remains of previous stumps. One large mound carries the sign – *'RIP, Mr. Bear (Xmas dinner 1999)'* whilst on a clump of smaller humps – *' RIP Mouse family (hors d'oeuvres).'* The roe deer skull is impaled on a twig above the *Home Sweet Home* sign outside the den.. On dog walks over the last few weeks, we have added to the den, dragging large boughs felled in the gales and enlarging the hole in the stump. Arriving for evening surgeries with Swiss army knife and bones in my pockets, and knees covered in mud, I have frequently pondered whether this is normal behaviour for a middle-aged woman.

After a tense moment while the boys decide who puts their gloved hand in the hole, the treasure is unearthed – sweets, small fossils and pound notes for the youngsters, and some novelties for the adults. Collecting bones as we go, including those carried by dogs, we set off home for a rest before the next event on the agenda – an evening ceilidh in Julie and Bill's village. Before then is time to play with the treasure, and send Rosie home with her grateful owner. The boys have come into the surgery with me to visit Rosie, and we fill in time before she goes by looking at a stack of x-rays. For eight- and ten- year-olds, they are astonishingly astute at interpreting the abnormalities. I suggest a master plan – they will go off to vet school, then take over from me in about twenty years. They appear to be mulling this over as we return to the house for a light tea. Everyone is flagging a little by now, but they have come to enjoy themselves -AND ENJOY THEMSELVES THEY WILL! Lounging around watching the television for the evening is just not on the agenda at all.

Before long, we set off for the ceilidh. Risking an outing after their colds, Julie and Bill arrive at the same time as we do. Together we bag a table and unpack provisions – wine, beer, soft drinks, crisps, nuts and shortbread. The visitors look bemused; they have not experienced a ceilidh before. We set the boys a task, a prize for the first one to spell ceilidh correctly (pronounced caylay – this is a mean trick to spring on English boys).

A good time is had by all. The dances are not hard to pick up for the uninitiated, and there are even enough of us to provide a full set for an eightsome reel. All clump around in one direction, intoning

'1 ... 2 ... 3 ... 4 ... 5 ... 6 ... 7 ... 8,

steps before repeating the process in the other direction, roughly in time with the music. Dashing White Sargeants, Gay Gordons, Military Two Steps, we do them all, the lemonade and snacks disappearing like magic as we fuel our way through the evening. Pete catches sight of a poster advertising tonight's event and triumphantly claims his spelling prize, looking horrified when we tell him he has won a dance with his Auntie Kate. I arrange my features in a Les Dawson pucker and chase him round the table. By midnight, the boys are flagging and we take our leave. They have done very well, two late nights and early mornings in a row. Tomorrow will be a day for recovery.

Hot chocolates all round when we get home then everyone wearily turns in. We are no sooner in bed than the telephone shrills. I stare at it incredulously for an instant for answering – I can't believe it, it's 1a.m. on the day after New Year, for Heaven's sake. This shouldn't be happening. The inevitable sinking feeling is made immeasurably worse by the owner's description of the problem 'My dog is trying to be sick and his stomach is all swollen up.' Damn and Double Damn! There is little doubt what this is – *a gastric dilatation or torsion,* a real emergency. Probably the one condition which small animal vets on call dread most of all. It occurs only in deep-chested dogs, usually after over-indulgence in food. For some reason, fermentation occurs in the stomach trapping large quantities of gas. This is serious enough, but a quirk of canine anatomy can allow the stomach to flip over on its axis cutting off its blood supply and sending the victim rapidly into deep clinical shock. Patients can die within half an hour of symptoms first appearing, and it is not unusual to get them DOA (dead on arrival) at the surgery.

Instructing the owner to come to the surgery as quickly as possible, I ring Julie and break the glad tidings. If the dog is not DOA, then we have a long night ahead of us. All thoughts of sleep have instantly evaporated. The weather is deteriorating as I pass from the house to the surgery, the wind making even that short distance an effort. There is just time to lay out the necessary equipment before both the patient, and Julie arrive together.

Our hearts collectively sink as we observe the torpedo-shaped Dalmatian being carried into the surgery, the stretcher party swaying alarmingly in the gale. A quick examination shows her mucous membranes to be white as a sheet, her feet and ears cold and her heart fast and weak – cardinal signs of shock. As we hurriedly install her on the operating table, administer oxygen by mask and prepare to set up an intravenous drip, I spell out the gravity of the situation to the owner. If we proceed, our first actions will be to combat the shock, followed by attempts to decompress the dog's stomach. We will try passing a stomach tube but this rarely helps. If the stomach has twisted, the tube will not pass. Even if it hasn't, in addition to gas and food, the stomach also fills with a viscous foam which usually blocks the tube. Plan B would then be surgery to empty the stomach and reorientate it in the correct position. This is a very risky situation, and there are many hurdles at which the patient may fall. If the shock, anaesthetic or surgery does not 'get' her, then there is the risk of peritonitis post-operatively. The overall success rate with this condition is about fifty percent survival, and Nan is eleven years old, a good age for a Dalmatian. The chances of her survival are probably less than that. It is a horrible dilemma for an owner, but she needs to know the facts.

After a hurried telephone discussion with her husband, she elects to go ahead with treatment, and tearfully leaves us to do our work. With fluid running full blast into Nan's circulation, Jay is recruited to assist while I try to pass a stomach tube, but as expected, the bottom two inches block with slimy froth. As I expected, surgery is going to be necessary.

Anaesthetic solution is injected via the catheter we have placed in a vein, then an endotracheal tube is inserted into Nan's trachea (windpipe) and connected to the anaesthetic machine administering anaesthetic gas and oxygen. Tipped onto her back, the dog looks like a beached whale, her distended stomach as taut as a drum. After speedy preparation of the op site, we are ready to begin. Julie monitors the anaesthetic closely while I carefully cut through the body wall. The massive stomach takes up the entire front end of the abdomen, bulging like a beachball. Immobilising the organ as much as possible, I make an initial stab incision into the interior. Foul smelling gas hisses out and the stomach deflates like magic. This is similar to the situation in cattle and sheep when a bloated stomach is relieved by insertion of a special instrument – *a trocar and canula.* The trocar punctures into the stomach and is then withdrawn, leaving the canula in place. In ruminants, methane gas is produced as a result of fermentation in the stomach. This leads to the much-quoted tale of the new vet wanting to impress the farmer with his extensive knowledge: explaining the fact that methane is combustible, our hero casually struck a match to demonstrate a jet of flame expressing from the canula. Unfortunately, the story goes, the demonstration worked rather too well, the flames igniting a pile of straw and burning down the barn. Whether this actually happened, no one knows but the tale has been added to the many veterinary legends used as cautionary tales.

Unfortunately, in dogs, releasing the gas is not enough, the stomach also has to be emptied. *Not* my favourite task, I grumble, investigating the depths. In all, we retrieve over half a basin full of semi-digested material chronicling Nan's extreme over-indulgence – peanuts, raisins, sweetcorn and other unidentified materials are all visible within a semi-digested porridge. The scene is almost biblical as we work – wind howls round the building and rain blasts the windows. The heat and smell in the room are almost overpowering. What a night to be ill. What a night to be a vet or vet nurse. Why could we not just work in an office? Once it is empty, I flush the stomach with saline and suture it, then close the abdomen and body wall. The stomach wall is severely stretched and inflamed, and we can only hope that it can recover. After over an hour of surgery, Nan is hoisted on to her Vetbed (commercial fleecy material ideal for patients. Any fluids pass through the fleece onto newspaper below keeping the patient warm and dry). Front or back end?' enquires Julie, as we prepare to stretcher the dog into her kennel. The front end person gets to manoeuvre the leg with the drip and carry the fluid bag between their teeth, while the back end reverses into the kennel, then scrambles out over the dog, emerging like Quasimodo on a bad day.

Once the dog is settled with drip running and blankets tucked in, the mammoth task of clearing up begins. This is a joint effort. I clear the operating room while Julie cleans and sterilises innumerable instruments. The initial instruments involved in handling the open stomach and its contents were replaced by fresh ones to prevent contamination on closing the site, so there is much sorting and bagging to be done before the packs are run through the *autoclave* (steriliser). The ops room is cluttered with discarded drapes and swabs, and the unavoidable bowl of stomach contents. All such material is packed into marked bags for collection by a firm specialising in clinical waste. Then the table, surfaces, walls and floor need cleaning. It is quite amazing where spots of stomach contents or blood have reached. Once we are done, the dog is conscious, but not moving under her blankets. Her temperature has improved and her extremities are now warm. 'She looks more human than she did two hours ago,' comments Julie with her usual twisted logic.

It is now 4 a.m., and we are both wide awake, running on adrenaline which will take time to dissipate. Bracing against the weather, we head for the house. Outside, the roar of the wind in the trees is all pervading, like a mighty waterfall. We start the winding down process with another New Year's drink of hot chocolate, then Julie goes home. I check the patient before setting the alarm for 8 a.m and falling into bed. If I'm lucky, that will be three hours of uninterrupted sleep. Not easy as the storm shrieks and wails outside, rattling doors and windows wildly in seeming attempts to demolish the house.

Eight o'clock comes all too quickly, and I struggle out off bed, professional concern fighting a duel with personal comfort. Nan looks surprisingly well considering last night's ordeal, and insists on moving round in her kennel. I want to give her more fluid but realise that the drip will probably become detached if she persists with her pacing. There is nothing for it but to supervise while the fluid goes in. Luckily, I am well prepared for attendance at patients' bedsides – a quick trip to the house for a mug of tea and a magazine, then I settle down by the dog on a luxurious cushion made from the first fleece sheared from our pet sheep. It is extremely comfortable, and saves the nether regions from the discomfort of squatting on the cold kennel room floor. With one hand stroking the dog, and the other holding either drink or magazine, I am in the ideal position to ensure that Nan's line does not become tangled or pulled out. An hour passes pleasantly enough while a bag of fluid enters Nan's circulation. She seems to have appreciated the company, but now I am leaving her to rest. The radio is turned on low to give the room a homely feel while I leave to attend to my own dogs. They both get big cuddles when I return to the house – it makes you really appreciate them being well and happy when you dwell on Nan's plight. Fear of gastric torsion makes me neurotic about feeding our two; they receive three modest meals per day, neither immediately before or after exercise, and we are both on the alert for any sign of a distending abdomen. It really is a supremely unpleasant condition.

The day passes peacefully, interspersed with trips next door to check Nan. Thank goodness this is also a holiday in Scotland and we have some chance to catch up on lost sleep. The patient seems remarkably well, and is allowed home in the early evening after another bag of fluid. Her owner has instructions to allow her to drink small quantities of water, and takes some tins of special post-op diet to offer her if she expresses any interest in food. We will see her at Clayfern surgery tomorrow. She is not out of the woods yet, but so far so good. This has certainly been a New Year we will not forget. I will always remember how we celebrated the Millennium.

Chapter 2

Back to normal working hours after the festive season. It feels as if we've never been away, although it has been lovely not having to walk the dogs at crack of dawn before surgery. At this time of year, dawn is only just breaking when we set off on our usual morning route – along the road and down the track through the field. The sky is full of birds 'commuting' to the day's feeding grounds. Ragged strings of geese fly briskly over the valley, their members honking plaintively in unison, while less compact, more relaxed flocks of gulls soar loftily overhead, scanning the fields for a suitable landing spot. A small fishing boat heads up-river, ducking and diving precariously in the heavy swell. It will be heading for Clayfern after a night's fishing at the mouth of the firth.

With many people still on holiday, morning surgery in Clayfern is relatively busy. Nan is doing well and has been drinking on her own, although she is not particularly interested in food yet. The last two cases of the morning surgery are a bald, scratching guinea pig, and a dog with colitis. Both conditions can be exacerbated by stress, and the festive season provides plenty of that. 'Lucky we're not guinea pigs or dogs,' muses Alice, 'or we'd all be bald and diarrhoeic by now.' Both of us feel shattered and agree we would rather face a lazy day on the settee than work. But today is our main operating day so I return quickly to Clayfern to attend to our list. In addition to some routine neuterings for the local animal charity, we have two cases which have been brewing since last week. The first is a whippet who has been losing small amounts of blood from her vulva, and, although not acutely ill, has been rather listless of late. A blood sample taken to the lab this morning confirms a mild anaemia and indicates that her white cell count is markedly elevated – a sign that the body is fighting an infection. I suspect a cystic ovary, and we set up a drip before beginning an exploratory operation. Opening into her abdomen, the problem is immediately clear, she has a large *pyometra* or infected womb. Each horn of the uterus is nearly eighteen inches long, thick as my wrist, and contains a soup of stinking pus. Once removed, the enlarged organ remains coiled grotesquely in the tray. 'No Cumberland sausages for me for a while,' comments Julie, describing the appearance aptly. I am quite surprised at this finding. There are two types of pyometra – open, where the cervix is open and pus discharges to the outside, and closed such as in this case, where all infection is retained within the womb. Usually animals with a closed pyometra are much iller than our patient today, and will be off food, vomiting and frequently virtually collapsed. Although not at her best by any means, our whippet must be a tough cookie to remain as bright as she was. Now that all the infected material has been removed, her outlook is extremely favourable.

Our final case is an old friend, Robbie McRobbie, an elderly dog who has been operated on before. He has an intriguing history, which begins when he first ran into problems over two years ago. The sudden appearance of a fast-growing lump on his neck resulted in a very sick dog. Supporting him with fluids and penetrative antibiotics, we operated to remove a horrible mass from his neck. The surrounding tissues were congested with fluid – almost like a jellyfish in texture – and within this material lay an area crisscrossed with fibrous tissue and haemorrhagic pockets – rather like a Swiss cheese. Suspecting a tumour or possibly a reaction to a foreign body, we sent a sample to the lab for microscopic examination. Robbie bucked up immediately post-operatively and never looked back. The lab reported '*Chronic cellulitis and panniculitis with no evidence of tumour*'. Translating – throughout the tissue was areas of haemorrhage and inflammation, with both muscle and fatty tissue being replaced by fibrous strands (the body's usual way of repairing damaged tissue). There was no clue as to what was causing the inflammation, although I always suspected that a foreign body had been involved. It is not uncommon for sharp objects such as sticks or even grass awns to penetrate the soft tissue at the back of the mouth, and wander in the throat and neck region causing tissue damage. Occasionally such a foreign body will stimulate a localised collection of pus and inflammatory cells which can burst to the outside, discharging the foreign object from the body.

I particularly remember the case of a German Shepherd with a swelling on his neck which burst and discharged matchstick-like pieces of wood over two days. His owner could dimly remember him chewing up a large plank during building work six months previously. In any event, Robbie seemed cured after the surgery, and lived happily ever after – at least until a year later when he reappeared with a smaller swelling close to the original scar. The lump appeared painless and his temperature was normal but he was miserable, off food and vomiting. Explaining that the lump might not be the reason for his illness, I took a blood sample to check for likely causes of vomiting. The results were puzzlingly normal – no increased levels of enzymes suggesting liver or kidney malfunction (quite common in older patients), not even an increase in tissue damage enzymes or white cell count – which might point to the lump causing problems. His owners remained convinced that his problems stemmed from the new lump, so with some misgivings, we operated again with similar findings.

His new scar, parallel to the first, promoted him to corporal and we hoped no more chevrons would be added to his collection. As before, lump removal produced total recovery and he was fine until a new mass appeared on the opposite side last week. Not wanting to bother us over New Year, the owners persevered until he took a turn for the worse overnight. It is a miserable, dehydrated patient who appears at the farm surgery this morning. I am shocked at how poor his condition is, and again mention the many causes of vomiting in older dogs, but the owners remain convinced that the new lump is yet again to blame, and are keen for us to operate again.

Robbie has deliberately been left until last. He has been on a drip all morning to replace fluid and electrolyte loss, and looks slightly better just as a result of that. Once again we go through the familiar procedure. Today's lump is his best effort yet – a horrible haemorrhagic, gristly mass whose boundaries are difficult to decipher. Far from being made up to sergeant, today's scar looks as if he has been partially decapitated. A polyurethane drain is stitched into the cavity before the wound is closed. It will channel secretions out of the neck into a large padded bandage. True to form, our boy is Mr Cheery when his owners collect him after evening surgery. They have brought his trademark outfit – a smart green body warmer, ideal for securing his bandage and preventing him tampering with the wound. Off he goes, dragging his owners down the path, lifting his leg at every available opportunity. After over two litres of fluid, I can't say that I am surprised.

Although Wednesdays are traditionally a quieter day, the next day bucks the trend by having a packed morning surgery. Several cases are follow-ups from the last few days. Nan, our gastric torsion Dalmatian, is doing remarkably well. She sits growling at other patients in the waiting room before stalking into the consulting room and taking up position next to our jar of doggie treats. 'Not yet, I'm afraid', I apologise while checking her over. She will have to be on very bland, easily-digested food until her stomach wound has time to heal. She is making such good progress that I sign her off until Saturday, dispensing food and antibiotics to be given in the meantime.

Next is our pyometra from the previous day. She is also extremely cheerful and *is* allowed a celebratory biscuit. She has always been a very fit dog, accompanying her owner on long hill walks, and I suspect this is what has allowed her to appear so relatively bright in the face of such a serious condition. Last is Robbie in his suave green body warmer. Unfortunately his drain has come out – rather shamefacedly, his owner admits that it caught in the body warmer zip. The gap where the drain was is luckily still draining and his owner has found yet another novel way to protect the area and collect the discharge –

round Robbie's neck is attached a disposable self-adhesive nappy. First a jacket, then nappies, this ex-working dog will be getting a complex. Completely unfazed by his new outfit, Robbie also accepts several offerings from the goodie jar. Three bits of good news in a row – that makes me rather nervous. It may sound strange for a professional to be so superstitious, but it frequently follows in this job that for every up there is a down – and, luckily, vice versa.

The icing on the cake would be if our planning permission arrived today, I think as I return to Fern. We have been eagerly awaiting the arrival of the first post since 30th December. The year 2000 promises to be a big year for Jay and me; our neighbours are moving and we are hoping to buy their house. Although we both love our little cottage, it is becoming increasingly cramped, and the larger house with outbuildings to accommodate both the surgery and Jay's business would be the perfect move, especially as it is only two hundred yards away. It all depends on us getting planning permission to convert an outbuilding into a surgery. The outlook seems hopeful – the new property has plenty off-road parking and no immediate neighbours to disturb – but planners do seem to be a law unto themselves, and we cannot finalise matters until we receive the official go-ahead.

There is no post on the mat when I reach home. This means that Pete is on duty today. He is a wonderful postman with time to chat with all the isolated inhabitants of our sparsely populated area, and lend a cheery helping hand for elderly or infirm householders living on their own. The only downside is that the mail tends not to appear until nearly lunchtime. This regime often works to our advantage, allowing time to take and package blood samples for collection before Pete comes. We have occasionally been caught unawares by the early arrival – and departure – of a relief postman before our 'victim' is even out of the kennel. 'Nothing today, Kate,' says Pete, leafing through our mail as he climbs out of his van, 'Shouldn't be long though, surely?' 'I really hope not, Pete,' I reply, quite disappointed, today seemed to be a lucky day. Still, there's always tomorrow. Our neighbours are ready to move, so it is only red tape which is holding us up.

Normally, I have a half-day off on Wednesdays, but the move and surgery conversion threatens to be hideously expensive so I am attempting to save some money by cutting this out. For a single-handed vet, any time off requires paying a locum to 'mind the shop'. However, my regular locum has recently moved away, and rather than look immediately for a replacement, I am trying to manage without for the quieter winter months. We do still try to keep the day free of any work between surgeries (except for emergencies of course) so it is almost like a day off.

The local hunt appear to be in our vicinity today so the dogs and I set off for a walk down by Peeswit Point out of harm's way. Dicing with death, we descend the steep, muddy path wending between the trees to the river. An abundant covering of mud and fallen leaves makes the surface supremely slippery. Fintry descends like a polar bear cub seen on the television recently – a mixture of wild galloping and sliding on all four feet as if snowboarding. Old Kippen plods slowly but surely, large hairy feet holding the surface like suckers. I am the least artistic of the trio, slithering, slipping and frantically grabbing nearby saplings for balance. Noise fills the air as we progress – the deep roar of the wind in the tallest trees, its hiss through the lower ivy and pines, and the slapping together of young saplings given room to grow by last year's timber operations. Nearing the river (which is almost a mile across at this point), waves bash against the rocky bank scaring Fintry the Wimp, who retreats behind me, tail and ears flat against her rotund little body. There are two directions in which we can go now – along the sheltered shingle beach to the east of the point, or the west beach in the full force of the wind. Kippen decides the latter and dashes into the water, is nearly bowled off his feet by the waves and retreats to beachcomb up by the trees.

The many stranded items here tend to come more from upriver than from the sea. I spot a propane gas cylinder last seen half a mile upstream. Although almost five foot high, and solid, the force of the water has tossed it casually over assorted tree trunks piled at the top of the beach. There is also a long wooden beam like a railway sleeper with bits of metal attached at intervals. Perhaps it has detached from a dock somewhere. I hope there wasn't a boat attached. There are no balls today, much to Kippen's disgust. After only minutes of battling in the teeth of the gale, we retreat towards the point. Waves scroll along the beach, white horses chasing each other like whirling dervishes. The dogs spot a lump of wood in the shallows; it looks as if it may be beached, but disappears silently back into the murky brown depths before they can rescue it.

Back home, I run into acquaintances from the local badger group. They have been checking up our hill for badger activity. I can tell them that all has been quiet in the setts in Fern woods. They only appear to be used occasionally when badgers pass through – usually in the spring when youngsters leave their home setts to become independent. The men have found a large active sett on a hill across the valley – a great excuse for an expedition in that direction soon. This is ideal badger territory, and they have been here in the past as some old place names testify – Brocksgate, Broxden – but persecution by gamekeepers and shepherds has greatly reduced numbers.

Once indoors, Kippen makes a beeline for the woodburner – going like a furnace in this wind. When he was younger, he preferred cooler places but in his golden years, he enjoys stretching out in front of the fire. He has even been singed once or twice. Fintry has taken the opportunity to lie on the old dog's Christmas beanbag in the kitchen. It is a wrench to leave for evening surgery in the gathering dusk but promptness is important today as I need to put my friend Sheila's ducks and hens away before it gets completely dark. The ducks are not keen to go in, and I do my sheepdog act round the pen. They really are stupid birds – the routine is the same *every* day, but there is always the usual panic-stricken quacking and rushing about. They would quack on the other side of their beaks if the fox got them. In the past, Sheila's dog Jonno could be called upon for help, but he is too old now and spends most of his day in front of the Aga. His walks with my lot are restricted to every two or three days, but tonight he looks so hopeful that I resolve to collect him tomorrow when we set off on our travels.

It is hard to believe that only one week ago was New Year's Day. It has been a busy week, but thank goodness, we get to the weekend at last. After morning surgery, Alice is helping me to collect some old surgical instruments which I have purchased from a nearby collector of military relics. Over the years, he has also amassed a collection of old military medical equipment including such gems as an entire regimental first aid kit *circa* 1940. This kit is packed in a wicker basket with straps for attaching to pack animals. Lack of storage facilities is forcing Dave to sell off this collection, as the military equipment takes up a lot of space. This is immediately apparent as we wend our way past an armoured car and a small tank parked in his garage. 'Come back in spring and I'll give you a ride in my tank,' he chatters airily as we rummage through dusty boxes in the depths of the garage. 'That would sort our parking problems,' muses Alice thoughtfully, 'And it might be fun too!' However, at only six miles per gallon of fuel, visit fees might be somewhat prohibitive.

Business concluded satisfactorily, we join Dave for coffee in his conservatory. Staring out on his garden featuring miniature tanks 'driven' by gnomes, we listen enthralled to tales of adventures into which his hobby has led him. Going in search of a World War 2 aircraft reputed to have crashed in the nearby hills, he found a farmer's wife still using the parachute cord for hanging out the washing. As we prepare to take our leave, he suggests we attend an enthusiasts' rally held later in the year. 'You don't have to restrict yourselves to military antiques,' he confides, 'One collector only brings his collection of blow lamps.' Mmm, y.e e.s! Still, could be a novelty, we agree as we head for home. Enthusiasts may be slightly mad, but they are always such interesting and charming people.

Once home, it is finally time for a BIG dog walk. The poor dogs have rather missed out this week. Tragically they are always active and wanting attention when Jay and I want nothing more than to sink onto the settee in front of the television. Today is a chance to make it up to them. After days of rain, it is at last sunny although the winds are still blustery. The dogs and I walk briskly along the hill to the 'thinking stones', my favourite spot for peaceful contemplation. While I gaze over the valley, the dogs prospect down the hill, following up intriguing scents.

My daydream is broken by what sounds like a pack of dogs barking – it is only Fintry scaring off a metal pheasant feeder, but the echo in the valley causes the noise to reverberate from all sides. This rapidly silences Fintry who obviously decides that pheasant feeders have powerful friends and are not to be trifled with. The racket revs up old Kippen who comes galloping down the hill in support. His stiff, arthritic legs make his progress resemble that of a rocking horse, and I make a mental note to increase his dose of anti-arthritic tablets tonight.

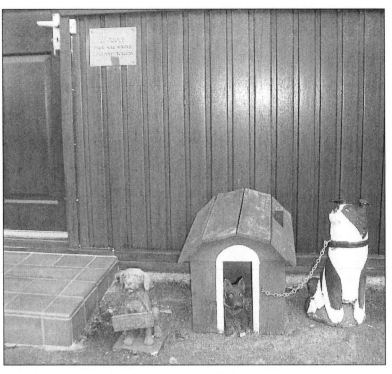

Welcome committee at farm surgery

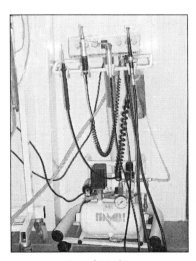

Dental Machine

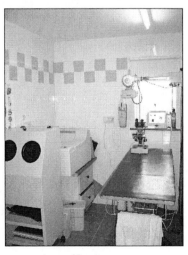

X ray room

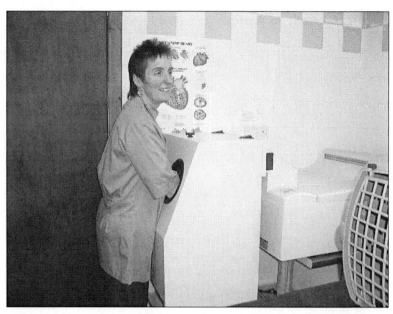

That x-ray is in here somewhere

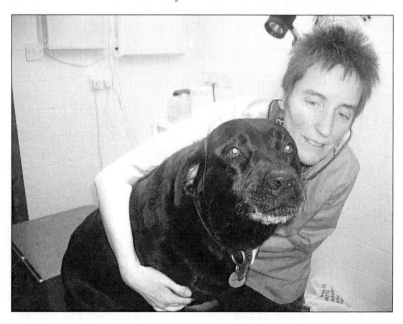

Oooh! that stethoscope's cold

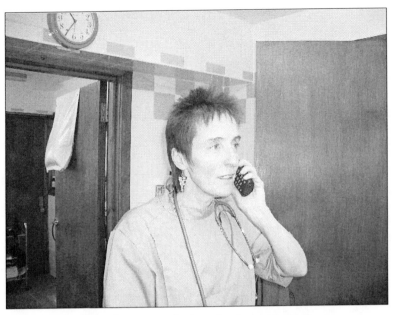

What do you mean there's another six cats tomorrow?

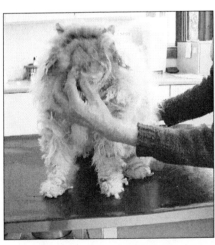

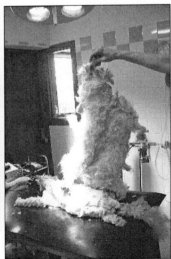

De-mat before (above) and after

iii

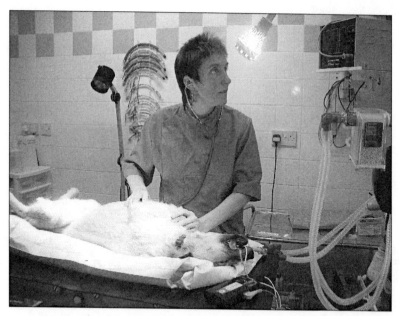

When I said I had a flash of illumination, that wasn't what I had in mind

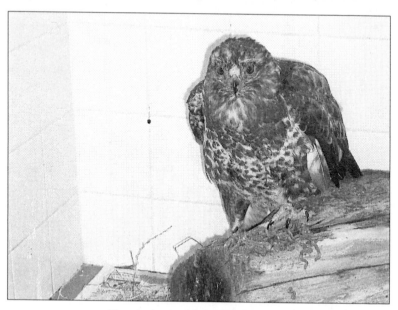

Very nice but I ordered the steak well done

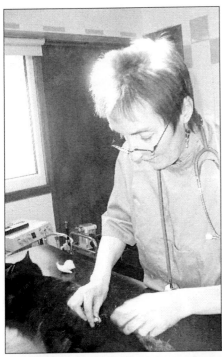

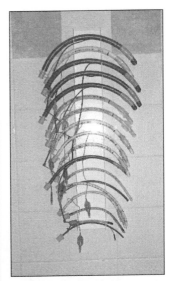

Above: Endotracheal tubes
Left: I need glasses for this cat castration
Below: Julie's clogs
– best anaesthetic there is

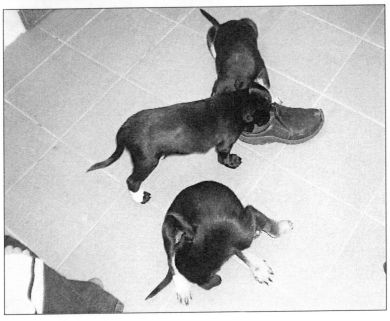

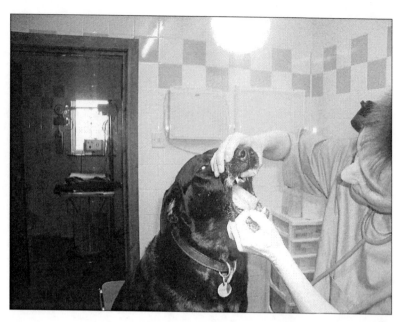

I know you ate something when my back was turned

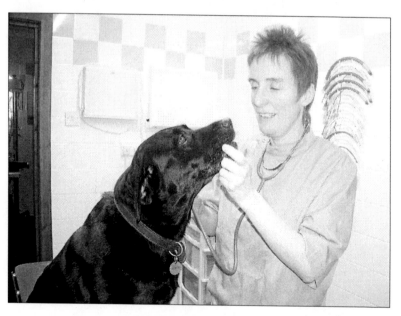

Friends again

Chapter 3

Another operating day rolls round. We have mainly bits and pieces today, a nice change from the usual neutering marathons that we undertake for the local animal charity.

First up is a young rabbit with an unpleasant head wound. She has sustained a slash extending from her forehead down the side of her face and on to the surface of the *cornea* (front of the eye). She is anaesthetised with a combination of two injectable anaesthetics and is placed on an insulated pad to conserve body heat. The loss of body heat during anaesthesia is significant for small creatures and can be fatal if not paid attention to. The damage to the cornea is not deep and should heal on its own – already small blood vessels are beginning to grow into the damaged area from the conjunctiva. The cornea has no blood supply of its own – healing depends on blood vessels coming from the sides of the eye carrying cells to heal the lesion then fading away once their usefulness is over.

My most important task is to mend the torn upper eyelid so the margin of the eye is once again intact. Eyelids are necessary to hold tear fluid within the eye, and to lubricate the eyeball whenever the animal blinks. If this mechanism is not working properly, the eye dries out and becomes susceptible to infections. It is also uncomfortable for the animal who will permanently feel as if it has grit in its eye. Carefully the two cut eyelid edges are joined using suture material no thicker than a hair. Then, I cut away damaged tissue above the eye and undermine the skin at the edges of the new wound to enable the defect to be closed. Luckily, it is possible to pull forward spare skin from the rabbit's forehead – almost like a facelift in reverse – and the wound is stitched closed without excess tension on the suture line. This bunny will have a lovely wrinkle free forehead for a while. Lucky bunny! I am pleased with the end result although the wound does look rather gruesome. The owner is made of stern stuff and is not put off by her pet's appearance when she collects her later. 'We've thought of a new name for her,' she announces, 'Bridie.' 'Something tasty in pastry?' I joke facetiously, referring to the Scottish version of the Cornish Pasty, 'No, bride of Frankenstein,' she counters quick as a flash.

Next we have another pyometra operation – as usual, similar cases occur in clusters, none for weeks then three in a row. 'Just like buses,' according to Julie. Today's patient is a very old chihuahua, no teeth, not much hair and parchment-thin, dry skin. As we get older, the skin's natural elasticity decreases, resulting in skin like Cherie's. Cutting into such skin is a somewhat unpleasant experience 'Like operating on a dead chicken,' suggests Julie. Although frequently lacking in finesse, Julie's comments usually hit the nail on the head. We both decide to redouble our own personal efforts with moisturising cream. Despite the unaesthetic quality of the op, it goes well and we remove a surprisingly large infected womb from the depths of Cherie's abdomen. Her drip continues to run when she is returned to her kennel, replacing lost fluids and flushing toxins from her system. Like many old locals, human and animal, Cherie has an indomitable spirit and is on her feet yapping and tearing up bedding in a remarkably short time.

Our final job of the morning is a cat demat belonging to Mrs Cassidy, our neighbour at Clayfern surgery. Another two indomitable old locals if ever. 'Would you also check her teeth and trim her nails?' asked Mrs Cassidy when she dropped the cat off at the surgery before continuing in the same deadpan tone – 'And if you find a brain button, would you switch it on.'

Although necessary, demats do not require the same degree of concentration as our previous operations, and as we work, we chat about the layout of the prospective new surgery and reminisce about the previous one. After running a three-vet surgery in a detached house in the city, starting afresh as a single-handed vet in a rural area was very appealing to me. When Jay and I moved to this area several years ago and decided to start a new practice, we proceeded with caution, not sure whether the idea of a veterinary surgery in Clayfern would catch on. The initial surgery was housed in an eight by ten foot wooden chalet at the back of the house. The chalet had a chequered history – having started life as a holiday camp chalet, it was then bought for use as an office on a building site. We purchased it when all the buildings had been completed and it was up for disposal. We worked successfully in the Green Shed, as it was irreverently called, for two years until confident that the surgery would support a modest living, and the present surgery – three times the size – was built on to the side of the house.

'Those were the days!' we reminisce. Of course the surgery was quieter then, but we still had our moments. Like pioneers, we remember days gone by: one memorable day in midwinter the water pipes froze in the Green Shed, reducing us to scrub up with thermoses of hot water from the house. Electric heaters ran continuously in winter as cool air blew in through gaps round the door and windows, and fans worked overtime in summer to combat the effects of direct sunlight. As space was limited, we tended to do one or two operations per day, rather than group them on dedicated operating days. Even then, our clients' notorious disregard for appointment systems would have us tearing our hair. One day we might be expecting a cat at 10.45 a.m., a rabbit at 11 a.m. and a large dog at 11.15 a.m. This timing was carefully worked out so that the small animals were safely ensconced in their kennels before the big dog arrived and could be dealt with immediately. Inevitably, the 11.15 a.m. appointment (i.e. big dog) would arrive at 10.45 a.m., and the others at anything up to 11.30 a.m., necessitating handling nervous small creatures on the table below which the big dog was tied. Hardly ideal for the patients, and not recommended for a stress-free life. Our working conditions improved markedly when we moved into the present surgery, but neither staff nor clients regard it with quite the same affection with which we looked upon the Green Shed. Much to Jay's dismay, I am determined that it comes with us when we move along the road. After all, even Abraham Lincoln had his log cabin.

An emergency call last night brought in a very distressed young cat, losing blood from both his mouth and nose. Wide-eyed and terrified, he was breathing through his mouth as his nostrils were blocked with blood. This is not a natural way of breathing for a cat and he was very close to panic, only allowing me to carry out a fairly rudimentary examination. The cat's ears and feet were warm, and gently dabbing blood from his mouth showed the colour of his mucous membranes to be reassuringly pink. This showed that shock was not a major problem as yet. A quick listen to his chest and appraisal of the rest of his body confirmed my suspicions that his head was the only part of his body injured in the inevitable traffic accident. He was showing no sign of concussion or other brain trauma; his nose did not appear broken, his main injury being a broken lower jaw. He might not have felt that way, but after an argument with a car, he had got off rather lightly. In such a case, painkillers, warmth and quiet are often of more use than protracted messing about, so the drugs were administered and our boy was ensconced in a cosy kennel overnight. Considering the relative sizes of cats and cars, it is really incredible that cats survive traffic accidents at all.

This morning, young Alfie is feeling very much more like himself although his jaw is still at an unusual angle. He checks out fit for an anaesthetic has received his premeds. During morning surgery, we ended up with another cat who also requires an anaesthetic. Over the telephone, his owner reported that the cat was having head tremors and was salivating as if having a fit. The only other information the owner could give us was that the cat was in a fight on Monday. These symptoms had me intrigued. Fits are not very common in cats, and I considered other possibilities – brain damage from the fight (rather unlikely), organophosphorus poisoning (again unlikely to be intermittent), even the terminal twitching of end stage kidney failure (yet less likely but still to be considered). When the cat arrived at the surgery, diagnosis was surprisingly quick and easy. After standing back for an initial look at the whole animal on the table, it is my practice to begin my examination at the front end and work slowly backwards. Head carriage, ears and eyes fine, next the mouth – problem solved. One of the cat's large fangs – a *canine* tooth – was loose and was lying crookedly across his mouth. The cat fight must have dislodged it. From time to time, the tooth made contact with his lower jaw and caused a judder of pain to sweep through the unfortunate cat's features. This shows so well how impossible it is to come to a diagnosis over the telephone: there is really no substitute for a patient being seen. What sounds serious on the phone may be simple, or worse, what sounds simple over the phone may in fact be rather more complicated.

So, although this week may be pyometra week, this afternoon is definitely cat mouth afternoon. Alfie first. Premedicated with a sedative and painkiller before I went to morning surgery, he offers no resistance while we trim up his foreleg and insert an intravenous catheter into his vein. First I inject an anaesthetic solution which allows me to pass an endotracheal tube into Alfie's windpipe and connect him up to the anaesthetic machine, then we connect a bag of fluid to the catheter. As Alfie has not been able to eat or drink since his accident, this will keep him going until he can manage on his own.

At last able to examine him thoroughly without the patient's interference, I can confirm that he has indeed sustained a fractured jaw. The lower jaw is broken at its weakest point – where the two halves of the jaw join at the front of the mouth. This area is called the *symphysis*, the lower jaw is known as the *mandible*, hence the cat has a *fractured mandibular symphysis*. It sounds very technical, but is in fact remarkably easy to fix. While the patient is under anaesthesia, a length of surgical steel wire is looped over the front end of the jaw behind the canine teeth and each end is burrowed through the tissues to meet up under the chin. Both ends are then twisted together to tighten the loop holding both sides of the jaw in place and cut to size leaving a small spike of wire protruding under the chin.

Alfie will stay on soft foods until the wire stitch is removed under anaesthetic in about a month. Sorted. It only takes a few minutes to sort out our other cat patient. His tooth is very loose and only requires gentle persuasion to come out. A quick check of the other teeth before a second patient is also recovering in a warm kennel. The next best thing to a quiet Wednesday morning is one with one or two easy cases, quickly fixed.

Now for some quality leisure time. For a keen walker, this is a marvellous area in which to live. There is such a choice of terrain in which to walk. We can amble leisurely through the fields to the river, and beachcomb along its shore; wander through either deciduous or coniferous woods; or, if feeling energetic, head steadily upwards until we encounter the heather and rock strewn landscape of the larger hills which run in a wide band throughout the region. It is seldom that we return from a walk without having seen or found something interesting – be it biological, geological or even archaeological.

Today is no exception. I have chosen to amble through the mixed woods at the top of the track leading to the far side of the hill. At this time of year, the undergrowth has died back allowing us to pass, and often revealing features not noticeable during the summer months. Below the pine trees, the forest floor is soft, a mixture of pine needles and moss-covered mounds. Our habitual high winds cause old trees to fall over with surprising frequency, either breaking the trunks clean through or yanking the roots out of the soil. This involves us in a degree of clambering either over or under large trunks until they eventually rot down and also become covered in moss. Some fresh branches from a large Scots pine have sheered from the top of the tree. This wood is almost terracotta in colour, and surprisingly smooth to the touch despite the scaly mosaic of bark. Looking afresh at the tall Scots pines, I can see that the lower trunks are dark and the bark deeply carved with crevices while further up the tree, the colour gradually lightens to the characteristic pink terracotta and the crevices become no more than superficial cracks separating jigsaw-like pieces of bark. Now why didn't I notice that before? A wren chunters its alarm call when Fintry chases a rabbit frantically through a tangle of fallen wood.

The wren itself perches at the front of a dense pile of branches. It is almost as if he is on his doorstep, and it is a nice but unlikely thought to imagine him hopping back into a comfy living room, dry and sheltered from the elements. The wren's call is surprisingly robust for such a small bird, a near-continuous throaty warble like a piece of machinery.

Something white shows up on a mossy stump. It is a skull. The study of bones and what they can tell us is an intriguing subject. From such remains, an expert can tell the species, size, age and sex of the complete creature, and often much more about nutrition, state of health and even cause of death. Fascinating. While unable to compete at that level, I amuse myself by working out what I can. The size and shape of this skull is similar to a small dog, with teeth which belong to a carnivore. The suture lines where the large plates of bone making up the skull join are easily distinguished so the animal was young, a fact borne out by examination of the teeth – most are present and in good condition with scarcely any wear or deposition of tartar on the surfaces. Of course it could have been a small dog, but it is more likely that it is a fox. On arriving back home, I compare it with another fox skull in the surgery. The latter is kept to demonstrate dental matters to our clients, and it is obviously an older animal, the skull is larger, the suture lines are less noticeable (these lines fade as the creature ages) and there are minute signs of wear on various teeth. Peculiar person that I am, such a 'successful' analysis helps to make my day.

Chapter 4

Our planning permission to change an outbuilding into a new surgery at our new house has come through at last. The good news is that permission is granted; the bad news is that we also need to apply for building control regulations, and possibly yet more planning permission to alter the front of the building. Argghh! For the last few days, we have had not only the usual activity associated with house buying – calls to bank, solicitor, insurance agents etc., but have also been meeting builders, electricians and plumbers to explain the alterations necessary to produce a working surgery. On top of this, we have been filling in forms (four copies of each) for the next round of planning requirements. My head is spinning, and I'm sure Jay's will be as well.

All the organisation alone could be a full-time job, but we have to fit it in around our busy daily work. Luckily, today is quite quiet at the surgery, but I have a sad mission to perform before having a restful day. Robbie – the dog in the body warmer – had initially done very well after his third operation, but this last week has seen a deterioration in his condition. He has always been such a vibrant chap and his owners feel that he is just wasting away. We could do further tests, but at fifteen years old , there is unlikely to be anything radical that can be done to halt his decline. Better to gently let him go now than wait until he is totally miserable.

As I walk in his kitchen door, the old dog barks and comes to greet me looking quite chipper – but it doesn't last, he licks my hand then returns to his bed by the fire. He has lost weight in the last week and his ribs are beginning to show clearly through. There is no need to trim up his leg for the final injection as he is still bald from last time. He is used to this procedure and doesn't stir. His owner cuddles him close and steadies his leg while I slip the drug into his vein. It is an overdose of anaesthetic, peaceful and painless; he will just fall asleep – a nice way to go. The drug takes effect swiftly and he is gone by the time I have finished injecting. I will miss the old fella – he really was a dog in a million. His owner will bury him on the hill overlooking the house, still in his green body warmer.

I take my leave and drive homewards, sad but satisfied that we did the right thing, and pleased that he went so smoothly and with dignity. It is the end of a chapter, and after a few minutes of remembrance, it is time to close the book so to speak and move on. Dwelling on the sad events which occur in this job is not a good plan. At home I gather my two dogs, collect Jonno from the farm and set off up the hill. It is a clear still day and we can see for miles at the top of the hill. Green fields of growing crops are interspersed with the deep brown of newly ploughed land. The beech tree behind the thinking stones is bearing buds making my thoughts turn to spring. Already we are seeing the effects of the lighter mornings and can find our way on morning walks without a torch. This morning was particularly beautiful, the stark trees on the skyline silhouetted against a violet sky, while a creamy dawn spread from the east. Geese flew honking overhead in the huge expanse which is our valley. It makes something of a change to be able to admire these effects without battling against the ferocious winds which howl down the valley so frequently in winter.

Arriving home at midday, something is different – we have the sun back. It is wonderful to see sunlight flood across the garden and through the windows after its two-month absence behind the hill. Today is such a welcome break in our dreich winter weather. Driving into evening surgery is also a spectacular treat. The sun is close to setting behind Clayfern hill painting the western sky a vivid orange and pink. The tide is out leaving herring-bone patterned sandbanks reflecting the orange glow, while in the distance, the snow-capped hills are bathed in warm pink light. As I drive towards the village the street lights switch on, many pinpoints of orange light adding to the breathtaking scene. A world away from the bright lights and glare of city driving which wild horses would not drag me back to.

After morning surgery the next day, I am off to my old friend Edith McNaughton's to pick up her oldest Dachshund, Mo, for some dental work. Mo is the only one of Edith's three dachsies not to have had surgery for slipped discs – a common problem in this long-backed breed. Both Eeny and Meeny have mercifully recovered from the worst of the condition although Eeny still walks with the jerky gait of a string puppet. When an intervertebral disc slams into the spinal cord quickly as Eeny's did, it causes more severe damage than a gradual extrusion, and although Eeny had emergency surgery very quickly, she has not regained her full locomotive function. Still she manages, and is happy to potter round Edith's small flat and garden.

Edith is doing a crossword when I go in. She is a game old lady, supremely happy with her lot in life despite being virtually housebound. She has a wide range of interests, and her little flat is lined with books, videos and paraphernalia related to her numerous hobbies. I fish two brightly coloured stones from my pocket to show her. They were picked up on a walk and I thought they might interest her. 'Well, that's an agate,' she exclaims, 'And that's a piece of jasper.' Apparently in her youth, she joined a lapidary group and one of their activities was gem-finding expeditions on the local farms. Is there no limit to this lady's knowledge? Little Mo is ever so excited to be going in the car; in fact, I rather fear she is over-excited as a foul aroma reaches my nostrils. Not looking forward to cleaning out the rear of the car, I am greatly relieved to spot a tractor in the field, spreading muck from the nearby barn. Sorry Mo, falsely accused.

At the farm surgery, Julie has arrived before me and is preparing for the day's work. Another dog is also due in for dental attention, so Julie is gathering the relevant equipment – the usual anaesthetic paraphernalia plus all the necessities for dental work. Newly sharpened elevators, extractors and hand scalers are laid out on a stainless steel tray, and Julie is preparing the ultrasonic scaler for action. This machine uses ultrasonic waves to vapourise water droplets delivered to the tip of the probe, the energy produced by this process dislodges tartar from the surface of the teeth. The water is supplied from a drum-like reservoir which requires 'priming' to pressurise the container thus delivering the water to the probe. To do this, a handle leading into the drum is vigorously pumped up and down. This always reminds me of the detonation boxes used when large buildings are blown up. After a few minutes energetic pumping, Julie is quite red in the face. Once Mo is anaesthetised, we quickly get underway. Mo has an endotracheal tube inserted into her windpipe; through which anaesthetic gas and oxygen are administered. The tube is vital in dental work; it has an inflatable cuff which produces a snug fit in the airway and prevents the inhalation of any debris or water produced in the scaling process. As the scaler produces a mist of water mixed with tartar and bacteria dislodged from the teeth, I wear a paper mask and goggles to protect myself. It looks a bit silly and I can see Julie smirking across the table as usual. Thus attired, it is hot, slow work to do a thorough job.

Mo has no teeth which require removing, but they are all caked with tartar – a mixture of bacteria and crystals deposited from saliva . As an adult dog has forty two teeth, this means that there are forty two outer surfaces and forty two inner surfaces to clean, and the process cannot be rushed. Once all tartar is removed then the teeth require polishing to leave a smooth, clean surface. A mechanical polishing device belonging to the same machine is used for this, and I operate both scaler and polisher by using a foot pedal. When our patients go home, they will have pristine mouths, but the process of tartar deposition begins immediately. It is important that the owners continue our work today with teeth cleaning at home. As for humans, regular brushing is best, but if the animal absolutely will not cooperate, then there are a variety of gels that can be applied directly into the mouth which reduce the rate of tartar formation. Chewing on specially designed dental chews or even raw vegetables and tough cuts of meat are also useful in the fight against tartar. I happen to know that Mo is particularly partial to chews so this gives her an golden excuse to legitimately be given treats.

Once our last dog – a bulky spaniel – is returned to his kennel, we have another procedure which promises to be taxing, a rabbit in for the removal of his misaligned incisor teeth. This is becoming an increasingly common complaint in veterinary life, and it appears that rabbits are becoming victims of our 'convenience' society. Just as we humans indulge in easy-to-prepare-and-eat convenience foods, so do our pet rabbits. In the wild, a rabbit will spend the majority of its time grazing on grass and other abrasive foods. Rabbit teeth grow continually but such abrasive materials help to keep them the correct length. In captivity, we tend to feed them mainly convenient concentrate diet which does not do the job as well. It has also been noticed that rabbits pick out the tastier constituents of such food, causing the ratio of calcium and phosphorus in their diet to become imbalanced and thus affecting the development of the tooth sockets. Certainly twenty years ago, a bunny with overgrown teeth was only infrequently seen, whereas nowadays, this is probably the most common condition seen in our rabbit patients. Treatment in the past has always involved trimming the teeth regularly with nail clippers. This is now frowned upon by veterinary dental specialists as the teeth splinter and cause the patient pain, and the rabbits are not at all keen on the procedure. It is preferable rather to trim the teeth with a dental burr, but a newer, more permanent solution is to totally remove all the creature's incisor (front) teeth. They manage to cope with their hay, straw and concentrates fine although vegetables require cutting into thinner pieces.

As with many advances in veterinary techniques, novel operations such as this are originally performed in the specialist centres such as vet schools or research centres before they filter down to the GP on the ground, so to speak. This procedure was not being used while I was at vet school, so, as with many new procedures, I am virtually self-taught. Reading texts describing the operation has been backed up by practice on rabbit corpses – courtesy of our friend Andy the shepherd. Unfortunately, no more practice sessions are on the cards since Jay discovered the corpses in polythene bags in the freezer. Over the years, my poor partner has had to put up with all manner of macabre finds in our freezer shelves, but now the worm has turned and the rabbits are no more. We have performed this operation several times now, and the tooth-removing procedure is in fact easier in rabbits than in dogs or cats, but the tricky bit is the anaesthetic. We routinely use injectable anaesthetic cocktails for our rabbit ops and top them up if necessary with anaesthetic gas by face mask. As we are working in the mouth for tooth removal, using the mask is no longer possible so we have to get the injection just right. Even when all goes well, rabbits are more likely to die under anaesthetic than dogs and cats.

Today's patient refuses to go adequately to sleep with the calculated anaesthetic dose and requires two top-ups during the procedure. We know this as while I operate, Julie is continually listening to the rabbit's heart through the stethoscope and reports any increase in rate which corresponds to any painful stimulus from my end. If this persistently occurs, we stop and administer more anaesthetic. After over an hour, we are finally finished but the patient still requires careful attention. He is wrapped in insulating bubble wrap, and placed on a warm water bottle after receiving injections to counteract the anaesthetic and to provide pain relief. 'He'll probably sleep for a week now,' comments Julie, always the optimist. After the intense concentration, we feel as if we could.

We both begin the cleaning up, chatting as we go. We discuss the coming weekend, when, in an attempt to make some money for our coming move, I am sharing a table with Julie at an antique fair. My collection of old medical instruments is ever growing, and it seems a good time to prune it in a good cause. I have spent any spare moments sorting through what I want to sell. 'How many things are you bringing?' Julie asks. 'Five, so far,' I mutter. *'Five?'* she shrieks, 'You'll need to do better than that.' Truth is, I don't really want to part with anything but needs must. I will harden my heart at the next sort out.

'The soda lime is getting exhausted,' comments Julie next, referring to the granules which 'scrub' carbon dioxide from the anaesthetic circuit, allowing us to re-use gas in bigger dogs. 'So am I!' I reply light-heartedly. While Julie replaces the old soda lime with new granules, I clean the dental instruments. On the field opposite the surgery are hundreds of Pink-footed geese graze, studiously ignoring the bird-scarer set to go off at regular intervals. They do cause some damage to growing crops but it is still good to see them. As we work, the sun streams through the ops room window. Staring along at our new house, I am disconcerted to see that it is still in shadow. It may be a case of 'Deal's off!' It does seem strange that for the last few years, we have stared along in that direction, but, after a month or so, we will be staring this way.

Surprisingly for an ops day, there is time for a reasonable walk after the ops are completed. Many such days we only finish just before I need to leave for evening surgery, so today is a welcome change. Considering where to walk, I decide to take a trip to the west end of the woods. When we ventured in that direction before Christmas, we found a recently dead roe deer under some bushes. I suspect the poor creature had been hit by a car as it had typical traffic accident injuries. It must have managed to escape up the hill before collapsing and dying. Wild roe deer often cross the road from the woods to graze in the fields, and several times a year, there is a knock on our door to alert me to an injured deer. The victim frequently is either dead or has vanished by the time I get to the scene. If they are still alive then invariably they require putting to sleep, usually with a gun which provides a quick, humane end. These wild creatures cannot be comforted like a domestic animal and the mere presence of a human causes them intense anguish, so the deed needs to be done as quickly as possible.

I am interested to see whether the deer has become skeletonised yet, but reckon that it is probably unlikely considering how cold and wet the weather has been. Although interesting in themselves, many of our walks take on the nature of expeditions – to see if the swallow chicks have hatched or fledged, if the stag has lost his antlers, if the fox earth is still in use, if the large damaged branch has finally detached from the tall pine tree. It is nice to have such intimate knowledge of one's surroundings and it makes life very enjoyable.

There is no sign of the deer corpse under the bushes, but the dogs find it half way down the slope. It has been dragged there by hungry forest residents and is not as intact as it was. As expected, it has not yet rotted down to bare bone. In warm weather, it would have by now – according to one textbook, in warm weather, the minimum time to total skeletonisation can be as short as ten days. Mentally booking in another trip to this corner later in the year, we regain the track and wend our way homewards in time to return to Clayfern for evening surgery.

The surgeries this week have been rather restful as they are the first this year not to have been interrupted by telephone calls regarding house buying or planning permission. Unfortunately, they have not been particularly lucrative. It is a prime example of Murphy's Law that when a good income is desirable (such as when you have just signed for a large mortgage) the surgery clientele responds either by staying away or by bringing in patients consisting almost totally of creatures in cardboard boxes. Obviously health is equally important for wee beasts such as guinea pigs, hamsters, gerbils, mice and rats, but from a fiscal point of view, they are hopeless at providing big money fast. For light relief, we receive a phone call requiring advice on a 'naughty' cat. 'What exactly is he doing?' enquires Alice, and only then do we realise that the cat is in fact 'knotty'. An appointment is made for him to come in next week for a sedative and demat. His knots will be trimmed off using the clippers – the safest way of dealing with them. After laughing at Alice with the 'knotty' cat misunderstanding, it was inevitable that I should also get caught. 'My dog's got a lump,' announces Jim Duff, fondly regarding his elderly Labrador. 'Where?' I enquire. 'On his left back leg,' comes the reply. After several minutes running my hands over the entire leg, I am none the wiser, '*Where* exactly is his lump?' I ask again. 'No!' exclaims Jim, 'Ah said he's lumping.' Ever felt a fool? Last December, Linda our Australian locum was also fooled by one of our 'broader' spoken customers who rang in with a query: 'Ah dinnae ken whit tae dae,' she began, 'Thir's a rabin that keeps bangin' on the windae.'

'Excuse me,' said Linda in her Aussie drawl, 'What was that again?' Ella's question was duly repeated and misunderstood twice more until the frustrated lady added more information, speaking loudly and slowly as if to a backward child – 'A *RABIN* ... wi' a reed breest.' At last the light dawned on a bewildered Linda. Poor Linda, not only has she to deal with the vagaries of our more eccentric clients, but at times she even needs an interpreter.

Almost the very next customer also raises a smile. I suspect that her itchy little dog is allergic to

something, and he has been referred to see a veterinary dermatologist for allergy testing. She has come in to report how the appointment went. 'The taxidermist was wonderful,' she enthuses, 'He dealt with Hamish so well.' As Hamish is a stroppy little devil, a taxidermist sounds like a good idea.

Chapter 5

February at last – January is always so long. The weather has been mild for this time of year and there have been signs that Spring is just round the corner – lengthening days and even buds on the beech tree by the thinking stones. However, a letter in the local paper today warns against being lulled into a false sense of security – apparently a mild January in 1947 was followed by snowstorms and sub-zero temperatures in February. Who remembers these things? I can't even remember what it was like last week.

It is certainly pleasant to see where you are going on the dogs' morning walk, I think, hopping over the stile into the back field. Its days as a walk are probably numbered as it will soon be ploughed up for planting of spring barley. We take full advantage today, ambling companionably along, me in one tram line and Kippen in the other. Tram lines are the tracks made by the tractor through the fields which make useful paths for walking through the crop.

The drive into Clayfern is also pleasant – snowdrops are emerging on the banking and yellow flowers are appearing on gorse bushes. The kestrel is sitting in his usual spot on the telephone wire along from the house. The sun is just touching the northern hills, highlighting the snow-capped peaks and reflecting the ripple patterns on the exposed sandbanks in the river. Sunlight is striking Clayfern for the first time this year, reflecting the warm colours of the sandstone walls and pantiled roofs. Observing the village nestling below the hills on the bend of the river, I realise afresh what an ideal site it was for early settlers – fertile meadowland, hills for lookouts and the river to provide food and transport. Driving past Abbeygate Farm with its millpond, I wave as usual to the covey of elderly gentlemen sitting by the barn and proceed up the High Street to the surgery, waving at friends and acquaintances on the way. An exceedingly civilised way to start the day.

In the surgery display window, our Christmas display has been replaced by our usual stopgap – a display of old veterinary instruments. Something about Clayfern produces longevity in its residents, and several older inhabitants have told us many a tale about days when such instruments were in daily use. On a quieter day such as this, it is our cue to revamp the window display. Luckily, February is Pet Smile Month so our topic requires no particular flashes of inspiration. Out come the 'before' and 'after' posters demonstrating the benefits of proper dental hygiene, and the props to hold the public's attention. Amongst the latter are the two foxes' skulls and assorted teeth removed from assorted patients. We sound like parrots about home dental hygiene, but a few minutes brushing per day backed up with suitable chewable treats can help to prevent the horrendous mouths which we often have the misfortune to deal with on ops days.

There is not much afoot at the surgery this morning, just as well really as our first patient is a guide dog puppy. These pups are homed with 'puppy walkers' for their first year. These volunteers have a brief to expose the pups to a wide range of sights and sounds, and to provide basic training. If they are shaping up satisfactorily at the end of their stay, then the pups return to the Guide Dogs For The Blind centre to continue their training. It is heartbreaking for the temporary minders to wave them goodbye, but they do get considerable satisfaction hearing about their future progress. They are usually lovely, extrovert pups – a joy to deal with, but they do come with reams of paperwork. First, information about the pup's weight and condition are entered in one book, then further details are entered on a treatment card. As I also fill in a surgery record card, the whole procedure does take longer than a routine consultation. Luckily there is nothing terribly wrong with young Gus, only a tummy upset which is easily treated.

Next a fairly new client with her old dog. She has moved from her last home where she lived next door to an old, long-retired vet who told her that nothing much could be done for her crippled pet with a mouthful of revolting loose, tartared-up teeth. When we first met last week, I disagreed, and we arranged an appointment for Dan to have a thorough dental under general anaesthesia. Many people are nervous of general anaesthetics in old animals, but the agents available nowadays are much safer than before and the risks are considerably less than they would have been twenty years ago. It is thoroughly miserable for such patients to have to put up with a stinky, painful mouth, and the slight risk involved with the anaesthetic is well worth taking to improve the dog's lot. Last week, Dan had his dental – twelve teeth removed and the rest scaled and polished, and he has also been on a modern anti-inflammatory drug to ease his arthritis ... and treatment has paid off; he is like a new dog. Much of his slowing down which was put down to aging has simply been due to the misery of living with a horrible mouth and sore legs. A friend of Jay and I says she is looking forward to getting old so that she can 'sit with her knees wide apart showing her massive drawers, and beat her way to the head of the pension queue at the post office with a knobbly walking stick!' For a brief minute, Alice and I indulge in a mental scenario of Kate as an ancient vet holding forth – 'Anaesthetics, who needs them – just stuff the patient down a wellie boot' (as was the method of restraining farm cats for castration not all that long ago). I ask Alice to shoot me if I ever get to the stage of dispensing out-of-date advice.

Alice is curious to know how Julie and I got on at our antique fair over the weekend. Rather sheepishly, I tell her that, after fifteen minutes, I was £30 down, tempted by two rather nice antique medical instruments on another stall. Fortunately, trade improved over the day and we both made a modest profit. In addition to being a part-time veterinary nurse for the surgery, Julie also runs a small antique shop. Both Jay and I enjoy visiting the many auctions in this area, and for fun, Julie is kind enough to sell our occasional purchase in her shop. Pressure of work has rather reduced our activity in this field, but I tell Alice about one of the funnier incidents that occurred last year –

viewing at an auction house one day, I left a bid for a rather elegant 'silver samovar ' (or so I thought). Delighted to find my bid had been successful, I returned to collect my prize to find it ignominiously described on the receipt as a 'tea urn'.

Today appears to be 'foreign body in stomach day'. There is nothing remotely infectious about this condition, but coincidentally, our first three patients either have had or might have a gastric foreign body. First in is a little cross collie who has been bringing up a little yellow bile first thing in the morning. Otherwise, she is perfectly bright and cheerful. There are many reasons for a dog to vomit, but nothing of any significance is apparent on a physical examination. This symptom occasionally occurs when a foreign body is lodged in the stomach. It is only when the stomach is empty that it causes some irritation and results in the early morning sickness. The owner and I discuss the case – the ideal solution is to x-ray the dog to see if anything can be seen, but the owner is due to go on holiday tomorrow. As the situation is not dire, I suggest she tries giving the dog a small snack last thing at night to see if that improves matters. If not, then she will book in for an x-ray on her return.

Next in is a young Labrador who has been having treatment for a bad ear. On his last visit, his owner mentioned in the passing that he too occasionally brought up bile in the morning. 'He brought up this stone on Thursday and hasn't thrown up since,' exclaims his owner, proudly displaying a round stone almost the size of a small egg. To complete the threesome, Brutus MacLeod comes in for his booster. Also a Labrador, he caused quite a stir several years ago. Also an occasional morning vomiter, one day he astonished his owners by bringing up a golf ball. They quickly rang the surgery to be told that hopefully this might signal the end of his problem. Alas, this was not the case, instead of vomiting less, he was sick four or five times that day and was quite dull when he was brought in the following morning. An x-ray showed not one but two more golf balls in his stomach, which I dutifully removed. Like the initial ball, one was white and appeared freshly eaten, while the second was a dirty green, indicating that it had been in the stomach for quite some time. Brutus recovered well from his surgery and has not yet repeated this trick. He lives next door to a golf course but his owners have resisted the temptation to hop over the wall, and now walk him in a totally different direction.

It is obviously going to be a quirky day, I think when I return to Fern and receive an emergency call. The patient is Emma, an elderly Labrador who was in the surgery only last week for her booster vaccination. At the time, I examined a small lump on her underside. Her owner assured me that it had been there for a while and did not appear to be growing noticeably. Many old dogs are covered in lumps and bumps of varying sizes, and it is impractical to remove them all. In general, if the lump is round or oval, painless, not growing into the surrounding tissues and only growing slowly if at all, then it is likely to be benign and should cause no problems. This does not mean that it should just be forgotten however – the owner should check it regularly, and allow their vet to have a look every so often as well. I certainly did not expect to see Emma again so soon. Catching herself on a sharp nail, she has somehow managed to shell out the growth entirely leaving an open pouch of loose skin. 'It would make her a handy purse,' I think irreverently as I examine the damage. John, her owner, has brought the lump as well, it looks like a small white walnut nestling in its bed of tissue paper. Luckily, she is a very calm dog and allows me to instil some local anaesthetic along the top end of the sac before cutting it off and stitching the resulting skin wound. I really can't decide whether this case of self-surgery has been good or bad luck. It has certainly saved us a general anaesthetic had we decided to remove the growth at a later date.

During evening surgery, a regular customer lifts her exuberant spaniel onto the examination table, 'We've got a feature', she pronounces. 'What kind of feature?' I reply facetiously – 'Ornamental, water ...?' 'No, a feet chewer.' Definitely a quirky day.

Chapter 6

The serious work begins at our new property this Saturday morning. We are still waiting for the results of the building control application, but we can at least begin some preliminary work. As the new surgery will need a water supply and drainage, Jay and Andy are to start by digging a trench from the house to the outbuildings, to locate and join up with the waste pipes from the house. Julie's partner Bill begins the proceedings by cutting a track through the tarmac using a special saw – a Stihl saw. '*That* would be useful for amputations,' Julie and I think as it slices its way across the yard like a knife through butter. By the time I return from morning surgery, the trench is three feet deep but still no pipes are to be seen.

The plans are repeatedly perused and anxiety gives way to relief when the familiar fire clay tubes are finally uncovered. Two pipes run side by side – one will be surface drainage, the other sewage – but which is which? Next follows an energetic half-hour of flushing toilets and inserting a hose in drains or other likely orifices, and watching and listening carefully by the septic tank for evidence of running water. Being the smallest, I am dispatched into the trench with a stethoscope to confirm the team's findings. Unfortunately fire clay is not as amenable to being sounded as flesh and blood, and try as I might, I can hear nothing at all. Never mind, the troops seem to be quietly confident, and the trench is left open for the imminent plumbing works.

Being a shepherd, Andy has the same brand of black humour as vets, commenting 'You could always fill the trench with your unsuccessful cases.' As Spring approaches, many shepherds will now be digging pits into which any lambing casualties are put. Like pet rabbits, sheep do seem to have a disturbing propensity to shuffle off their mortal coil at the least opportunity. For Christmas we gave Andy a mug – the picture on it depicts a sheep standing on a bale addressing the surrounding flock – *'Now it's Spring girls, we need to vote on who has the privilege of dropping dead for no apparent reason!'*

Luckily we are nearing the end of the outdoor work when it begins to snow, lots of it, delivered horizontally for much of the afternoon. Leaving the workers preparing to clear out the outhouses, I sneak off to walk the dogs. At five hundred feet up the hill, the snow is thick underfoot, scrunching satisfyingly as we troop along. No creatures have been out before us, and a virgin blanket of whiteness stretches as far as the eye can see. More snow begins to fall, large wet flakes which cling to every surface – the dogs have white jackets and even the stag's antlers are coated. Avoiding the harsh wind, we return through the trees. In the woods, the world is two-tone – only the white of snow and the grey-brown austerity of winter trees. Unfortunately, the snow is not lying below the trees, so it is with regret that I leave the silent woods behind and descend to the bleak wetness of the valley.

Amazingly, by evening the skies have cleared, leaving a starry moonlit night. Jay and I set off to paint at the new house, taking Kippen and Fintry with us. It will be their new home too, and we are anxious that they are used to it before we finally move in. The world is defined in shades of silver, grey and black as we walk along the road, our shadows keeping us company. Fintry's looks like a plump wart-hog, while Kippen's is a hairy wolf. Wimpy Fintry is not at all keen on a house with a moat, and needs much gentle persuasion before she plucks up courage to hurdle the trench. While we make a start on painting, the dogs excitedly explore the house and garden. The house is really not in a bad decorative state – it was the previous owners' pride and joy – but some sort of primitive, territory-marking behaviour makes us want to put our own seal on the place. As Julie says, painting is more socially acceptable than weeing in the corners as our patients would do. We shall miss our ex-neighbours, they were fun and sometimes gently eccentric. My favourite memory is of the late night phone call from Morag – 'Just ringing to check you're okay.' 'We're fine Morag, why shouldn't we be?' 'Well, I was looking your way and all the outside lights suddenly went out.' 'They would do, we switched them off when we went to bed.'

After a fruitful night's decorating, we stand quietly in the garden admiring the peaceful scene; myriad stars puncture the sky, moonlight glimmers on the river and the lights of distant homesteads twinkle on the far hillside. An owl hoots from the edge of the woods, answered moments later from deeper within the trees. Arm in arm we stand as the happy dogs snuffle in the bushes – yes, we can be happy here.

Chapter 7

It is a beautiful frosty morning and encouragingly light at 7.30 a.m. when the dogs have their early walk. There are sounds of geese flying overhead but no sign of them on the fields. This tends to happen over winter, sometimes they are here in their thousands, while at other times there are none to be seen. They will be massing on land on the far side of the valley. On the way to morning surgery, I spot our feral sheep by the roadside. I thought she had gone when the flock were collected, but she must have been on the hilltops and has been left behind. She looks quite contented grazing on the verge, and seems to have some road sense unlike most sheep, waiting patiently for cars to pass before crossing to the other side.

Preliminary work has at last begun on the new surgery, but Clayfern surgeries this week have been quiet while locals recover from the triple whammy of gas, electric and telephone bills all appearing at the same time. It certainly makes us appreciate the clients that do come in – we fall on customers in to buy flea products or dog food like manna from heaven. Mrs Cassidy comes in to buy some food for her cats. She drops the change and, as she bends to retrieve it, a rude noise rents the air. 'Oh, *excuse* me!' she exclaims, extracting the dog's squeaky toy from her pocket. Alice asks why she is out and about so early. 'I must be ready by 11 a.m.' she replies, 'I'm going to the *'Introduction to computers for pensioners'* course at the community centre. I can reassure her that it's well worth it, I went to the last one. I hasten to add that I am <u>not</u> a pensioner, but the community centre show genuine community spirit when allowing all and sundry on to their courses. I have also been to *'Painting for the unemployed'* and *'Pottery for single parents,'* despite being unqualified for either course. In fact, the centre is being uncharacteristically coy in referring to pensioners – they already run two clubs flatly called 'Clayfern Old Men's Club' and 'Clayfern Old Women's Club' so are well used to calling a spade a spade.

Luckily for the ailing surgery bank balance, there is a busy day lined up at the farm surgery. My neighbour Sheila (the cat lady) has been active again and there are twelve feral cats to be neutered. These come from a farm where the numbers have got out of hand and the owners have requested Sheila's help. Her particular expertise is in trapping feral cats – she instinctively knows where to set her traps and has unlimited patience – she has been known to wait almost all night to capture an elusive individual. Once today's cats have been neutered, they will be returned to the farm where they will become a stable colony and will continue to earn their keep by catching mice and rats. Some people have the idea that neutered cats will not hunt as well as unneutered ones, but this is a complete fallacy. Unfortunately it leads to the uncontrolled population increases with which we are so familiar. Cats are very successful at breeding and numbers will multiply at alarming rates. Food then becomes short, and disease, fighting and interbreeding occurs, with sick or dying cats being seen with increasing frequency. Many dog and cat welfare problems are caused by indiscriminate breeding producing – 'Too many animals for too few good homes.' If numbers were controlled then dogs and cats would become a valued commodity and would be treated well. As it is, it is all too easy for bad owners just to acquire another pet as it suits them and charity shelters are always full.

First, I have to pop in on Edith McNaughton , and resolve to mention the computing course to her. I am convinced that she would take to the Internet like a duck to water. The visit is something in the way of a social call – Sheila does a brisk trade in car-boot and jumble sales to finance her cat rescue work, and passed on to the surgery a smart knitted coat for a small dog. It will be ideal for one of the dachsies. It is a coincidence that it is the same colour as the nurses' uniform – bottle green with white piping. As Alice is a 'cold' person, I offer it to her first as a balaclava. Ever aware of our precarious financial position since buying the new house, Alice helps matters by rationing heat to the surgery. We have five minutes of fan heater in each room in addition to our oil-filled radiators and that is our lot. Both of us turn up for work in layers of clothing like the little man in the Michelin tyre logo. The locals are a hardy lot and seem not to notice the cold, and are often to be seen tripping along the high street in sandals and T-shirts on the days when we are swathed in fleeces and heavy boots. Of course, the farm surgery is always piping hot for ops and if we have in-patients. This tends to involve much putting on and removing of layers but we are used to it by now.

Edith is a little subdued this morning, she is bruised after a fall in the kitchen. Since a bad traffic

accident, she has suffered from narcolepsy and is quite likely to black out at any time. I have always been terrified that she will collapse while I am there but so far this has not happened. Her garden is as unsuitable for a narcoleptic as you could imagine, sloping at a near vertical angle. Before her worsening health more or less confined her to the flat area at the bottom, I would frequently observe the results of her latest plummet from the heights; 'I had a wee fall today,' she would say in a matter-of-fact tone, displaying livid bruises on arms and legs. Fortunately she must go limp when she blacks out thus preventing more serious injury. She promises to give the computer course some thought, but at two sessions per week, it may be too frequent for her to cope with.

On the way home, I call in at the new house to see how the work is going. The joiner has battened the walls and is cutting out two windows to provide more light. The air is thick with dust. Luckily I am not needed, so escape. Sheila and her cats are not due until the afternoon, so I collect the dogs, pick up Jonno from the farm, and head up the hill. Perched on the thinking stones, I observe the scene; the overall colours are muted – the coconut- matting brown and dour green of the forest is relieved by the occasional buttermilk white slash of a freshly broken bough. The meadow is predominantly the fawn of dried grass with only a glimmer of fresh green. Something interesting has caught Fintry's attention. First she stands with erect posture, chin tucked into chest as she eyes a tussock, then she proceeds to poke into the depths with short, sharp jabs of the muzzle. Kippen has noticed this activity and ambles over. Like a raw student, Fintry backs off and allows Kippen – the learned professor – to inspect her find. He passes on after only a cursory sniff, and she skips away in search of further mischief, reassured that nothing exciting has been missed. Moving on round the hill, we catch the full force of a snell, north wind coming fresh from the snowfields of the highlands. There is more colour in this direction. The sapphire-blue river is fringed by golden swathes of reeds which look like idyllic sandy beaches from this distance. The deep green of the cereal crops is backed by icing sugar snow-capped mountains. A pillar-box red tractor is spraying fertiliser on a field – from up here it looks like a matchbox toy. Turning to go back, the dogs head for the water trough for their usual drink but find it frozen solid. I lift out a half-inch thick sheet of ice and throw it to them. Fintry has great sport crunching and carrying chunks of ice. What it is to be young and have good teeth. Into the woods, more devastation has been wreaked by the gales; a long pine is lodged in the Y of a beech tree, and a massive branch is held horizontally in the 'arms' of a sycamore. The noise in here during the gales must have been incredible. Jonno is becoming increasingly deaf as he gets older – he is nearly thirteen now – and I need to keep a sharp eye on him or we lose him. He then stands stock still looking gormless until I retrace my steps to find him.

I now have the luxury of an hour with nothing particularly pressing to do. I have plans to research a topic which has been intriguing me since we bought the new house ... or in fact, before that, when we set the treasure hunt. In the midst of the woods, not far from The Beast's Lair, Jay and I noticed a pile of moss-covered stones set out in a roughly rectangular shape. Further observation revealed faint tracks leading across the hill towards the neighbouring farm. Jay bought me a metal detector for Christmas, and we had a vague plan to investigate the area when the weather improved.

In the meantime we were somewhat diverted by the purchase of the house. It is quite strange how separate strands of daily life often tie up – a prime example occurs here. The new house is called 'The Laigher.' The previous owners were not sure why, but some preliminary investigating suggests that the name may well derive from the Scots word *laich* or *laigh* meaning low. We felt satisfied with this explanation as the ground is certainly low here. The two historical strands might have remained separate if not for a chance conversation with friends who mentioned that there was once a old road in this area that ran over the top of the hills. The present road was only built to accommodate more modern transport which could not cope with the more direct up-and-over approach of the original routes. Perhaps our new house's name in fact referred to the new road; perhaps the pile of stones was an old dwelling alongside the old road ... the scene was set for an intriguing project.

First on my list is to carefully peruse the old map which hangs in our office. It dates from 1800 and shows the area of the lair as being afforested, with a track alongside. The present day road appears to be in position at this time. I log on to the Internet in a search for earlier maps, locate some and order them by e-mail. Browsing through items of local history, I move from local parish maps into parish records for the 1840s. I can't say exactly what I intend to find – name: *x*, address: *pile of stones above Fern* – but the records make fascinating reading. Although our surgery is in Clayfern, Fern Farm in fact belongs to the parish of Duncraig. The most striking aspect of the records is the number of inhabitants that lived in this area. Fern farm itself boasted six ploughmen, whereas now there is only one who drives a tractor, not a handsome Clydesdale horse. We have a collection of horseshoes found on the farm and these horses were certainly big beasties. Duncraig parish also gave homes to millers, wrights, weavers, hostlers, a coachman and even a watchmaker. It is rather sad to see how the population has decreased with the advent of mechanisation. In those days, farming might have been tough but at least it was sociable. Today, farming is quite a lonely business. Sometimes progress is not all it is cracked up to be.

Before long Sheila arrives, and we are plodding through the feral cats when the telephone rings. It is the architect involved in the new surgery conversion with the results of the latest planning application. The powers-that-be think that we should have a disabled toilet in the surgery. At first I think he is joking – such a toilet would take up one of the four rooms that we are planning and for what? We only see a couple of clients a day at the farm surgery, and if they are caught short, they use the toilet in the house. This arrangement has worked very well for the last decade in which possibly one person a year has availed themselves of our facilities. After enduring ten minutes of my incensed rambling along this theme, the architect backs off, promising to see if the planners will accept a compromise. As a parting shot, he mentions that they also require more plans for us to alter the entrance to the outbuilding and these will take another three weeks. My day is now ruined, and poor Sheila has to put up with my disgusted mutterings for the next few hours.

You would think we were building the Millennium Dome, not a small rural outpost of Clayfern surgery. How much worse can we make the front of the building than the present battered metal door? In any case, the property is in a dip and is hardly visible from outside; our nearest neighbours are two hundred yards away ... etc. etc. So we now have a delay of a further month in which no work can be done on the new surgery, another month of maintaining two houses

I am not a happy camper, and desperately want to harness up the dogs and disappear up the hill again, but as luck would have it, every cat turns out to be female apart from one, and the neutering session seems to drag on for ever. There is no respite after evening surgery as instead of sulking by the fire, I am instead called upon to deal with two emergency cases.

The planning department's decision has really been a bombshell, Jay and I agree as we fall into bed. For once, we both feel bruised and defeated, and totally disenchanted with the whole concept of moving house.

Chapter 8

It is a jaded pair that greet the dawn this morning. The continuing planning permission saga has fairly taken the lustre off our life. We have both lost all enthusiasm for the whole project. At the end of the day, all we are trying to do is to provide a decent service for our customers in the shape of a very small, rural surgery, but because we are a business, all the rules are carried out to the letter. The surgery receives fewer visitors than our neighbours who belong to a large family and routinely have nine or ten visitors per day. Even when we first started the surgery in the famous wooden shed, we needed planning permission, and one visiting official even suggested chopping down an avenue of three hundred-year-old beech trees to improve visibility for cars arriving at the surgery. All that for two to three customers per day. Minute details of type and colour of external finishes, and size and position of windows were required in our application for the present surgery to preserve the environment , yet local farmyards virtually all feature one or more fields filled with piles of rotting metal and old machinery. Life can be very unfair sometimes. Jay is more pragmatic about the situation, but mere mention of the subject now incites me to complete hysteria.

Some relaxation is badly in order so we both get up early (we can't sleep anyway) and take the dogs for a peaceful walk. It is a sunny, frosty morning and yesterday's washing is frozen stiff on the line. Serrated ice lies in tractor tracks like shark's teeth. There is no wind, and sounds carry over long distances – from a hundred yards away, we hear the slightly muffled bird song from the cow barn along with the occasional cough, and clanking of the water troughs. Coming closer, we can see sun streaming through the perspex roof panels catching dust particles in its path. An owl is calling from the woods and suddenly we hear the first green woodpecker call of the year – a distinctive sound like a falsetto, manic giggle. Cheered up, we bid each other goodbye and head towards our respective day's work.

After morning surgery, my mission is to track down Jock the electrician and threaten or beg him to come to the new house before tomorrow. Since the planners delayed all work on the new surgery, we have taken the opportunity to transfer our slightly disgruntled joiner into the house. It seems a good idea to get essential work done before we move in. Brian the joiner worked over the weekend, but can go no further until the electrician does his bit. He was expected yesterday, but did not appear. Brian is coming tomorrow to complete the work so we need Jock urgently. I drop into the shop to be told that I have just missed him, he has gone off on an emergency. With a sinking heart, I leave entreating Bunty his assistant to try to send him our way. Clayfern tradesmen do a wonderful job but have no sense of urgency – there is a definite sense of 'manyana' that pervades the entire community. If Jock does not appear before tomorrow, Brian will be annoyed and will probably go off again, Jay will be annoyed ... and yours truly will be piggy in the middle as usual.

There will be no more time today to chase up Jock as we have a marathon neutering session lined up for the local dog charity – fourteen pups in all, two litters of seven. The optimum age at which neutering should take place is an extremely controversial subject amongst vets. I have been neutering pups and kittens from eight weeks of age for various animal charities for over fifteen years now with no apparent ill effects, and fail to see why some folk are so totally against it. No one has yet brought an animal back saying ' You neutered this at eight weeks old and look what has happened to it.' They have all led as healthy lives as those neutered at a later date. Early neutering, as it is called, has tremendous benefits for the charities as the animals they home are not able to reproduce and add to the considerable numbers of surplus and unwanted ones. Some charities home unneutered pets requesting the new owners to have them neutered when they are older.

Unfortunately, not all do. It is also pleasant for the new owners to be presented with a *fait accompli*, and not to have to endure the worry of having their pet anaesthetised and operated upon.

We enjoy our puppy days and revert to what our last locum (a lecturer on animal care at a college) scornfully referred to as 'Puppy cuddlers'. This apparently is a term of derision used at the college to describe students who have no interest in learning, or the more realistic facts of animal care, but just want to play with the animals. One litter is asleep in each large kennel, ready sedated and injected with routine painkiller. Julie extracts a dozy puppy from the sleeping doggy pile. We quickly anaesthetise him or her, perform the surgery – which is very simple and atraumatic in such a small creature – and return the patient to the group. Within half an hour, that puppy will be as awake as any of its not-yet-done littermates.

The first operation of the day is a quick castration – Alice suggests that we send the removed organs to the planners with an anonymous note 'Next time it'll be you!' We have complained so much about planners over the last twenty four hours that if any go missing over the weekend, we will be prime suspects.

Last on the day's agenda after the puppies are two ferret spays. Ferrets begin to come into season in spring and remain in season until mated. If they are not mated, the prolonged season can result in serious health problems. Ferrets are not to be trifled with – today's pair are mercifully friendly, but are still not impressed at being restrained and injected with anaesthetic solution. They have small heads with very sharp teeth, long snake-like necks merging into long bodies, with four sets of sharp claws on the end of each leg, and are extremely difficult to immobilise, experts as they are at squirming and twisting out of trouble. The key seems to be speed, and as soon as Julie pounces on an unsuspecting victim, I rapidly inject the drug then the annoyed creature is swiftly returned to her box. Both of them have been noisily attempting to dig out for the last two hours so it is a relief when they are finally sedated and quiet. Explaining our theory of ferret handling to a young colleague once, I mentioned that they have necks like the Loch Ness Monster – only to be greeted with looks of incomprehension. In the same vein, instructing a nurse attempting to lift a swan – 'Just hold it like a set of bagpipes' – fell on deaf ears. As I was working in England at the time, I suddenly felt like a stranger in a strange land. As with all small creatures, the ferrets are swathed in bubble- wrap and kept very warm until they are fully recovered. Heat loss is a serious consideration when you weigh less than one pound.

As always, the post-op patients are watched closely – an added hazard on puppy days occurs when one patient tries to lie on top of another, as puppies' natural instinct is to cuddle in together – and we frequently need to separate tangles of warm puppy bodies. Not a totally unpleasant task. By mid-afternoon, all pups have recovered and playing happily in their pens, none the worse for the experience. In fact, I am sure that it is less stressful for them going through the procedure with their littermates than it is for an adult dog who is left alone in a kennel, anxious after being parted from his or her owner.

We quickly fall into our familiar routine; anaesthetising, preparing, cutting, stitching then returning to kennel and grabbing another. As I reach over to switch off the anaesthetic, Julie throws a wet swab into the bin behind me. It whizzes past my legs with scarcely an inch to spare. Before I know it, I am indulging in another of the 'flash fantasies' which befall us on ops days. Working for so long together in the confined space of the ops room, we unconsciously modify our movements to avoid collisions ... I explain to Julie that we could be a veterinary version of the Red Arrows – the Red Vets perhaps – movements synchronised and flawless. While Julie returns a pup to the kennel, I bend past her to collect the next, straightening up before she backs out. She accepts the pup on the move – like a rugby pass – while I step to the cupboard to collect an injection ... and so on, in a strange veterinary ballet. Sending a display team to church fetes could be tricky however, we both agree.

As we work, we endeavour to keep costs down by using just as much materials as is necessary. In my first job in a large practice, the boss would sneak up on young assistants being extravagant and grill them – 'Do you know how much that catgut costs per foot ... cotton wool per ounce etc ...?' Once alerted to this habit, we assistants made it our business to memorise all the costs so we could cockily answer back – 'Yes, £2 per foot ... 50p per ounce.' With his thunder stolen, the boss would return muttering to his office while we giggled in triumph. *Now* I see his point.

By mid-afternoon, we are finally finished and all pups are recovered and cheerful, ferrets too. Time for a late lunch, joined in the kitchen by my two dogs, pleased to see us after a boring day on their own. To ease my conscience, I am generous with their rawhide chews so their day is not all gloom. In fact I suspect they quite enjoy Chewsdays. We have a long running joke on the topic of chews and everyone tries adding to the list which goes something like this – What's the dogs' favourite fish? – chewna; favourite musical instrument? – chewba; favourite country? – chewnisia etc. etc. Julie has a cold today and triumphantly asks 'What's their favourite sweets? ... chewnes.'

There is just time for a short trip up the hill with the dogs. The frosty start has transformed into a sunny but windy afternoon. Finding a sheltered corner, I indulge in the first sunbathe of the year. It is surprising how much heat there is in the sun so early in the year.

Driving to evening surgery, I pass the horses at Abbeygate Farm who have been outside for the day but are now being taken in before it goes dark. Smart in his waterproof rug, the first trots along the road in front of the car, tail and mane streaming in the wind, while his companion hangs over the fence, ears pricked, watching his departure. It will be his turn next. Before too long, they will be able to dispense with their coats and stay out overnight as well.

Chapter 9

Life has fallen into an unvaried routine – work, liase with joiner, electrician or plumber, eat, paint and go to bed. After morning surgery, I pay my daily call to the electrician's shop. He did turn up on Tuesday night, finished part of the job then had to leave on another call. The joiner couldn't come on Wednesday as arranged, but on Thursday instead. He is supposedly returning tomorrow, so yet again Jock is being stalked. As a friend says, our tradesmen could do with a calendar let alone a clock. The work always gets done in time, but the laid-back approach is deeply stressful to one used to working to a tight schedule. It is quite frustrating to have to forget about the house now and attend to veterinary work. It would be nice to have some time off to press on with the renovations ... but we need to work to earn the money to pay for it all. Probably the best plan is just to let everyone just get on with it and stop worrying.

Today we have only two operations. First is an overweight bitch for spaying. Faced with her or a pup, there is no contest as to which we would prefer. Neutering a fat bitch is more difficult and potentially more dangerous for the patient. Fat has a good blood supply and a disconcerting habit of disintegrating at the merest touch. The operation involves tying off the blood supply to each ovary then removing the entire uterus after ligaturing the cervix. With the ovaries buried in thick wads of fat, securing the ovarian arteries is rather like lifting up a strip of jelly from a bowl and tying a thread round it . The suture 'cheesewires' through the disintegrating fat, hopefully tightening round the blood vessel before the whole caboodle breaks up altogether. The operation is quite stressful and we are both relieved when it is satisfactorily completed.

Next we have to remove an ulcerated mammary tumour from an

old bitch. The tumour has grown rapidly and will probably be malignant, in which case it will be a gamble whether the dog will survive for more than a few months. Mammary tumours have quite a high probability of metastasising (spreading) elsewhere – usually to the lungs or liver, and the usual scenario sees the patient returning to the surgery in three or four months with further symptoms.

Unfortunately, veterinary chemotherapy is not particularly useful against mammary tumour metastases so the poor dog ends up being put to sleep before she suffers further. If the owner wants to know the type of tumour, we can send a portion to the laboratory for microscopic examination but this dog's owner says she would rather remain in the dark – 'What will be, will be,' she says philosophically. Neutering before a bitch has a first season virtually eradicates the chance of her developing mammary tumours – yet another reason for neutering young. As usual, the 'bits' from both operations are bagged up and put in special containers for collection by a specialist firm. We have separate containers for used needles, out-of-date medicines, old syringe cases and even the used bedding out of the kennels – whether it is soiled or not. This special disposal service is not cheap and adds to the many costs involved in running the surgery. This is a sensitive subject today as both the drug bill and the VAT bill are due to be paid. As always, a late rush of busy surgeries and today's operations has provided the necessary cash – for which I am eternally grateful, although it would be rather nice to reach one's target just a few days before absolutely necessary and ease the anxiety of the last week.

After the day's ops, my in-tray needs mucking out. I need to run through it whenever possible to be sure nothing vital gets overlooked. After an hour of arranging its contents into further piles, I decide that a break is in order and set off towards the river with the dogs. Along the track, the hedgerows are alive with singing birds beginning to pair up for the breeding season. Yellow-headed Yellowhammers are doing their usual trick of imitating flocks of budgies. All makes and sizes of birds are singing their hearts out and darting from bush to bush. The sky is alive with skylarks – mere fluttering dots against the blue sky as they hover overhead performing their sweet song, a complex mix of melodious warbles and trills to advertise their virtues to potential mates and rivals.

The spring barley is now three to four inches high, the field like a sward of lush grass. The early growth is very attractive to the dogs who lag behind, grazing avidly by the side of the track. Looking towards Clayfern up-river, I can see the white shape of the feral sheep also grazing on the next farm's field. On the willow trees bordering the stream are miniature versions of the sheep – the fluffy white catkins which are the willow's flower. As children, my friends and I used to paint little eyes on them with ink, and keep them as 'pets' in matchboxes. I suppose they were the crude forerunner of the electronic '*cyberpets*' which are popular nowadays. Ours were considerably cheaper.

By the riverbank, I pause while the dogs forage happily on the beach. Unfortunately the tide is out, and they return with stockings of dark, evil-smelling mud. There follows several moments of chaos while I persuade them to jump in the stream for a rinse. Clean water is obviously not so attractive as the muddy variety. There is as yet no sign of the luxuriant clumps of daffodils which set the banking ablaze in spring. They should be blooming soon, an excuse for another trip here later in the week.

The dogs are now rootling through the reeds on the riverbank. I watch Kippen carefully – like Jonno, he too is getting rather deaf and might get lost in unfamiliar surroundings. It was only by chance that Jay and I realised how deaf he was; Fintry was in the surgery with me getting her nails cut when Jay came home unexpectedly and was able to open the door and walk right up to Kippen before he realised someone was there. Usually there is a chorus of barking from both dogs when the gate opens – but we now realise that the old dog has been following Fintry's cues. It is amazing how skilled animals can be at masking disabilities. A remarkable example was a blind fox cub contained within a pen with several others due for release into the wild. This fox cub would gallop round the pen over and under fixed obstacles looking exactly the same as the others, and was only caught out when an obstacle was moved to a new spot or another added. Diagnosing deafness in animals can be quite difficult as they will often see movement or sense vibrations. The scientific way of assessing the extent of deafness is by *BAER* testing. This stands for *'brainstem auditory evoked response,'* and involves using electrodes attached to the head detecting electrical activity in the inner ear and auditory pathways of the brain in response to stimulation. However, Kippen compensates well by making full use of his other senses, and his sense of smell nets him a prize today. Back he comes through the reeds, proud as punch, carrying a tennis ball in his mouth. This has made the old dog's day. Never happier than when he is carrying something, the battered old ball will be carefully carried all the way home and will be tucked in a secure space deep in his bed.

Ambling homewards along the tramlines, I can see John the farmworker with his tractor in the field behind the house. The bucket on the tractor holds various stakes and coils of wire – he is mending the fencing. This is bad news for dogs and humans. It will not be so easy for us to slip through loose sections on our travels across the farmland. Hoping for rain to put him off, I head back to my still bulging in-tray.

There is no sign of Jock by late afternoon so I crack and phone again. 'He's not here,' says Bunty, fortunately slipping in quickly 'but he's on his way.' Sure enough, as promised, he arrives just before evening surgery so I leave him working away when I head into Clayfern.

After months of travelling home in the dark after evening surgery, it is pleasant to be going home when it is only dusk. At Abbeygate Farm, the geese are roosting in the middle of the road – not a good plan for survival of the species, I think, chivvying them carefully into the farmyard. Geese are frequently used as watchdogs on farms and are not to be trifled with. An angry goose will dash towards you at full pelt, extending its long neck horizontally and pecking ferociously at all parts of the body. This attack is accompanied by loud honking, thereby alerting all within a radius of at least quarter of a mile. It is lucky that their wild brethren do not get the same idea, or the fields would be no-go areas for at least six months of the year.

Passing the Laigher, there is no sign of Jock's car so I stop off to see what has been done. There is a particular behaviour pattern with some Clayfern workmen – when you increase your demands, they will appear, do some work then vanish again. This is done to all customers in a bid to keep everyone happy. Like a juggler, they keep several punters in the air at once, and it must require considerable skill and effort merely to keep track of where each job is up to. With a degree of trepidation, I open the door and observe the room. I should never have doubted him – the work is on schedule. Heaving a sigh of relief, I relax and head homeward for supper.

Chapter 10

After an uneventful Saturday morning surgery, it is a case of a quick change into painting clothes before joining Jay at the Laigher. We take the dogs with us these days. They investigate the garden and wander from room to room, familiarising themselves with their new territory, while we work. Fintry is no longer scared of the trench and hurdles it with panache. The joiner has telephoned to say he cannot work today, but Jock appears to continue where he left off. 'Looks as if electricians are more reliable than joiners,' he laughs, disappearing into the roof space to trace some wiring. There will be no living with him now. All the same, I make some excuse to go to our cottage, then park behind his van on my return, blocking him in – at least we will know when he is leaving this time!

The painting proceeds slowly, but the sun streams through the windows and we chat as we work so it is not an unpleasant task. A small bird is singing energetically atop the nearby bush – 'Isn't that sweet!' I exclaim, thrilled that our garden has a decent population of wildlife. Four hours later, the birdsong is not quite so sweet, and the bird is in danger of meeting a sticky end if it does not quieten down soon. We begin to tidy up and wash our brushes before setting off on an exciting mission. The boiler in the new house is geriatric and there are grave doubts whether it will totter on for much longer. We heard on the grapevine that the engineer at Drumdurn has a Rayburn stove which he is converting to run on oil. After a few enquiries, it appears that this stove not only acts as a cooker, but will also run the central heating system. We are off to discuss the finer details of fitting and costs.

Sheila has a large Aga which sits benignly in her kitchen belting out heat, surrounded by a covey of contented cats and old Jonno. We have both always hoped that, one day, we too might acquire one, and the dicey boiler is giving us the very opportunity that we need, much sooner than we ever thought possible. 'Our' Rayburn is an attractive racing-green colour, and careful measuring shows that it will fit in the kitchen alcove where we hoped it might. Getting down to the nitty-gritty, the engineer informs us that the stove will be driving the central heating and the cooker all the time. In very cold weather, it may be concentrating so much on the heating that the ovens and hot plates will be cooler than usual. In summer, the only way of reducing the heating will be by using thermostats on the radiators. I have a sudden mental picture of us draped out of open windows in summer in a desperate attempt to cool down, or huddled by a pan of soup for hours in the middle of winter – either cooked or starved, what a future. 'You need to learn to work round the stove, not vice versa,' advises the engineer gravely. Our friends have a similar set-up in their home, and don't look unduly flushed or thin, so I'm sure we will manage fine, but it will obviously be a challenge getting used to it. I am comforted by the vision of old Kippen, Fintry and Piggy the cat all relaxing in front of this marvellous source of heat, and Jay and I coming into a warm house with lashings of hot water and a fragrant stew cooking in the oven since morning.

There is quite a saga leading up to my activities later this afternoon. Yesterday, I received rather an odd call from some clients concerning a hen. The story really begins with the Scotland – France rugby match last Saturday. Our clients travelled to the game, meeting up with their son and his French friends. After the match (which Scotland unfortunately lost), the ecstatic French contingent presented Anne and Phil with a package, thanking them for their hospitality then disappeared into the local hostelries to celebrate. The package was found to contain a rather bewildered French cockerel – the mascot of the French side. Being quite fond of hens, Anne and Phil took their package home and installed the bird in a pleasant run. However, in conversation with a neighbour the following day, a disturbing fact came to light: the neighbour had read an article in the local paper pointing out that French cockerels had entered the country illegally and were liable to be impounded. Being law-abiding citizens, the pair dutifully telephoned the number given in the newspaper and were connected to an official at the Ministry of Agriculture who spelled out the situation. If they wanted to keep the cockerel, then a restriction notice had to be served on him effectively placing him in quarantine for the next thirty five days. The bird must be kept in isolation and inspected by a ministry-approved veterinary surgeon both now, and again in thirty five days. This is where I come in. Already a local veterinary inspector for small animal export (that is, appointed by the government for export certification), I have temporarily been promoted to cover import of birds. Listening with amusement to the sorry tale, I joke with the Ministry vet 'Mrs Black would have been better just keeping quiet about him.' *Not* the correct response at all – 'I can assure you that we knew about the existence of this bird,' retorts the vet stiffly, '…and it's not the *only* French hen in Scotland,' he mutters darkly. Bang go my chances of any career in the Ministry.

So on my day of rest, I am charged with the responsibility of inspecting the said bird. This involves a fifteen mile trip to the village of Finlogie. It is a gorgeous day – blue sky with a light, warm wind – and the promise of a relaxing drive followed by a simple task sounds just the ticket, a pleasant break from painting, if I'm honest. As at Fern, the birds are active, flitting from bush to bush with mouthfuls of building materials, or proclaiming their territory to all who will listen. Two buzzards soar lazily on the updraughts from Fingle hill. Snowdrops and crocuses blossom by the roadside, and the first lambs trot jerkily after their mothers in the fields. They are very young, with the knobbly knees and big heads common to all young creatures. Someone has really made an effort with the scarecrows watching over the crops – they sport swirling capes and hold curved branches aloft like cutlasses warding off all comers … or pigeons and geese at least.

Leaning over the fence at the Blacks' hen house, I catch my first sight of the cockerel. He is a very handsome bird, tan with red, blue and green highlights, and appears healthy, staring at us with bright dark eyes. 'We've called him Ici,' says Anne, 'as Phil used to work for ICI.' 'That's a particularly apt name,' I reply, 'Especially as he has to stay *ici* for the next five weeks.' Summoning my schoolgirl French, I chatter to the bird while catching him for a closer look ... 'Bonjour mon fils, comment allez- vous?' cuts no ice with the bird, and there is the usual frantic scrabbling and squawking before he sits subdued in Anne's arms. He looks the picture of health and is returned swiftly to his pen. The main health risks are those of Avian Influenza and Newcastle Disease, neither of which are present in the UK at present. These infections can cause heavy losses, so it is important to make all efforts to keep them out of the country. If there are no signs of disease in thirty five days, then the cockerel is home and dry. 'It looks as if Customs were not doing a good job,' I comment as we adjourn inside for a coffee. 'Och, I think they just looked at the mountain of beer crates in the bus's luggage compartment and gave up,' comes the dry reply from Phil. 'What are you going to do with him when he is payrolled?' I ask with interest. 'We will get him a couple of lady friends,' replies the cockerel's guardian angel. Perhaps Julie's Ever Ready, the ex-battery hen, would be suitable ... just think of the names available for any offspring – Duracell, Astra, Vidor and Longlife spring immediately to mind.

Chapter 11

I have a conscientious objection to any emergency calls before breakfast, so it is with misgiving that I answer the insistent ringing at 7.30 a.m. – 'Excuse me, I'm sorry to bother you', trills a pleasant voice.

'No problem, how can I help you?'

'Could you tell me the name given to a male and a female beaver?'

'Sorry, I have no idea.'

'Well, thank you anyway, goodbye,' and I am left staring bemusedly at the receiver. What I really meant to say was – 'You silly woman, what sort of time do you call this for your inane question, you have woken up the entire household', but being a well brought up girl, I responded in kind to the polite caller. It is not uncommon to receive similar queries, and I suppose it is something of a compliment that the public regard the surgery as the fount of all knowledge regarding all animals, but crack of dawn is a little extreme. Not only has the caller upset our leisurely morning start, but the query drives me mad all day – no one I have asked has any idea what a male and female beaver are called.

However, it is a gorgeous mild sunny day, so it is a joy to be awake. The birds are singing, and daffodil stems are pushing their way up through the snowdrops and crocuses lining the roadside. Morning surgery in Clayfern is uneventful apart from Alice and my temporary disappearance to move our cars to the sanctuary of our neighbour's driveway. The good weather has tempted out the traffic warden on his weekly visit to the village, but luckily, we have an efficient bush telegraph which alerts the local shopkeepers.

Mrs Cassidy is our good fairy, and, pausing on our doorstep after our parking trip, we watch her progress along the street, popping briefly into one shop after the other. Within a minute of her call, a flustered shopkeeper will appear clutching car keys and casting furtive glances in the direction of the yellow peril. In passing, Alice catches a glimpse of our window display, clamps her hand over her mouth and collapses with helpless giggles. Following her gaze, I see the problem. As rabbits are so topical these days, we have followed our pet smile window with a rabbit display. Correct feeding and management are the main topics covered, and Sheila kindly lent us a bagful of rabbit toys from her jumble to make the display come alive. Seeing all the cuddly bunnies invading the window, we added an information poster advocating neutering to prevent rabbits breeding, well, like rabbits.

An unknown window-dresser has manoeuvred a large black rabbit and a smaller white one into an extremely compromising position in front of the display. It certainly illustrates the point, but as this is a family window, we have no option but to separate them. In future, we will need to keep a sharper eye on the occupants of the waiting room.

Full of the joys of spring after an untaxing surgery, I decide to fit in a visit on the way home. We have a couple of ops due, but are not starting until 2 p.m. as Julie has a doctor's appointment. Albert Guthrie – one of the unkindly-named Glaikit Guthrie brothers – has requested a call to cut their old collie's nails. The elderly pair have had to give up their car, and Meg only exercises in the field by their cottage.

Responding to a worried call from the brothers several months ago, I revealed the cause of Meg's recent lameness to be an overgrown toenail growing directly into her pad, easily mended but excruciatingly painful for the patient just the same. I had pencilled in a reminder to visit again in April, but am really pleased that the brothers had enough presence to call. They are both becoming increasingly demented, and are scarcely able to care for themselves let alone a pet, but Meg has been with them for years and they love her dearly. The home help and neighbours keep an eye on things, and I try to pop in if I am in the area. With luck, Meg will die peacefully of old age before social services decide that enough is enough, and cart the boys off to a nursing home. Today is one of their better days, and they appear simply gently eccentric rather than barking mad. Anxiety always makes them worse, but they are relaxed today and triumphant to have remembered Meg's nails. The old dog lies beside Alfred (the elder brother) on the settee while Albert holds each leg for me. The nails are getting long but are not yet growing into the flesh so the procedure is accomplished easily.

'A cup of coffee?' suggests Albert hopefully. 'Why not, that would be lovely,' I reply. While Alfred rewards Meg with a digestive biscuit, Albert bounds to the cooker to prepare the drinks. Making a drink is something of a production for the boys, but I have time in hand today. I need to be back at the Laigher by 12 o'clock for a delivery of building materials, but a glance at the kitchen clock tells me that it is not yet 11.30 a.m. All the same, I become slightly anxious as minutes tick by without much discernible progress. Some kind soul prepares flasks of coffee for the brothers each morning so the task should be easy, but this is not good enough for Albert. Milk is poured into a pan and heated on the stove; this is then stored in a thermos while the pan is washed. The coffee is poured into the pan to warm and set to simmer while Alfred boils the kettle. This water is put into the mugs to warm for a few minutes while the cupboard is inspected for edible treats. By this time, I am almost at screaming point, but you cannot rush a master. There is evidently not sufficient coffee in the pan now, so yet again the kettle is laboriously filled and boiled. This is like watching paint dry, I think while attempting polite conversation with Alfred who is at the stage of repeating his earlier tales, and, rather disturbingly, seems to be mistaking me for the doctor.

At long last the drinks are made and transported shakily on a tray to the settee. Alfred waits until now to search for the card table, casting aimlessly round the cluttered kitchen. Patience hanging by a thread, I lunge across the room for a nest of tables, briskly saying 'This will do.' It is now quarter to twelve – five minutes to drink up then a dash home to meet the lorry. A scalded mouth later and I am on my way.

The brothers wave me off from the doorway looking vaguely hurt. They don't receive many visitors so this was an event for them. Feeling guilty for leaving, and with my burnt tongue stinging, I race home only to kick my heels until the lorry finally appears at 12.30 p.m. I will definitely visit the brothers again soon – but not unless I have a good two hours free.

Up the hill with the dogs instead of lunch, I find a sheltered spot and stretch out for a sunbathe. The sky reverberates with skylarks' songs and the plaintive scream of the buzzard. I notice the first bumble-bee and ladybird of the year as I relax on my comfortable mossy bed. The proportion of tan to green is changing on the meadow, everything is growing. A horrible thought strikes – we have two gardens to maintain until we move. I have put the metal detector in the car, and after lazing in the sun, the dogs and I set off into the woods to investigate the old farm rubbish dump – largely grassed over, but still with intriguing shapes visible under the surface.

Success with the very first pass – a strange-looking bucket. The galvanised bucket has a solid top about two inches down from the rim, apart from an elliptical gap nearly three inches across. Corresponding to this open segment, the rim itself has a narrow lip. At the bottom of the bucket are two struts on the same side as the open section. Bearing my find down the hill, I puzzle over its purpose – could it be some sort of butter- or cheese-making equipment? Luckily, Andy is at the Laigher when I arrive, dropping off a crowbar for Jay. 'Och, that's a hen pail!' he exclaims, 'you fill it with water then lay it on its side with the struts to steady it. The lip then holds a constant supply of fresh water for the hens to drink.' Well, of course. Having vivid memories of tottering along with fresh clean pails of water for Sheila's hens, only to watch them muck up the water in seconds, this seems like an excellent piece of kit. I shall mention it to Sheila when I next see her.

We appear to be having a rabbit day today; there have been two rabbits to see during morning surgery, and back at Fern surgery, two more require attention for their teeth. Teeth problems are probably the most common reason for rabbits to be brought to the surgery. This morning's patients illustrate two conditions which crop up all the time. Rabbit number 1 has overgrown incisor teeth – these are the long teeth at the front of the mouth. The teeth curl as they grow, and both of the upper incisors are growing into the side of the rabbit's mouth. He cannot eat and the wounds caused by the teeth will be intensely painful. There are various ways of dealing with this problem, the oldest method being to trim the teeth with nail clippers during a routine consultation. This is far from ideal – the rabbits do not like it and often object strenuously, the teeth split and the gums can become infected from the trauma.

Plan B is to admit the rabbit for sedation and trim the teeth down using a burr on a dental drill or a diamond disc. The latter looks like a small circular saw with fragments of diamonds embedded on the cutting surface to provide the necessary hardness. This equipment produces a much better finish, but both techniques are usually temporary measures and require repeating every time the teeth regrow, although changing the diet can slow the rate of regrowth. This rabbit, Benji, has had his teeth burred down on two previous occasions but they persistently overgrow, so he is in today for Plan C – total removal of all the incisor teeth. Much care needs to be taken during this procedure, the teeth are fragile and if the root breaks before it is extracted, there is nothing for it but to attempt the procedure again when the tooth regrows in about six weeks. We can usually tell that the extraction has been successful as the root end of the tooth is hollow, rather like a dried reed.

It takes over half an hour but the job is finally finished satisfactorily, and Benji is swathed in the obligatory bubblewrap and gently placed on a warm hottie. He has been given a small drip under his skin pre-operatively – this simply involves injecting warmed fluid directly below his skin where it will be absorbed into small blood vessels and thus make its way into the circulation. The surgery has taken a while, and rabbits are often quite slow at recovering from anaesthetics – it is a long time for such a small body to do without sustenance. Unlike dogs and cats, we do not ask for rabbits to be starved prior to surgery, and ask owners to bring in a dish of food to be offered post-operatively. The subcutaneous fluid helps to prevent dehydration, and when a rabbit patient is discharged, we will routinely give the owners a syringe with instructions to dose the rabbit with a mixture of glucose or sugar and water if he does not eat when he gets home. Small creatures have little energy reserves, and even a few hours without food can bring them seriously low. The effects of such a solution on a wee beast can be almost miraculous – 'just like WD40 on my car', according to one impressed customer.

The second rabbit has overgrown molar teeth (cheek teeth). Sharp spikes form on the edges of the teeth causing damage to the tongue and side of the mouth. Knowing how painful a small ulcer can be in a human mouth, it is hard to imagine what agony these poor patients must endure. The rabbit will suddenly stop eating and the only clue to the problem may be saliva staining of the mouth and chin. A vet can usually confirm the diagnosis by inspecting the cheek teeth using a scope, but an anaesthetic is required to allow us to fully examine the mouth. Rabbit mouths are not built for easy access, but specially designed instruments make the job easier. After the rabbit is anaesthetised by injection, a mouth gag is fitted over the front teeth and adjusted so that the mouth is open. Then long-handled clippers are used to clip off the spikes and any rough surfaces filed with a diamond file. It should be mentioned that all this diamond-edged equipment does not come cheap. I check the mouth by inserting my little finger alongside the cheek teeth: in an untreated case, the spikes are sharp enough to draw blood, but these are once again nice and smooth.

In the evening, we drive over the hill to Duncraig to attend a talk. The steep road past our neighbouring farm is quite hazardous at this time of year – it is covered with frogs en route to their breeding grounds, and much zigzagging is necessary to avoid them. They sit erect like tiny gargoyles, daring cars to touch them – definitely creatures with attitude. Luckily most locals know of this seasonal migration and do their best to miss them From a distance, this makes their driving appear very eccentric to say the least. The frogs are early this year due to the mild weather.

The talk discusses the many semi-precious stones to be found in the region – just up our street, we have hoards of attractive finds spread around the house. The lecturer concludes with a brief summary of the methods used to transform the rough stones into ornaments and jewellery. This involves cutting with diamond saws and polishing with abrasive pads. A thought strikes me – another use for our expensive rabbit dental equipment.

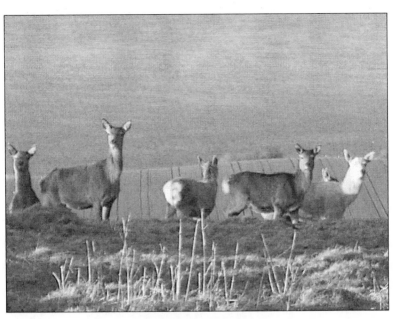

Have you brought the carrots?

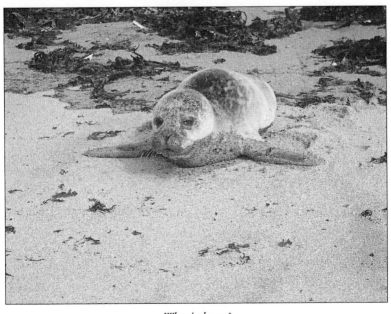

Where's the sea?

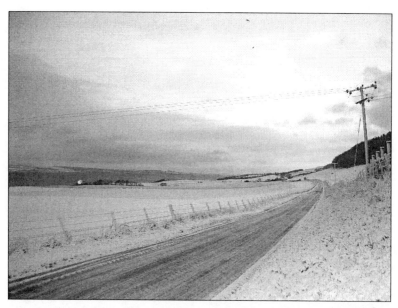

In the bleak midwinter

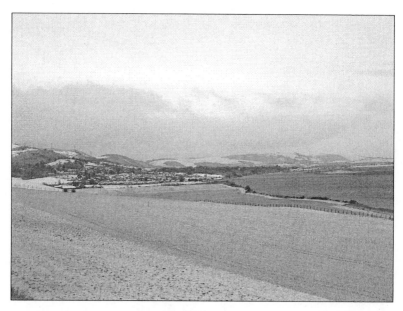

Clayfern in winter

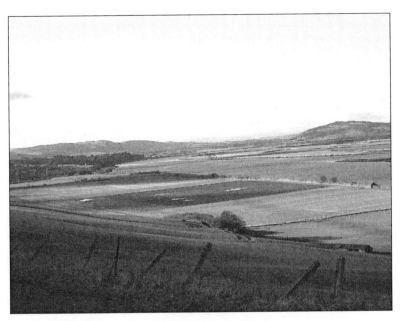

Clayfern in summer

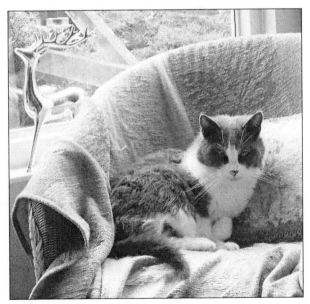

It's my chair

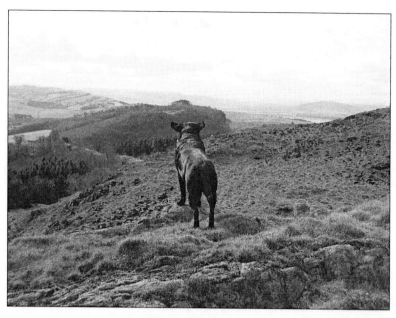

Queen of all she surveys

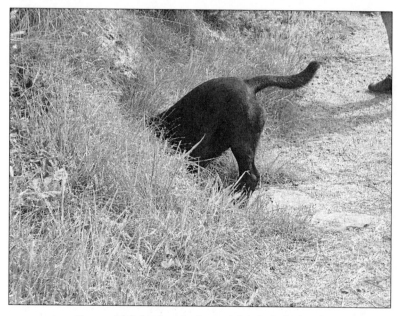

I'm sure I left that bone in there – definitely the back end!

Chapter 12

Taking advantage of the pleasant weather, I take the dogs up the hill before work. There is no wind and a slight frost coats the grass. Birdsong pervades the air – tits, finches, skylarks and green woodpecker all add to the continuum of sound. Wending our way through the woods, I note the vigorous new shoots on the dried bramble and raspberry canes, and realise that soon this walk will not be so easy. Arriving back at the car, Fintry is with me but there is no sign of Kippen. He really is getting so disobedient, ignoring my calls to do his own thing. Amusement turns to irritation to anger – 'Where is he, we're going to be late, I'll kill him' – to concern (what if ... he has fallen, got lost ... etc) to worry, then panic. I am about to summon help when he shambles into view looking sheepish. Having imagined all sorts of scenarios, I am so pleased to see him that I cannot be angry – I'm sure the sly old devil banks on this response.

Giving up all hopes of another cup of tea, there is just time to leap into the car to head for Clayfern and morning surgery. Our first patient is a canary – seemingly delicate little birds, but I have known them survive supremely adverse circumstances: one hung upside down for hours, leg caught in a piece of wire; an escapee recovered despite being caught in a reflex clapping-together of hands when it flew directly at our rugby-playing veterinary student. The expression on the student's face as he slowly opened his hands was a picture. More to the point, I have seen canaries survive chases round the surgery which have virtually reduced hardened vets and nurses to tears. The ceilings and windows at Clayfern surgery are very high, and recovering escaped birds can be a nightmare involving climbing laboriously on to handy items of furniture, only to have the bird fly off as one gets within striking distance. Luckily today's patient has been brought in his cage. This is always useful as it allows the vet to examine the bird first from a distance before it gets upset from handling. Like many wild animals, birds' instinct is to mask any sign of weakness from potential predators so if they look ill, then they *are* ill. This bird sits fluffed up looking the picture of misery. There are no obvious clues as to his problem – no swellings or discharges, breathing seems fine, the droppings in the cage look normal although perhaps sparser than usual. The next step is to take a closer look which this involves catching the bird – a risky business on two counts: firstly, the bird may escape into the room necessitating a chase; secondly, even handling these small birds can be enough for them to die in your hand – always an embarrassing moment. Cradled gently in my hand, this one feels roughly the correct weight, not too fat or too thin. Using my free hand to open his mouth then move over the rest of his body, I find nothing to explain his symptoms of lethargy and reluctance to eat. Popping him back on his perch, I begin to cast the diagnostic net wider – is there any change in his circumstances recently? ...

Has the food changed, has he been moved, is any building or decorating work being done in the house, any new pets? 'Well, yes,' says his owner, 'I moved him into the living room last week ... in fact, he seems better during the day, but goes off in the evenings.' Further questioning reveals that, after tea, the family lights the gas fire in the living room and settles down to watch the television. I suggest that the canary is moved back to where he was, and that the family arranges to have the gas fire serviced – after all, canaries are very sensitive to noxious substances and were used in coal mines to test for the presence of toxic fumes. It would make a lovely story if the canary had saved the family from carbon monoxide poisoning.

Next, one of my less favourite jobs – a kennel cough vaccine to be given to a boisterous spaniel. Kennel cough is caused by a coalition of several viruses and a bacterium. Protection against some of the viruses involved in kennel cough is already provided by the regular routine vaccination which dogs receive every year, but for added protection against the bacterial component of the disease, a specific kennel cough vaccine must be given. The problem with this vaccine is that it requires to be given directly into the nostrils. Not surprisingly, this is not at all popular with our patients. The vaccine vial is in my pocket warming up, a small refinement which sometimes makes the job easier, as warm fluid being trickled into the nose is marginally less unpleasant than vaccine straight from the fridge. This is the spaniel's first kennel cough vaccination so she is not forewarned. With her owner on the far side of the table holding the dog and reassuring her, I gently loop my free arm round her neck to lift her head against my body and slowly inject the warm vaccine into a nostril. The procedure goes better than expected, and the rather baffled dog is swiftly lifted onto the floor and offered some tasty biscuits to take her mind off the ordeal. After some low key snuffling, she is easily distracted by the treats and recovers her composure. A lot easier than some.

The last patient is an old friend – an elderly Labrador Don. Two years ago, Don had a large growth removed from his leg and a special biological tissue produced from the inner layer of pig intestine was used to bridge the extensive defect in his skin. For over three months, he came to the surgery every two to three days for a dressing change and careful monitoring of the healing wound. The excitement amongst vet, nurses and owner when the wound reduced to postage stamp size was quite something. Unfortunately, the cure was not as absolute as we would have liked. Every so often, Don attacks his leg with a vengeance producing a fresh wound which painstakingly heals over the next few weeks. His owner is accustomed to the situation now, and redresses his wound herself. Although disappointed that we have not gained a completely healed leg, I am still glad that we undertook the surgery, as the growth was undoubtedly painful and prone to infection. The superficial defect which we have from time to time is fresh and clean, and does not bother the dog at all. However, Don is doomed forever to continue wearing his trademark collection of protective socks on the affected foot. He does not mind at all, and it adds interest to our day to see which sock he is sporting on his occasional visits to the surgery. He is here today for a different reason. For the last week, he has been coughing frequently and is a little off-colour – not that you would think it, seeing him rush into the consulting room and position himself below the jar of dog treats. I privately suspect that he keeps messing up his leg just so that he can visit his friends at the surgery. Anyway, I diagnose a touch of bronchitis and send him home with a course of antibiotics, an expectorant to help loosen the secretions in his airways and instructions to leave the kettle on occasionally for fifteen minutes and allow him to breathe the steamy atmosphere. No doubt to his satisfaction, he will come back for a check-up in a week.

As with old people, old dogs not uncommonly get bronchitis. To work out a rational treatment, it is necessary to understand a little of how the respiratory system works. The airways look very much like a tree – one large trunk (the trachea or windpipe) branching into successively smaller tubes. Throughout the bronchial tree, there are mucous glands in the lining of the tubes, and microscopic finger-like projections which jut into the hollow centre. The mucous traps foreign material – debris, dust, bacteria etc. – and the wave-like movement of the tiny fingers move this material up and out of the bronchial tree. This mechanism has an impressive name – the *muco-ciliary escalator*. As we get older, the mechanism becomes less efficient and secretions sludge in the tubes which become inflamed and infected. Treating any infections and loosening the mucous is often sufficient to improve things greatly, although other drugs may be necessary as the condition progresses over months to years.

Later in the day, the phone rings as Sheila and I work through another batch of feral cats. It is the architect, the last planning application has been granted, work can at last begin on the new surgery. This is truly good news, and after the operations, I examine our home with a critical eye. Luckily, refurbishment of the new house is nearly finished, but we must begin moving some possessions along.

Once the new surgery is completed, all our time will be taken up with transferring equipment and fittings in as short a time as possible so that we are ready for emergencies. It would be just like Murphy's Law for some poor animal to require urgent attention when the surgery is in transit. There is Clayfern surgery, but it is not really equipped for major surgical work. Both Jay and I are hoarders and it would be a nightmare to shift all our belongings in one go. In addition to the usual household paraphernalia, many nooks and crannies are filled with our 'treasures' – attractive stones from the beach, old pheasant eggs and a swallow's nest, the stag's discarded antlers (for the last five years) and so on. Yesterday's trophy still sits on the kitchen table – two pheasant feathers, eighteen inches long and gently curving, chestnut-brown edges fading inwards to greenish-grey with dark brown stripes crossing the entire vane. Jay spent many happy moments teasing Fintry with one last night, despite which the feather has survived unscathed.

No time for packing today however, there is a blood-donating session in the community centre and my presence is required. It should be compulsory for all medical workers – both in the human and veterinary field – to occasionally find themselves on the other end of a needle. It certainly makes us more sympathetic towards our patients. At the hall, there is an embarrassing moment for me and a hilarious moment for everyone else – as I roll up my sleeve, a flea hops smartly off on to the side table. Being more used to this scenario than the nurse, I briskly dispatch the stowaway with a quick smack, then we both dissolve in hoots of laughter. This is something of an occupational hazard for vets, and I remember the probable source of my infestation – a flea-bitten old stray cat with multiple medical problems who I put to sleep after Sheila's neutering session. Like rats leaving a sinking ship, fleas soon sense when their host has expired and make for fresh pastures. We usually pre-empt this mass exodus by treating the body with insecticide, but this flea was obviously too quick off the mark.

The occasional flea is only one of several veterinary occupational hazards, but luckily they do not like living on humans and will only cause the odd bite. Conditions which can be passed from animals to humans (and vice versa) are known as zoonoses. Examples are diseases such as scabies, brucellosis, tuberculosis, ringworm and quite a few more. It is the veterinary surgeon's job to be aware of these possibilities and advise clients and staff accordingly. Another risk in our workplace is the danger of injury from the patients themselves, and the vet must assess every situation and take precautions to prevent damage either to themselves, assistants or owners. Most vets and nurses develop a sixth sense which tells them when an animal is likely to be troublesome. I am seldom bitten nowadays, but if I am, it is usually my own fault.

On my wrist are two puckered scars – a reminder not to be careless. I was examining a large German Shepherd dog belonging to a small lady. The dog had been licking and rubbing his rear end – a common symptom when the dog's anal glands are blocked. These glands are lodged within the muscle ring surrounding the anus, and to totally suss the situation out, it is necessary to perform an internal examination. This involves the delightful task of inserting a gloved finger into the rectum.

So there we were on the floor, owner holding the dog's front end while I gently eased a lubricated finger inwards. I could tell that the dog was getting agitated and his owner was having trouble controlling the head but foolhardily thought *'I've started so I'll finish.'* Bad decision. In the twinkling of an eye, the dog shook off his owner, whipped round and sank his teeth into my free wrist. With the other hand 'indisposed,' there was no way to ward him off or even spring out of the way. To add insult to injury, as I stood there trying to staunch my bleeding wounds, the dog's owner crooned gently to her charge – 'It's all right, pet ... don't be scared, the vet didn't mean it.' I recount this tale to trainee vets to explain the client's psyche – the average owner is not interested in the vet's well-being, only that of their pet. A more dramatic example is that told by a colleague: ending up in casualty with a broken leg after a DIY mishap while on duty, he was awaiting the results of an x-ray when his emergency mobile phone rang – 'Is that the vet? My dog hasn't been himself all day.' Explaining the situation, he was interrupted before suggesting a call to the neighbouring surgery 'Well how long will you be, I don't want to have to drive in the dark' delivered in an irritated tone.

Evening surgery sees a visit from Hector, a retiring soul who lives in a simple cottage high in the hills. Until a few months ago, he had only one dog, Lena, his faithful whippet, but he has recently inherited his father's two border terriers, Wilbur and Flora. Visits to the surgery form an important part of Hamish's social round and I am often hard-pushed to find anything wrong with the dogs when he brings them in. Ever mindful that he may not always be crying 'wolf,' I always try to give the dogs a thorough examination. Today's visit does seem to be something of a coincidence – he attends an evening class in Clayfern on Thursdays, so it is rather fortuitous that all three dogs should have chosen a Thursday to develop their (wildly differing) symptoms. Each dog gets a thorough going over anyway and a vitamin injection for all keeps Hector happy. There are some subtle features to a vet's role in society and treating sick pets is not the full story. The surgery sometimes provides important social contact for lonely people. Bringing a 'sick' animal for a consultation may be the only human contact that some poor souls have, but it can be a minefield for the vet trying unsuccessfully to find a problem with the animal – is this some obscure condition, or is the owner crying 'wolf'? This is all part of the art of veterinary surgery, there is

much more to the job than simply diagnosing and treating disease. I suppose that is why we 'practise', it really isn't possible to get it right all the time.

Chapter 13

Yesterday's rain has produced a surge of growth in the surrounding vegetation. There is a flush of green shoots on bushes and trees, early blossom has flowered and the daffodils are in bloom along the roadside. Today it is warm again, and as I leave the house for Clayfern, I hear the constant hum of the large fly population sheltering in our roof space. In hot weather, they come out to bask on the south-facing side of the building.

The joiner is working away as I pass the Laigher. Like Jock, his times of attendance are erratic but at least the day's work has begun.

Morning surgery is not stressful, just two vaccinations and a stitch removal. The final patient is Tippie, a pretty little sheltie. Tippie has a novel problem. For the last three days, she has been collecting all the family's mobile phones and secreting them under the table. If one rings, she becomes extremely agitated and refuses to allow anyone to answer it. The diagnosis is straightforward – poor Tippie is suffering a false pregnancy. This occurs several weeks after a season when a hormone imbalance fools the dog into thinking she is pregnant. Bitches in this state can do some pretty strange things – one ripped down the living room curtains to make a bed – and a common symptom is to become attached to a toy and carry it everywhere, but collecting mobile phones is a first. Perhaps the ringing tone sounded like a puppy's cry to a hormone-befuddled brain. Most bitches suffering a false pregnancy seem quite miserable and confused, so some treatment is in order. A drug is given to counteract the hormone imbalance and Tippie should be back to normal in a day or so. This is not the first time that she has had a false pregnancy, and her owner decides that enough is enough. We will arrange to spay her when the symptoms subside so the problem will never recur.

Ops day today. As we operate, both Julie and I stare along at the new surgery. We have become adept at recognising the cars and vans of the various tradesmen involved in the project. Brian the joiner is still there (blue van) and I am gratified to see that Jock is also in attendance (white van). Any unidentified vehicle is guaranteed to produce a swift trip along the road to investigate.

Most of today's work is routine neuterings. At the end of the list, we have an unpopular task – an anal gland flush. Both dogs and cats have these glands which appear to be involved in scent-marking and serve no useful purpose in the body's working. There are two glands embedded in the doughnut-shaped ring of muscle surrounding the anus, one at each side. Each gland is like a small sac with a narrow duct opening on to the surface of the anus. When the animal passes faeces, a small amount of anal gland secretion is deposited on top providing interesting information to other animals.

Occasionally there are medical problems with these glands. The duct can become blocked causing irritation for the animal who rubs its bottom on the ground and may turn repeatedly to lick or nibble the area. It falls to the vet to pull on a glove and empty the glands, often with a finger within the rectum. Understandably, this is unpopular with both vet and patient. The secretion has a powerfully unpleasant smell which lingers forever if it gets on to clothing. It is a truism between vets that anal gland cases always seem to come in before one is going out for the evening.

From time to time anal glands become infected and produce an even fouler aroma. This is the problem with our patient, Ben the boxer. He has been into the surgery several times for the glands to be expressed and has had a course of antibiotics, but the infection is still present. Plan C is to flush the glands with an antiseptic solution or saline before instilling antibiotic directly into the sac. In most healthy dogs undergoing this procedure, I would use a drug cocktail to knock them down, then follow with the antidote to bring them round after the job is done, but boxers and other short-nosed breeds can show idiosyncratic responses to sedatives, and a normal dose can profoundly reduce their blood pressure resulting in fainting.

With Ben, my plan is to give a small dose of sedative which may or may not be sufficient to keep him relaxed during the flush. If he is still unmanageable, then he will require a full general anaesthetic. This is always a dilemma in boxers who Murphy's Law has decreed to be among the most boisterous of our patients. Luckily, the dose takes the edge off him sufficiently for us to get to work. Even more luckily, Sheila happens by to collect some medicines and gives Julie a hand restraining the dog. Julie steadies the front end and Sheila holds his tail aloft while I thread a thin canula into the gland and flush it using syringes of saline. The muscle at the anus 'winks' in affront, and it is quite an art to find the opening of the gland and insinuate the fine tube into its depths, hold it in place while connecting the syringe to the end, and squeeze fluid into the sac. The canula is removed, the gland is emptied and the procedure is repeated until no discoloured material appears, then a tube of antibiotic cream is emptied into the sac. Hopefully that should do it, but we will warn the owners that this may require repeating. Not the most glamorous side of the job, I admit. Sheila beats a quick retreat leaving us in the foul-smelling surgery.

We always leave the dirtiest procedures until last to avoid contaminating cleaner ops, so after a thorough clean-up, we are free to escape for lunch. Even with using gloves, and after a handscrub in the surgery, I feel unimpressed at the thought of handling my usual cheese sandwich so while Julie prepares our repast, I disappear into the bathroom for repeated scrubbings feeling rather like Lady Macbeth ('Out, out dammed spot'). Not a bad day all in all; work is carrying on at the new surgery and there is time after the operations to take the dogs for a long walk up the hill.

However, regarding the building work, it seems that we have relaxed too soon. There is a site meeting this afternoon with the joiner, architect and building control officer ... oh, and Jay and me. The joiner has spent the last three days battening the roof, cutting sheets of polystyrene insulation and fitting them into the roof two layers thick. This apparently is wrong – there should be a continuous space in the roof for ventilation. The joiner will now spend the next two to three days poking out one layer of polystyrene. Worse is to follow – as this makes the roof space too big, we need to buy more thinner sheets of polystyrene for Brian to manoeuvre into position. Listening to the discussion with increasing anxiety, sensing yet more delay and expense, I butt in '*Why* do we need a space in the roof?'

With the exaggerated simplicity used when explaining to a child, the architect replies 'Because otherwise you will get condensation and the roof will rot.' 'But if it's my roof and I don't mind ...' 'Regulations,' parrots the building inspector in an end-of-discussion tone. Jay stares at me meaningfully, the vibes all too clear – '*For goodness sake, don't antagonise him.*' I subside into disgruntled silence. Phone calls are made to order more polystyrene and Brian begins to poke out the superfluous layer. The material which we purchased only a week ago begins to pile up in pieces, useless rubbish which requires disposal. Like all building projects, this one seems to be costing twice as much as originally planned and taking twice as long.

Passing a gloomy day reflecting on fiscal matters, evening surgery fails to provide the light diversion required. Don returns for a check-up, his cough is slightly better but not as much as I had hoped. I dispense more expectorant and add some bronchodilator tablets for good measure, requesting his return in a week's time. After all the work with his leg, it seems unfair to be heading towards another marathon treatment run. Let's hope that these drugs do the trick.

Another unwelcome sight follows on his heels, Benji the bunny, the same rabbit who had his incisor teeth removed at the beginning of the month. The present problem sends a chill of dread through me – Benji has an abscess in his neck. Rabbit abscesses are bad news, they are filled with a thick, tenacious pus not unlike cream cheese, and are not amenable to the draining procedures which we carry out on dog and cat abscesses. The best method of dealing with a rabbit abscess is to remove it unopened, as if excising a growth. Unfortunately, Benji's abscess has already burst onto the surface of the skin. Investigating further, I can see more creamy pus oozing from within the depths of his neck. As I examine the rabbit, I carefully begin to convey to the owner the seriousness of the problem. We will flush out as much pus as possible and administer antibiotics, but this is more problematic than a similar case in a dog or cat. Unlike those creatures, rabbits actually ferment their food and have a supply of helpful bacteria in their digestive tract. Too much antibiotic can affect these bacteria and upset the rabbit's digestion causing more problems. Thick rabbit pus does not drain easily from wounds and what frequently occurs with such cases is that the infection persists despite all efforts to abolish it. The end result is usually that the rabbit is put to sleep – either because it becomes ill with the infection, or because the owner can no longer cope with the constant unhygienic and unpleasant discharge. This poor rabbit seems jinxed. In his short life, he has been a frequent visitor to the surgery, first with a parasitic infestation, then for castration, a myxomatosis vaccination next, then two episodes of tooth rasping before the eventual removal of his incisors. Deciding to go for broke, I suggest that Benji returns each day this week for antibiotic injections, and give his owner a dilute solution containing antibiotic for flushing of the wound. Luckily for Benji, he has a very committed owner – this is a vital part of the equation if he is to survive this latest mishap.

Chapter 14

We have had a pleasant spell of mild, balmy weather – birds singing and grass growing. For days, the locals have been absent-mindedly musing 'Something is different, what *is* it?' The answer is – no wind. Although drier than other parts of the country, this region is notorious for its ferocious winds. We have all learnt to live with them, and are used to battening down anything which might blow over or away.

Today, the first of April, is the traditional start of the lambing season for Andy's upland flock. Typically the weather changes abruptly – the wind returns with a vengeance, and hail stones and snow flurries batter the hills. For Jay and me, the weather does not matter today as we are doing another antique fair to thin the abundant stock which will require moving to the new house – and to make a little extra cash to help pay for the ever-lengthening list of materials for the new surgery. Who would have thought that a mere outhouse conversion could cost so much.

As usual, I am on duty today but the fair is in Stramar, only twenty minutes away. One regret about my job is that other fairs are inaccessible except for the few times I am off duty. Morning surgery has to be done, but the later Saturday consulting times allow Jay and me to set out our stall first. Driving to Stramar, there are early lambs in the fields by the river. They stand in a line by the hedge as if queuing, backs hunched against the wind and ears dejectedly drooping – there is no sight so dismal as a chilly lamb. Poor wee souls.

At the fair, we greet Julie and Bill, and arrange our shared stand. If there is a veterinary emergency after morning surgery, Jay and Bill will be left to their own devices. As we are sited next to the cafe, this should not be a problem. Within minutes of our arrival, two other dealers seek us out to show off old medical curios which they think I might buy. 'Remember we're meant to be economising,' hisses Jay as my ears prick up. Fortunately, there is nothing special and I resist temptation without too much trouble.

Having a commitment elsewhere while on duty is tempting fate, and I almost expect an emergency to appear during morning surgery and tie up the afternoon, but it is surprisingly uneventful. Don returns for his check-up, still not as improved as I would have liked. In fact, his chest sounds rather noisy. I am a little concerned that there may be a degree of emphysema present. To explain what I mean to Don's owner June, I do a little drawing on paper. She is familiar with my explanation of the bronchial tree – the large windpipe branching into two bronchi which in turn branch into smaller tubes and so on ... so we move on to lesson two. At the very end of the smallest bronchial tubes are very thin-walled sacs known as alveoli which are lined with fine blood capillaries. They fill up all the lung tissue around the tubes (rather like the leaves on a tree) and it is at this level that breathed-in oxygen is absorbed into the circulation, and waste carbon dioxide is passed out. If the animal is breathing in with an effort, some of these little sacs can rupture, allowing air to escape into the surrounding tissue. This compresses the remaining alveoli and bronchioles causing more breathing effort which in turn leads to more alveoli rupturing. The condition becomes a vicious cycle causing ever-worsening breathing problems. Listening with a stethoscope to the lungs of an emphysematous patient reveals a characteristic sound much like silver paper being crinkled in someone's hand.

Don's chest does not sound quite that bad, but there are some noises which should not be there. Extra fluid in the chest can sound similar to early stage emphysema, so I dispense some pills for Don. These are diuretics – a drug which causes excess fluid to be dragged out of the tissues and passed out as urine. We also discuss an x-ray if he is not improving when he comes in again on Tuesday.

Benji, the rabbit with the abscess also comes in for his daily antibiotic injection. It is hard to say how he is progressing – there certainly is less pus discharging from the wound, but some can still be expressed when the cavity is investigated. He remains cheerful and is eating well which is something in our favour. His owner is coping well with the difficult and unpleasant task of syringing out the cavity at frequent intervals.

It is said that rabbits can be 'hypnotised' into immobility by gently turning them on their backs. This is because prey species such as rabbits feign death to put off would-be attackers – but this gambit no longer works with Benji who struggles vigorously. This is undesirable for several good reasons – firstly, rabbits have delicate backs, and unsupported kicking with the back legs can result in a paralysed rabbit. Secondly, a kick from a rabbit's back legs is best avoided – the powerful blow can rake their sharp claws through skin like a knife through butter. Before Benji's abscess can be dealt with, he requires trussing up securely in a large towel. I dispense some antibiotic liquid to see him over the next few days, and am finally free to return to the antique fair.

Jay, Julie and Bill are looking rather glazed on my return. The fair has not been busy and bored traders have been visiting each other's stands. They are all very friendly; some are interesting, while others can bore for Scotland. A champion borer has just left our stand after a monologue lasting half an hour on the trader's early life and times. My three comrades are wedged against the wall with the distinct appearance of rabbits trapped in headlights. Six hours in a large hall with other antique dealers and members of the public is an interesting experience for people-watchers. Business is quiet so we spend our time nicknaming our fellow traders. In the corner is 'The Gorilla,' a squat, hirsute, little man with long arms, an exceedingly large rump and an unfortunate walk which clinches his resemblance to our primate relatives. Across the room are 'The New-agers,' a young couple sporting multi-coloured flowing clothes and abundant body jewellery, peddling their wares of intricately crafted necklaces and bangles.

Goodness knows what the four of us might be dubbed, sitting in a row beneath pictures of the city fathers.

At the end of the day, after paying for our pitch and refreshments, we have only broken even, but we are not too despondent. A veterinary colleague who works in research refers to his occasional locum work as his vaccination against general practice. Similarly, antique fairs are our vaccination against other means of making a living. Other jobs can appear beguiling compared with our own work, but, after a taster, we are only too glad to scuttle back to our respective corners.

When we return home, we are met by two disgruntled dogs so we come to an agreement; Jay will unpack the car and prepare supper while I walk the dogs. The weather has thankfully reverted to a calm, misty afternoon. Staring across the field, we have to laugh – the farmer has placed brightly coloured cloths on sticks to deter the geese, but there is presently a large flock clustered round the gaudiest of the lot, posing, looking rather like the old pictures of arctic explorers clustered round the flag when they have reached the pole.

I have come out best in the deal – the walk is a veritable wildlife safari. Three roe deer – a buck and two does – are grazing on the rough ground at the top of the hill. Rabbits bolt for cover in the woods giving the dogs much sport. As I sit on my stone relaxing, two buzzards hove into view high in the sky, approaching from different directions and meeting above my head. In turn they flap their wings like fury then freewheel, gliding ever closer to each other then soaring apart in a spectacular aerial ballet. This may be a mating dance. As they pass overhead, they talk to each other in gentle clicking sounds, not their usual strident cries. I watch mesmerised as they glide their way across the sky, gradually fading from view against the rays of the evening sun.

We return through the woods where the dogs have another thrill – first one squirrel then another bolt across the forest floor and up a tree. For intelligent dogs, they have a mental block about squirrels and will stand at the base of the tree, staring fixedly upwards, seemingly unaware that the squirrels are half the forest away. One is a grey squirrel, but I am pleased to see that the other is a red – a more delicate creature with marked ear tufts. Both species co-exist in these woods but seeing the rarer reds is quite a thrill. They have been active on the ground too as large dug-out holes testify. The dry stalks of bramble and raspberry are sprouting thorny green shoots, the nettles are stirring too, and I sense that our days of rambling through the heart of the woods will soon be over until the end of the year. With antiques still on my mind, I spy pieces of what could be Delft pottery lying on a tree stump. Closer inspection of the delicate blue and white fragments shows them to be the inside of a snail's shell. Some clever bird has been using the stump as an anvil on which to shatter the shell and get at the tasty morsel inside.

The icing on the cake tonight is a grandstand view of a fox heading down the banking. This serves as a reminder that we are on duck duty for Sheila tonight. With young fox cubs to be fed, the ducks will certainly not survive a night in the open.

Chapter 15

The third beautiful day on the trot. It is the weekend at last and Saturday morning surgery is fairly quiet. The kids are off school and families are obviously taking advantage of the good weather. One patient is a budgie with long, curling nails. It is a finicky job to hold the bird with one hand, unfurl the toes one by one and trim the nails without cutting into the sensitive quick. The bird is very disgruntled with this treatment and pecks ferociously at my finger, sometimes hanging on for moments for added effect. This causes much hilarity amongst the budgie's owners – the obligatory family of mum, her two children plus their assorted friends – who are obviously unaware how painful this can be. At the end of the consultation, my poor finger is bright red and mottled with dents inflicted by the sharp beak. Give me a savage Rottweiler any time! It is depressing being the morning's entertainment for a bunch of kids at a loose end – I hate when they are off school.

Miracle of miracles, Benji the bunny's abscess actually appears to be drying up. I am deeply suspicious of this, and exhort his owner to continue with her stalwart efforts at bathing the area, and to return for yet another check-up in a week. Rabbit abscesses can usually be relied upon to be trouble, we seem to be getting off rather lightly here. A suspicious vet – what an advert. Don the Labrador is also in tonight. He too has responded well to his last treatment – the diuretic tablets. Relieved but not totally off-guard, I dispense more drugs and also request his presence in a week's time. These two are getting to be a double-act. Even the owners recognise each other now, and spend their time in the waiting room updating each other on their pet's progress.

The farm surgery is also quiet, only two cats to neuter for Sheila then peace. Off up the hill the dogs and I go. I find a secluded corner for a sunbathe, while the dogs forage nearby. Kippen starts his usual trick of ripping up a fallen branch and settling down to chew it to bits. Fintry grabs a smaller twig and follows suit. She copies all his mannerisms – when he eventually passes away, so much of him will be left in her. My finger throbs uncomfortably – you get no sympathy after being savaged by a budgie. Lying with my eyes shut, the wind gently ruffles my hair and the background sounds fill my mind – birdsong, dogs foraging, hammering-in of fence posts in the distance. I am nicely relaxed when I become increasingly aware of itchy areas on my legs and back. This jolts me back to full alertness especially when I discover I am lying by a colony of ants. This is a timely reminder to force me back home to deal with my filled-to-overflowing in-tray.

Two hours of paperwork is followed by an hour of carrying boxes of possessions along to the new house. My aim is to transport several boxes per day in the hope that this lightens the load of the final move. The Laigher started as a wonderfully uncluttered house, now both houses look like proverbial tips, rooms full of cardboard boxes. We really must try to stop accumulating junk. The sun is still beating down mid-afternoon so I muster the dogs again and head for the farm. The tar is blistering on the road, just like in summer. I know Sheila is out so Jonno will especially appreciate an outing. Towards the river we go, along the track by the oilseed rape crop. It has fairly shot up in the last week, reaching heights of nearly three feet and just beginning to bloom. I sit on a rock by the shingly beach while Kippen and Fintry fling themselves into the water. Jonno paddles but will not be persuaded to venture into water any more than six inches deep. The geese are massing on the next field; it seems odd to hear them on a hot, sunny day – I associate their cries more with bleak, winter weather. Today has been a welcome oasis, a taster of summer days to come.

Sunday sees us up bright and early, both of us determined to spend a good day working at the new house. A brief walk with the dogs before I retire to the surgery to see cases ongoing from yesterday. As usual, poor Jay gets lumbered with the breakfast dishes. We have planned a quick trip to Stramar to pick up supplies – paint, sandpaper and so on – before getting an early start on the house. No such luck – the pager shrills just as we arrive on the outskirts of the town – an old dog is collapsed and needs urgent attention.

Back we go to Clayfern post-haste, no time even to quickly get the shopping. The old dog is really not well. He has been sick all night and now can barely stand. Examination leads me to suspect a prostatic abscess or tumour. To confirm this, further investigations would be required, but not until after aggressive treatment had improved his present state. This produces a dilemma: his owner confides that recently his legs have been causing trouble, he is severely arthritic and has real difficulty in getting about. If we were faced with one or other condition in isolation, it would be bad enough but today's crisis has rather forced the issue. Even if he were to recover from his acute illness with intensive care, further work would be necessary to investigate his prostatic problems which might well be incurable. On top of that, there is the worsening legs situation.

After much soul-searching and talking things through, his owner comes to the conclusion that it is better to call it a day. This echoes my sentiments, so we gently put the old boy to sleep. Jay understands that such a consultation cannot be rushed, but is now frothing at the bit – it is nearly ninety minutes since we left home and we have not even bought our shopping yet. A frantic dash back to Stramar sees us in the checkout queue when the pager goes off again – a heavily pregnant bitch is in trouble. So off we hammer back to Fern. At least Jay can start work while I see the patient.

The tale told on the phone is that the bitch is due to whelp any day now, but for the last few hours she has been falling over and she appears distressed. Waiting in the surgery, I run through possibilities in my mind. After questioning the owner, it does not appear that the bitch is actually whelping yet but these symptoms sound worrying.

There are several life-threatening conditions which occur near full term – conditions such as eclampsia which initially causes incoordination, and can be fatal if not treated promptly.

When the patient appears, I have to laugh – no one mentioned during the telephone conversation that the little bitch has only three legs. With a body like a barrage balloon, of course she is likely to fall over! As she is not coping with her massive load, and as she is beginning to whelp, I decide to help her out by performing a caesarean section. A quick phone call summons Julie from her Sunday afternoon gardening and we proceed with the caesar.

Our patient, a Jack Russell terrier, practically offers up her leg for injecting in relief and the op is soon underway. Jay makes the mistake of popping in while collecting some nails and is co-opted onto puppy revival duties. While the vet is busy operating and the nurse is monitoring the anaesthetic, it is very handy to have extra pairs of hands to care for the newborn pups. Jay summons Andy who is waiting in the car so we have the luxury of two extra helpers.

The terrier is very large and looks like a giant pear lying on her back on the warm positioning pad. I cautiously cut into the abdomen, taking care not to damage the turgid womb lying just below the surface. It is desirable to manoeuvre it out of the incision before delving into its depths. Much blood and fluids are released from the womb during the caesarean, and it is preferable that they do not flood into the open abdomen.

'Everyone ready?' I ask before opening into the womb and fishing for the first pup. They come fast and furious after that. I quickly clear birth materials from their mouths and detach the umbilical cord before passing each pup to waiting hands. The helpers' job is to check each pup's mouth and nose, and then to gently but firmly rub the little body with a towel. The latter activity simulates the action of the bitch's tongue washing the pup and encourages it to breathe. Once the pup is breathing satisfactorily, it is placed in a warm basket lined with Vetbed under which a hot water bottle nestles. These pups are keen to come out, and aggrieved squeaks split the air as the helpers rub away. We all smile to each other – this is such a satisfying sound.

Eight pups later, the womb is finally empty – no wonder the terrier looked so large. After our bitch is stitched up, she is placed in a warm recovery kennel while we contemplate the scene of devastation before our eyes. Jay and Andy hastily excuse themselves, desperate to do some work along the road. Julie and I begin the big clean-up. The table and floor are soaked with birth fluids, the instruments are dirty and a pile of soiled puppy revival towels lie in a heap in the corner. Julie sets to with the instruments while I dispose of debris, load the washing machine and clean the operating table, all the while keeping a watchful eye on the bitch and pups.

The bitch is soon awake, responding dozily to the puppies' squawks. Once satisfied that she is reasonably compos mentis – I cautiously introduce her to a pup. This step needs to be taken carefully – it is not unknown for a drowsy, inexperienced bitch to harm her pup. No problems with this girl however; within seconds of her first sniff at the pup, she is washing it furiously. It squeaks in protest and crawls in the vague direction of her teats. Newborn pups are thick, I think as I rescue it from a fruitless search under her tail and reposition it in the right place. After a few false starts, it finally gets the idea. One by one, we add the others into the kennel so they can drink some all-important first milk rich in antibodies and goodness. Eight is really too many for such a small dog so I will suggest that the owners assist their pet by also feeding the pups with a milk substitute, then weaning them as soon as possible. Julie and I have our celebratory cup of tea while awaiting the owners' arrival. They depart after receiving their instructions for the days to come and Julie mops the floor while I zoom along the road to see how work is progressing at the Laigher. Time is pressing on, and we will be lucky if we have time for an hour's work outside before it goes dark.

For once, I have a key role in today's agenda. In order that plumbing work for the new surgery can proceed, it is deemed desirable that we locate the old manhole mentioned on the original house plans but now buried under a layer of tarmac. Simple, you might think, but the plans have not always conformed to our actual findings. Nevertheless, I spent some time yesterday perusing the plans and working out distances and angles with ruler and protractor (the first time I have handled such instruments since school). Armed with measured lengths of string, protractor and metal detector, I am quietly confident that I can find the manhole. With Jay and Andy holding the string ends, I am gratified to see that they converge on a small area. The final touch is to use the metal detector to confirm the cover's presence beneath the tarmac. Unfortunately, here I come to grief. The detector detects metal in several spots in the yard but not in the targeted area. Of course, all the nails and bits from the joiner's work. After a quick discussion, the unanimous decision is made to dig anyway. Pleased with the vote of confidence in my plan-reading abilities, I am decidedly nervous – the yard is beginning to look as if it is infested with a particularly hardy species of mole and yet more holes will not improve its appearance. 'You can't make an omelette without breaking eggs', I mutter in an attempt to comfort the workers as they set to with picks and crowbar.

My role is to bring brains to the operation, brawn I leave to the others. Three feet down and one foot across from our target area, the crowbar hits something with a dull thump. Could this be our manhole? Ten minutes more digging reveals that indeed it is, but it has become terminally damaged, probably when the tarmac was laid. And the reason why the metal detector failed to locate it? – It is a very old cover, made entirely of stone.

Chapter 16

No charity neuterings this morning, only three fairly minor ops and a cat demat. One of today's owners has a good laugh at the description for her pet's operation ... on the consent form, guinea pig castration is abbreviated to GP castration. This could be worrying for her husband as he is the local GP.

Our final patient is the cat demat. As usual when we are doing a non-taxing procedure, Julie and my minds move off on flights of fancy – 'We could start a fashion by doing a bit of topiary on these demats,' Julie suggests. That is all it takes for our imaginations to run riot. 'What a marketing opportunity,' I warm to the theme, then, after a pause 'We could call them cattoos' ... 'Or dogoodles,' Julie follows up triumphantly, 'People would home from far and wide to customise their poodles and persians – your money problems would be over.' After a brief consideration of the technical side of producing such cattoos – and a dismal failure on the first attempt, we settle for giving the unfortunate cat a once over with the number five clipper blade and thus salvaging its (literally) tattered dignity.

Taking advantage of the prompt finish, I decide to nip to Stramar to drop off a blood sample at the lab and to do some shopping. Vaguely remembering that Sheila's car is in the garage for repairs, I drop in at the farm to see if she needs any provisions. 'I'm glad you've dropped in, I want to ask your opinion on something,' she says, turning to pick up a jar from the shelf. A slim worm is thrashing around in the water. 'That came out of the tap this morning, do you think I need to worry?' 'I really don't know,' I reply, 'but I'm off to the lab, I'll see if they can identify it.' So at the lab, I collar one of my unfortunate colleagues for his considered opinion. After a moment's concentration, he gives his answer 'Och, its just a harmless nematode

... it's when they're dead that you need to worry.' We have been having very heavy rain recently, so I suppose this might be why the poor beastie ended up in our water supply. We are more likely to do harm to it than it to us.

The final examination of the French cockerel is scheduled for today, so yet again, I drive across the hills to Finlogie. The baby lambs of five weeks ago are bigger now and spend many hours playing in groups. In danger of arriving before my client comes home from work, I draw up by a field and watch the lambs' antics. They seem to play three main games – 'Tag' where one runs like fury with the others in hot pursuit; 'King of the castle' where one lords it over his mates by standing on a hillock or even his mother; and 'Breakdancing' where one starts jumping wildly up and down, soon to be copied by the rest of the gang. After a relaxing interlude, I continue on my way to Finlogie where I certify the cockerel to be in good health. Now his fun begins, as his owner has already got two wives lined up for him. If nowhere else, the 'Auld Alliance' will be alive and kicking in Finlogie.

Back home, I fax my final report to the local Ministry offices and the restriction order will be lifted. It is always a relief to be finished with Ministry matters – I must admit that filling in forms makes me nervous. In my role as a Local Veterinary Inspector, it falls to me to deal with export of dogs and cats for my clients. Each country varies in their import requirements which must be followed to the letter. My recurrent nightmare is that I do something wrong, and some poor pet is turned back at the border. After all the necessary vaccinations, blood sampling and health checks, the penultimate step is the signing of the official export certificate which is then endorsed (in red ink) with an impressive stamp bearing the legend – *Local Veterinary Inspector, Ministry of Agriculture, Fisheries and Food.* The owner is then presented with their document and sent off into the wide world.

The rest of the afternoon is now free to be devoted to moving more along to the Laigher. From the attic, I drag down such diverse objects as radio-tracking equipment from my badger radio-tracking days,

Christmas crackers, the stand off our old x-ray machine, Halloween outfits (Jay and I make a mean Frankenstein and his monster), antique medical instruments and antlers – Honky, the white stag's offcuts for the last few years. Tottering down the attic steps with a boxful of the latter, I manage to impale myself on last year's set. This is sharp enough to break the skin and bruise a rib, and is really quite painful. I wonder idly about which risk of infection is more likely, that from the antler itself, or from the covering of dead flies which blankets everything left in the attic. Deciding that I'll live, I steel myself to deliver all the gear along the road.

The new surgery is dragging on, every day some new problem. The latest concerns the air vent requirements for the back wall. The architect specifies six vents, each of six-inch length. 'The wall will look like a current bun,' comments the joiner in disgust. This kind of impasse is what I dread because of what happens next – I telephone Jay with the latest query, Jay calls the architect who calls the building control department then calls Jay back. Jay relays the pronouncement to me, who goes to tell the joiner ... who then says something like 'But what about the RS 2000 overlay?' The whole process then begins again. Not in the mood today, I play my trump card: presenting Brian with my mobile phone and the architect's number, I leave them to sort it out between them, while I peacefully rearrange the latest load in various nooks and crannies in the house.

Back at our cottage for another load, there is a message from Julie on the answering machine – 'Don't worry if you see a yellow van at the house,' runs the message, 'Bill has arranged for a mate of his to deliver some tarmac to mend your trench.' 'But we haven't got the pipes in yet,' I panic, desperately punching Julie's number into the phone ... *That* would be really popular, I think I'd have to leave home. Fortunately, the delivery is not imminent, and Bill is primed to hold off his friend until we need him.

Time for a relaxing dog walk, I think after evening surgery, nerves fragile after the build up of minor irritations during the day. We climb up the field behind the house towards the woods to check on the primrose banking there. It is a tribute to the resilience of these tiny plants that they still appear in their droves despite the major tree-felling operations last year. They are initially quite difficult to spot amongst the debris of discarded branches and shavings, but once my eye is tuned in, I can see that the whole of the hillside is covered in yellow flowers growing amongst the clutter. Beautiful.

We continue up through the woods disturbing a roe buck on the way. It is possible to recognise different family groups of roe and notice how far they range. This single buck was last seen at the far end of the west wood. A family of three frequently graze on the appetising spring barley field, but there is no sign of them there today. We disturb them later in a corner of the west wood, a secluded spot with mossy banks, tall Scots pines and rusty ferns. Young sycamore leaves are unfurling like half-open umbrellas and clumps of comfrey are sprouting under the trees. It seems just the ideal spot for a family of roe deer to hide.

Wending round to our side of the hill, I emerge through the trees above the Laigher. Something is happening below, I recognise the Rayburn engineer's blue van – our Rayburn must be here. Speedily chivvying the dogs back to the car, I whizz down the track to the new house. There in the yard is the little beauty, sitting squarely on two wooden rollers.

We wondered how it would be moved into the house. Made of cast iron, it is far from light, and although he is quite burly, it seemed rather a tall order for the engineer. He has brought an accomplice today, and I watch in amazement as they slowly move the heavy oven across the yard and into the house, moving first one roller then the other. Jay arrives as it nears the door and also watches its progress into its designated position in a corner of the kitchen. An historic moment.

I think we should name the beast, and suggest Shergar – as its colour is racing green. 'Not after what happened to Shergar,' points out Jay, 'What about Anna?' (after Anna Raeburn the agony aunt –

very funny). The engineer will return in a few days to install Shergar/Anna and leaves us looking proudly at our new toy which will no doubt become the heart of our new home.

Chapter 17

Over an early breakfast, we divide the day's extra-mural tasks. We are rising earlier and earlier to fit everything into the day. Jay is going to work, but will pick up plumbing supplies and shopping later so we can eat. I will see the electrician, pick up the drill, buy milk – oh, and take the dogs out. In a rare peaceful moment before departing for our respective jobs, I stare out of the window towards the river 'The swans are on the field,' I report to Jay in the kitchen, to be met by sudden chuckling and the shouted reply, 'Out of context, that sounds like code – am I meant to say "The more the merrier" or something!' For some reason, this strikes us as incredibly funny and we share a few precious moments of light-heartedness. Everything seems so serious these days, although the move is the Right Thing To Do, I am sure that we both occasionally wish that the opportunity had never arisen.

The river is invisible this morning, obscured by billowing mist. Up the hill with the dogs it is sunny, but only isolated church spires and tall buildings are visible above the sea of mist. I watch it slowly engulf a lone cottage, tendrils creeping stealthily up the valley and surrounding it. I wish Jay could be here to see it, but we both need to take on as much work as possible to pay for our move. Honky appears out of the gloom, looking a little weedy. I suddenly realise that it is not Honky but Charlie his son, so called as he is the Young Pretender. A bare-headed Honky is on the far side of the field – he has shed his antlers. Being younger, Charlie will not lose his until later in the year.

The hunt is now on for the discarded headgear to add to our collection. The antlers need retrieving relatively quickly, as they seem particularly attractive to foxes who chew them like dogs chew bones. A preliminary patrol round the top of the pen draws a blank, so the next few walks will need to case the remainder of the field.

Morning surgery is very routine until five minutes before the end when Alice takes an emergency call. Why do they always crop up after we have already been here for an hour and are just about to close? The story is that the parrot's cage has been very close to the mynah bird's cage, and the owner has just discovered that there is lots of blood in the mynah's cage – and over his beak. She is panicking as she cannot see his tongue and wonders if the parrot could have bitten it off. While we wait for her to bring the stricken bird in, I ponder the situation – *could* the parrot rip out a tongue? Could the mynah manage without it? I consider consulting a reference book but falter at what to look up – nutrition, gastrointestinal tract or musculoskeletal system (as the tongue is muscle tissue). Giving up, I wait to see what appears.

When the mynah bird arrives, I fish him cautiously out of the cage. He squawks with encouraging vigour, and fastens his beak round his owner's finger. 'I can see his tongue!' she exclaims happily, ignoring the pain. While owner and Alice immobilise his legs and wings in a towel, I grab the back of his head with one hand and gently prize his beak open with the other, freeing the mangled finger, before gently swabbing the blood from his beak. A crack into the sensitive quick tissue can bleed profusely but there is no sign of any damage there. Meantime the owner is bleeding profusely in sympathy but waves away our offers of assistance, casually wrapping a length of kitchen towel round her injured digit. Alice directs a light on my progress as I unravel wings and part feathers, looking for a bleeding point. Working down to his feet which are enmeshed in the towel, we hit paydirt; one nail is pulled clean out. Such an injury can bleed like a stuck pig. To prove the point, blood suddenly gushes from the damaged extremity. Handling the bird has raised his blood pressure and encouraged bleeding. As gently as possible, I hold a damp swab on the area for several moments to reduce the flow before touching the bleeding point with a silver nitrate pencil. This substance coagulates the blood and helps to seal the wound.

After the bleeding has stopped, we re-install him in the cage whereupon more blood floods over the perch. Repeating the procedure, I talk through the possibilities which come to mind – bandaging is possible but rather finicky and birds don't like it. The bleeding had actually stopped when the bird first arrived at the surgery and it is only with our investigations that it re-started. Further handling is only going to stress him more. I think it is best that we leave him in his cage in a darkened room. Birds become inactive in the dark and I am fairly confident that the bleeding will again stop. His owner is happy with this analysis of the situation, and departs to do the honours. She has been quite happy ever since we discovered his tongue was still intact. Mopping up the bloody table, Alice and I marvel at how long such minor (mynah?) incidents can take – it is nearly an hour since the phone call came through.

The remainder of the day is spent as most of our free time is these days – moving more stuff and

considering work to be done. The talk recently has been mainly of plumbing and there has been much staring into holes discussing the next move. Jay and Andy are doing the plumbing for the surgery as we simply cannot afford the quotes which we have received. They plumbed in the present surgery and we have had no problems, so they are confident of doing the same again. It appears more complicated this time as the building regulations have obviously been tightened up, and we need to comply with all the current requirements, but I'm sure my very own Botchitt and Scratchitt will win through in the end.

It doesn't take long for the day to come up with its quota of complications and annoyances related to the Laigher. Jay and Andy finally connected up all the drainage pipes, and Jay has informed the building control department who confirm Wednesday as the date for the drains to be pressure-tested. Unfortunately, they do not provide a testing kit – this is normally supplied by the plumber, and is therefore a problem for us who have not used a plumber. Luckily, to Jay's disgust, I have just arranged for a plumber to visit this week to fix thermostats to the house radiators ('Silly waste of money, we can do it ourselves,') and my first extra-mural task of the day is do what I am best at – the stupid-woman-grovelling technique to prevail upon him to (a) come tomorrow to check everything out, and (b) bring his test kit with him.

Next stop is Jock the electrician's shop. My pre-surgery visit to the Laigher to see the joiner confirms that Jock said he would be there this morning. 'The tiler and I cannae get on tomorrow if he disnae come,' is the mournful response, so I aim to nail our errant electrician after morning surgery which fortunately ties in nicely with his tea break. 'I didnae say I'd come Monday, did I?' he says absent-mindedly. '*Please* Jock,' I wail in stupid-woman-grovelling mode again, 'Even if you could just do the sockets in the back room.' '*Someone* will be disappointed,' he murmurs, casting sidelong glances at Bunty who is apparently expecting him to do some work at her home before her decorator starts tomorrow. Luckily, Bunty recognises a fellow customer on the verge of a nervous breakdown and concedes that I can have him first. Emotionally drained already, I speed off home to neuter some feral cats for Sheila, not usually my favourite task but a better option than all the hassle of attempting to get the surgery finished before our savings and patience are totally depleted. Cat wee and vomit will almost be a welcome change after all these shenanigans.

The week drags on with more of the same. P-day, pressure test day rolls round surprisingly quickly and the tension in the air is noticeable as we eat breakfast. The building inspector is due at 11a.m. so I pray there will be no hold-ups during morning surgery. We have an early meeting with the plumber Arghhh! There is some problem with the drainage – I'm not sure what, but it gives all the workmen the opportunity to huddle together around the trench giving their opinions. There are many doleful expressions and fishermen's tales of even worse horrors encountered on other jobs when building inspectors are involved. This is highly stressful for Jay who is of the 'What is the problem and what do we need to do to put it right?' mentality, but it is impossible to get to this stage before 'Well, you can't do A because you would need to do B and C ... and if you do C, then you can't do D etc.' After much debate, decisions are finally made and Jay departs at speed to buy yet more plumbing supplies while I dash into Clayfern arriving horribly late.

Luckily, Alice is holding the fort admirably. Poor Alice and Julie are also living through all the drama associated with the new surgery – so far, we have had the air vent incident, the disabled loo situation, the polystyrene fiasco and now the pressure test debacle. This project has taken over Jay and my lives, and turned what should have been a pleasure into something of a bad dream. Time and costs are mounting inexorably, and there is absolutely nothing we can do to avoid it. Far from looking forward to settling into a spanking new surgery, my most fervent ambition is to vanish on a long holiday. We want our lives back – to continue with building up Jay's business, and to investigate heaps of stones, high roads and other projects.

Morning surgery is peaceful as Wednesdays frequently are. Don is in for a check-up. His owner has been giving him his diuretic tablets as necessary but his cough has been rather worse over the last day or so. As his chest sounds quite harsh, I dispense some corticosteroid tablets and a powder. He sounds like a typical bronchitic old dog today. Hopefully the steroids will lessen the inflammation in the lining of his bronchial tree and the powder will loosen and mobilise the secretions in the tubes. In old animals, the bronchial secretions become thicker and stickier, making it more difficult for the body to keep the tubes clear. He is well enough to take his usual quota of doggie biscuits with alacrity and threatens the usual lifted leg on the way out so I am not unduly concerned about him.

Just before I leave for home, a client rings to discuss a behaviour problem ... 'My dog will not come back when he is out on a walk.' 'Well, first of all, you need to keep him under control until you start to train him properly.' ' And how do I do that then?' 'You need a long lead or line so you can reel him in after a run when you call him.' 'I haven't got a long lead.' 'Well what about a clothes line?' 'I've only got a rotary clothes drier, will that do?' Not in the mood for this conversation today, I pass the buck, suggesting that the lady telephones one night when our part-time nurse Cath is on duty. Cath has a special interest in behaviour matters and is attending a course of weekend seminars as well as studying at home. This is extremely useful for the surgery; although all vets have experience and knowledge of behavioural problems, dealing with them is extremely time-consuming and can be hard to fit into a busy day. Cath is still young and enthusiastic enough to enjoy spending time and effort on such cases. I think this particular lady will be a challenge for her.

Rushing back to the Laigher for the test, I am greeted by Jay sporting a wide smile. The dreaded test has been something of a damp squib – the building inspector rushed in saying that he was on his way to an emergency, had the plumber tested the drain? When Jay replied that he had, the inspector gave the okay to fill in the trench. So, for the first time in several months, we no longer have a moat. To celebrate, we have lunch together before Jay goes back to work and I saddle up the dogs.

Feeling light-hearted for the first time in a while, I head in an uncommon direction, westwards to where the forest meets the field. We have not come this way for ages. The entire banking is all rabbit warren, and we follow a well-trodden path – the M1 of the rabbit world. One rabbit sits quietly under a bramble bush unnoticed by the dogs, huddling in, ears flat back against his body. Others hop quickly down the nearest hole. They are more than a match for the dogs who range excitedly in all directions following scents, but not spotting the stealthy furry bodies disappearing in the opposite direction. The far end is a pleasant corner with mossy banks, overgrown tree stumps and lots of grass – a rabbit paradise. Wild cherries blossom overhead and a steep-sided stream burbles nearby, its banks dotted with primrose plants. Last spring, we came across a dead sheep in a hollow beside the stream, and now all that is left are some bones. I would quite like the skull for comparison with the deer skulls, but it is nowhere to be seen.

Come to think of it, many skeletons seem bereft of the skull, and most that I have found have been in splendid isolation. The skull must be a particular prize for the many scavengers which spread the remains of dead creatures far and wide over the forest floor. Possibly it is best not to dwell on why this is.

The feral sheep is two fields along in the spring barley, and we surprise a roe deer who gallops the length of our field, over the road and up the hill into the woods. What energy! I pause while dogs snuffle by the burn, watching the tractor spreading fertiliser on the neighbouring crop. It is approaching ever closer to the two swans who raise their heads to observe the interloper. From our angle, the tractor moves worryingly close before the swans ponderously take off and glide out onto the river. It is quite an effort for such heavy birds to become airborne. The dogs return from their investigations with beads of water perched on their noses. The natural oil in their coats is repelling the water just as my gore-tex waterproof coat does. Heading homewards, the distant hills are capped with snow: two neighbouring peaks bear an uncanny resemblance to a dog's premolars, I think, at the same time mentally noting that this may be a sign that I am working too hard.

Chapter 18

After weeks of much activity yet little visible progress at the new surgery, things are at last beginning to happen which hint that the end may be in sight. The windows were put in yesterday, and the joiner is transferring the kennel frames today.

Alice and I spent some time yesterday locating and recalling our collapsible wire kennels from households where they have been out on loan, and they are now standing rather forlornly in place of our smart kennels. I have been packing non-essential surgery items – of which there are surprisingly few, as anything may suddenly become necessary depending on the circumstances. Both Jay and I vividly remember a surgery move when we were at our city practice – no sooner were kennels dismantled than patients appeared out of the woodwork needing kennel space. A piece of equipment used once in a blue moon would suddenly become vital and would require fetching back from the new place. It is a similar story with household items – in a rash moment, I transported the entire contents of our drinks cabinet to the Laigher, only to retrieve a bottle of single malt after a particularly stressful day.

Having a foot in both camps is far from easy – we have just ordered more fuel for the Laigher, and our oil is running ominously low at our cottage. The weather has been cold, wet and windy, not the best time to run out of heating. But today is a gorgeous sunny day – unusual for a bank holiday weekend. This gives us a chance to get work done outside, and we make a start on painting the front of the surgery. Now the Rayburn is fully installed, we have to learn how to 'drive' it. There is a thermostat setting, and a baffle plate which diverts heat either to the water tank for central heating or to the oven for cooking. Today is for experimentation, and in-between sections of surgery front, I dash in to alter settings and check the results. It takes me back to when we were learning to use the woodburner. Both it and the Rayburn are like ships – it takes time for them to alter course after a correction.

A starling has nested in a defunct chimney stack opposite the surgery, and our painting efforts are accompanied by a considerable racket from above. The adult bird has mastered the sound of a telephone ringing and causes several false moves, even though the telephone is not yet connected at this house. The day passes peacefully enough with little snippets of interest to keep us amused. We discover a wasp byke (nest) while clearing out a loosebox. The interesting thing about it is that it is cherry-coloured, just like the shade of creosote used on the walls. The first swallow of summer appears on the telephone wire and keeps us company all day. It should not be long before his companions turn up to entertain us with their aerobatic displays.

Leaving Jay painting, I escape with the dogs for a short outing. It is dry enough to walk through the growing barley field towards the river where the blackthorn and wild cherry are flowering in a shock of white blossom. Absently checking that my pager is still attached to my pocket (an unconscious gesture which I perform throughout the day), I realise to my horror that I have left it behind, the reassuring weight in my pocket is a tape measure. I am seldom without this these days as I stand in the new surgery, working out where worktops and cupboards are to fit. There is nothing for it but to return to the Laigher to locate the pager which is sitting innocently on the car seat beside my keys. There have been no calls so I return to the painting while the dogs recover from the shock of being frogmarched home at top speed instead of our usual leisurely stroll. Poor old Kippen is becoming slower and slower, ambling doggedly in my wake, and needs to be watched carefully as he has a tendency to suddenly veer off the path to follow an interesting scent. Being very deaf now, he gets lost easily. This does not bother him much as he knows his way round the hill and would reappear eventually, but is a problem when we need to be home in time for surgery. When moving through undergrowth, I feel that I should have brightly coloured table tennis bats for signalling purposes.

Anyone watching our progress these days must wonder about the strange woman waving her arms and shouting at the top of her voice. When the equally deaf Jonno comes too, I feel like Joyce Grenfell – '*Don't* do that Kippen; this way Jonno ... No, *this* way. Leave that disgusting thing alone Fintry.' At this time of year, our walk options are rather limited; the crop and hay fields are only passable if bone dry, the woods will soon be off limits with nettles and brambles, and the cattle are now out in the grazing fields. We are soon to be restricted to the tracks until after the harvest when we range far and wide over acres of golden stubble.

Part of this afternoon is to be taken up with some work for Sheila. In a weak moment, I promised to fit them in. What should have been routine operations have proved to be oddities. The first cat spay appears to have only one uterine horn. This is a nuisance, as only one ovary can be easily located, attached as it is to the front end of the single uterine horn. Normally, cats have two uterine horns which lead into a short uterine body so the whole arrangement is V-shaped. There is an ovary at the front end of each horn. During the operation, the surgeon first locates the horns then follows them to find the ovaries. Each of these is tied off, the uterine body is ligated and the entire reproductive tract is removed in one piece. Has this cat only got one ovary, or is there another nestling free in the abdomen? If she was left as she is, she certainly could not become pregnant, but a remaining ovary could still produce hormones which would lead to her being pestered unmercifully by all the local tomcats. There is nothing for it but to stitch up the small incision in her left flank (the standard approach for cat spays), prepare her abdomen and open her up from this direction to enable a better view into the abdomen. Lucky I did, as an ovary is remaining on the hornless side attached only to a short fibrous cord which peters out one centimetre from the ovary. What should have been a quick operation lasting about fifteen minutes has taken almost an hour.

Just as well developmental abnormalities such as this are very rare. In over twenty years of working as a vet, I have only come across one or two other cats with the same abnormality. It is easy to imagine my horror when the next cat has exactly the same problem and takes the same length of time. By the time I move onto cat number three, I am decidedly twitchy. 'They are all related to each other,' mentions Sheila, so we decide to take no chances with this one and open her up through the abdomen. Typically, all her reproductive gear is present and correct.

After such an odd operating session, there is scarcely time to take the dogs out before evening surgery so a quick trip along the field will need to do. The world is yellow and green these days, green crops and grass contrasting nicely with yellow daffodils, primroses and gorse – and of course, the overpowering oilseed rape. With a fine instinct for making a bad day worse, Fintry finds and rolls in some fox dirt. The stench is appalling and there is nothing for it but to bath the little horror. As the remaining moments before evening surgery tick by, the dog and I wrestle over the shampooing procedure. We end up with a clean dog – and a soaked, stinking vet.

There is some light relief during evening surgery. Filling a gap between patients, Alice and I examine a new product brought in by a drug company representative. It promises to be the answer to a harassed owner's problems as vomit, blood, urine and *other secretions* (as it coyly mentions on the label) are immediately inactivated by a sprinkling of the tub's contents. When the special crystals come in contact with such unpleasant offerings, they solidify the liquid presumably allowing it to be tastefully picked up and disposed of. The concept causes us much amusement 'What an opportunity for the joke-shop market,' Alice exclaims, 'A clump of solid vomit – or worse – would be every schoolboy's dream.'

Chapter 19

Work on the new surgery has built to fever pitch in anticipation of the final inspection and drains test next week. I cannot remember being so nervous even before final exams. The surgery telephone is being transferred to the new house the following day, so it is really important that everything goes smoothly.

Last night Jay and Andy worked almost until midnight plumbing in the sinks, and today we have electricity and water. The central heating radiator in the present surgery was disconnected yesterday, and this morning Brian the joiner removed the double-glazed front door to fit to the new surgery and replaced it with a solid door. The old surgery feels quite claustrophobic now ... and rather sad, as if our lovely house and surgery which have served us so well are gradually running down and dying.

The evenings are still taken up with painting the new surgery, interspersed with trips indoors to see what the Rayburn is doing. Yesterday evening Jay and I sat for a while in the garden after work. The dogs were rootling in the bushes, blossom flourishing on the fruit trees and the stream burbling in the background. Swallows swooped overhead and nesting birds sang energetically. Basking in the honeyed evening sunshine, we came to the conclusion that the move *may* after all be worthwhile.

Today is another beautiful day, I wish we had time to enjoy it, but a busy morning's operations are scheduled, culminating in quite a tricky procedure. Solo, an old black and white cat, has had an inflamed patch on one side of his nose for several years but his owner has noticed that it has become raw and sore recently. The area in question is right on the outer edge of his nostril where the fur is white. I suspect that this is a *squamous cell carcinoma*, a malignant skin tumour increasingly commonly occurring on the extremities of white cats. Just as in humans, exposure to the sun can cause skin cancer, especially in fair skinned individuals. As Solo is very old, his owner has been reluctant to allow surgery and we have tried a variety of treatments to slow the cancer's growth, but all have been to no avail and she now appreciates that the best chance of improving matters lies with surgery. I have explained that I cannot guarantee that we can completely cure the cancer, but at least, it will be greatly reduced in size and will buy Solo more time. My hope is that the tumour is only involving the skin and is not invading the underlying tissues. There is not a lot of spare tissue to play with in this site.

As with many challenging procedures, I anticipate it with a mixture of excitement and anxiety. First, Julie and I anaesthetise the cat. After his pre-med injections of mild sedative and painkiller have taken effect, I insert a catheter into his leg vein and inject enough anaesthetic to get him asleep. As cats have a sensitive larynx, I spray local anaesthetic on to the area before placing an endotracheal tube into his windpipe and connecting it to the anaesthetic machine. A drip is then connected to the catheter to keep the cat supplied with fluids while he is unconscious.

Many old animals survive with kidneys which are not working perfectly, but a long spell without fluid intake can tip them over into kidney failure. Thus prepared, we are ready to begin. Using fine instruments, I carefully cut round the lesion, trying to include a margin of healthy skin. Some tumours require a margin of two to three centimetres to be removed with them to prevent tumour recurrence, but this amount is not possible in this site. I need to take care not to damage the underlying cartilage which forms the outer wall of the nostril and prevents the opening from collapsing. Once the abnormal skin is removed, some fiddling is required to close the defect. A skin flap is freed from the surrounding muzzle and swung into position, then stitched to the edge of the cartilage using fine suture material. I use a synthetic suture material known as *Vicryl*. It is related to polyethylene and will eventually lose strength and fall out, but not until the wound has healed. This seems a sensible option – Solo might not be cooperative enough to allow permanent stitches to be removed from literally right in front of his nose. *Vicryl* is also a softer material than the nylon which we usually use for skin stitching and will be less likely to irritate the cat. Even so, he will need to wear a special collar – known as an Elizabethan collar – to prevent any rubbing or tampering with the wound. The nose has a good blood supply, and I suspect that post-operative bleeding might be a problem. It would not be sufficient to cause danger from excessive blood loss, but could do an excellent job of pebble-dashing walls or a pale carpet. For this reason, his owner was pre-warned that he might need to stay in overnight, but the wound hardly bleeds at all, so Julie can tell the anxious lady that, yes, she can take Solo home tonight.

Seeing vehicles moving at the new surgery, I whizz along to see what's doing. Hooray! Jock has finished and hands me his completion certificate, and the builder and his mate arrive to harl the front of the building. Having spent the last week carefully varnishing the wood, I would dearly love to stick around and supervise – I'll kill them if they pebble-dash any of the windows or wood – but I need to go into Stramar to seek out a replacement pager, the present one having gone into terminal decline. For emergency cover while out and about, it has been necessary to transfer the surgery phone to my mobile phone. This is an uneasy state of affairs as reception in this area is far from brilliant.

I dread changing any communications equipment. It may be a sign of age, but I find the ever-more sophisticated instructions difficult to master, and stick steadfastly to what I know. Displaying my old pager in the shop and asking if they stock any like it raises a stifled titter from the young sales assistant. Evidently, it is obsolete, indeed something of an antique – she has heard about them but has never seen one herself. She points to a vivid yellow and green object as the most likely replacement, and, seeing my anxious look, mentions speedily that it also comes in a more professional silver and black.

Comforted by her reassurances that it can be worked by a child barely out of nappies, I hand over the cash and bear it homewards. In the old days, acquiring such equipment necessitated taking out contracts and paying monthly fees, nowadays they are only expected to last a short time before you throw them away and buy another. That's progress.

Sitting in the car, I unpack the device and scan the instructions – seems straight-forward enough, only one hurdle to go, the recording of new messages on the surgery answering machines giving the new pager number. 'It will be fine,' I assure myself, 'For goodness sake, you can perform complicated surgery on living creatures, surely you are not going to be beaten by a mere machine.'

Another evening devoted to painting ceilings in the new surgery before the tiling work continues. I was a little anxious that tiles might make us feel as if we were working in a public toilet, but Jay has chosen a pleasant pastel green to be interspersed amongst the white wall tiles, and non-slip green floor tiles, so the overall effect is both smart and relaxing. It will certainly make the surgery very easy to keep clean. Miraculously, veterinary work has been quiet out-of-hours, allowing our extra agenda to continue uninterrupted. I wonder occasionally when our luck will run out, but so far so good. I leave Jay to finish off the ceilings and spend the remainder of the day cleaning and packing more from the old surgery. All my drugs are now in cardboard boxes as the wall units are transferred along the road. In between tasks, I try to compile a list of agencies to be notified of our imminent move gas, electricity, poll tax, TV licence, insurance ... the list seems endless. I don't know whether to behave as a householder or as a vet these days. Yet again, our diet deteriorates in the evening. With no time or inclination to cook, I make the familiar trip into Clayfern for our tea – fish suppers all round.

As dusk is falling, I carry out my dog-walking 'chore.' In late autumn, winter and spring, the dogs and I tend to spend about eighty per cent of our time in the west wood. It is a mixed wood containing Scots pine and larches, also beech, sycamore and ash, and becomes very overgrown in summer. Around this time, in May, we transfer to the east woods which are mostly conifer with less undergrowth. As they are further away, we stop at the stones to allow Kippen a rest. The solitary beech tree behind us is on the point of blooming, green leaves still furled in their brown holders like little trumpets. Passing the deer pen, I see that young Charlie has finally shed his antlers. Another project for the next few days.

Once in the woods, we pass along a green grassy ride spotted with violets and wood sorrel. Another break is in order to laze in the setting sun. At ground level, the grass is a hive of activity. A ladybird climbs along one blade of grass and on to another; a black beetle bumbles through on the floor while small round-bodied spiders and ants busily move through the fronds. All this is suddenly absorbing, and I could sit here all day, but I feel guilty at the thought of poor Jay working on alone. Meanwhile Kippen takes a break from demolishing branches and rolls on his back – hairy, plate-like feet waving in the air, open-mouthed with joy. He really is getting hairier as he gets older; he reminds me of a reindeer with his furry feet and shaggy neck. Tufts of hair sprout on his head giving him eyebrows and sideburns like Worzel Gummidge. My reverie is brought to an abrupt end by the arrival of Fintry bearing a rabbit leg. There is nothing like being nudged with a bit of a dead creature for getting one to one's feet in a hurry.

Chapter 20

The day of the final inspection finally rolls round. After all the hype, we are now fairly numb. It will either pass or it will not. Jay and I arrive in force to greet the building inspector. Over the last few weeks, we have learnt the best way to deal with this gentleman. Any irritation must not be displayed, abject grovelling is the best tack to take.

Much as it sticks in our throats, we grovel for Scotland. Nothing escapes his beady eye. After the (successful) drains test, the emergency lights are tested, fire doors inspected and emergency exit used. Then we repair to the house to check the downstairs toilet. A removable ramp provides access into the house and the toilet has been fitted with a support bar in case a disabled person requires to use it. This was all necessary before the planning authority dropped the idea of a disabled loo in the surgery itself. All seems well, and the inspector is on the point of leaving when he suddenly veers off towards the front door of the surgery, the double-glazed door transferred from the old surgery. 'Is this safety glass?' he queries, inspecting the glass for a confirming mark. Resisting with difficulty the temptation to say 'Lets see!' while pushing his head through the door, instead I stutter an explanation, 'It will be; it was specially made for us at the last place.' 'That's all right then,' is the somewhat grudging reply. At last, at last he passes the surgery, we can move at the weekend as planned. After he goes, Jay twirls me round in celebration – and we go for another lunch.

The changeover itself is planned like a military exercise. The next day, the telephone is switched off at our cottage and transferred to the Laigher. No going back now. I have already taken the answering machine along and connected it up in readiness. Although we are still sleeping there, the heart has really gone out of the cottage now. It feels strange to be there without the insistent ring of the telephone. Nearly all my clients know that we are in the middle of flitting and will only call in emergency cases. No routine operations are scheduled for the next few days, so, unless there are any emergencies, the old surgery has seen its last customer. Julie joins me and Jay this morning after Clayfern surgery, and we move the remainder of the equipment along the road. I have been spending time just standing in the new surgery, visualising where furniture and equipment should go, and at last things are beginning to fall into place. Only the extremely heavy hydraulic operating table is left in the old surgery. It will be moved on Saturday when a posse of hefty friends will be helping us with the final move.

The previous two surgeries have had wooden walls, easy for banging in nails and hooks to support a variety of equipment. I need to co-opt Jay to drill some holes to take screws for hanging clocks, and hooks for suspending bags of fluid. It takes some thought to accurately position all these aids, but I think I have covered everything. Gradually the new surgery takes on the comforting air of familiarity. Standing in position by the table, I mentally cover our routine – reach for clippers hanging on a hook to my right; position operating light to illuminate animal's mouth; pick up catheter from trolley on left; insert catheter, inject anaesthetic, reach for and connect drip; connect animal to anaesthetic machine in front of table; watch clock above operating light to check time before patient breathes, and to check heart and respiratory rates. Yes, that'll do.

Tweeking the new surgery into shape has to stop for a while when I receive a slightly worrying phone call from my old friend Edith McNaughton. Two out of her three dachshunds have had spinal surgery for slipped discs, and recovered after many anxious weeks. I was a frequent visitor during both dogs' recuperation, as they both had acupuncture sessions twice a week. Whether it made a difference is hard to say for certain, but both Edith and I thought it produced some improvement. Today Edith reports that Eeny is again tottery on her hind legs and sometimes loses power altogether, collapsing into a heap. I know that there is no way that Edith will countenance further surgery, and fervently hope that she is exaggerating Eeny's symptoms. There is the usual squeaking of excited dachsies when I enter the hall of Edith's neat cottage, but Eeny is not in front as normal. She brings up the rear, still on her feet but lurching from side to side, hind paws knuckling over badly. She does not seem to be in any pain, just frustrated that she is not in prime position. After an examination, we decide to try acupuncture again combined with cage rest. Edith sits on one end of the settee holding the front end while I carefully place my needles into the target areas.

When carrying out acupuncture, one is aiming for specific points. Some of these points are quite large while others are minute. When the needle is in the right spot, there is a distinctive feel when manipulating it – a resistance or drag. Today there is tremendous drag on all the needles, and when they are finally removed, many are bent or twisted almost at right angles. It is said that acupuncture frees channels of energy which have become obstructed so I hope that this is a good sign. Promising to return in a few days, I help to load the disgruntled Eeny into her wire cage, dispensing a meaty chew as a consolation for being locked away.

After a very long haul, moving day finally arrives, planned for a Saturday to minimise interference from the surgery clientele. We are both up early, packing the remaining items in well-used cardboard boxes

One big worry about the move is whether our cat Piggy will take to the new house. She is a semi-feral cat who adopted us nearly nine years ago. She graduated from sleeping in the shed to occasionally venturing into the kitchen if the door stayed open, and over the years has worked herself up to sleeping on the settee in the living room. We cannot approach her too closely without her bolting for cover, but *she* can approach *us* – usually if one of us is sitting quietly with a newspaper. It is then quite hard to get rid of her as she rubs round your face and tramples the newspaper to shreds. Typical cat policy of awkwardness. I have brought a cat cage along to transport her to her new home, and all that remains is to catch her. Unobtrusively, we shut all the living room doors, and try to chat aimlessly while I casually move towards the settee, pretending to glance out of the window. I swear that cat has extra-sensory perception. Not fooled for a minute, she suspiciously watches my every move.

'She's going to go,' warns Jay. 'I know,' I gasp, launching myself at the cat and clutching her in a rugby tackle. The little body goes rigid and hisses ferociously as I transfer her quickly into the cage. To her credit, she has never actually attacked us, only hissed dramatically when crowded. Once in the car, the hissing changes to a mournful yowling which is kept up throughout the short drive along the road. I install her in a kennel in the surgery, already decked out with her bed, a litter tray, water and a plate of her favourite food – prawns. Huddling on the floor behind her bed, she glares out malevolently. I will be in the doghouse for the foreseeable future.

Having carried out my important mission, I leave for morning surgery, hoping fervently that the fates are kind and I can return smartly to continue with the flitting. It is another beautiful day which helps. On my way to Clayfern, I install the dogs in the garden at the Laigher so they can watch the proceedings from a position of safety.

The house is a hive of activity when I return from Clayfern, luckily with no emergencies in tow. My friend Ann and her husband Richard are in the house, tidying endlessly while more and more is brought along by Jay, Andy and a clutch of friends. 'Where do you want this?' Ann asks as I enter, clutching an ornamental otter in her arms. 'Oh, wherever you think,' I reply. Through lack of space, that otter has been cheek by jowl with the toilet duck in the bathroom, so anywhere will be an improvement. I am in time to observe the most impressive part of the day's activities. Unable to manoeuvre the wardrobes up the narrow stairs in the house, Jay has rung our neighbouring farmer who has appeared in his forklift tractor. The wardrobes are going over the balcony on the first floor. There is a distinct carnival atmosphere as we all congregate on the balcony to receive the furniture. Balanced precariously on the forklift prongs, the wardrobe edges ever closer as the hydraulic arms extend heavenwards, then sideways towards our waiting arms. I wonder idly if the insurance would cover any mishaps at this stage. Many hands do make light work and the wardrobes are soon installed in their new home.

Ann and I make endless cups of tea and sandwiches while more and more stuff appears, then rack our brains about where to put it all. The hydraulic operating table comes last. It sorts the men out from the boys as it is immensely heavy. I suspect everyone thought Jay and Andy were exaggerating when they explained how hard it was to install in the old surgery, but everyone believes them now. Unfortunately it leaves a trail of oil behind it which I manage to remove with liberal applications of white spirit. 'You are definitely settling in,' Jay comments, smiling at my aggrieved expression when my new territory becomes messed up. Not known for my housecleaning skills, any soiling of surgery premises is not tolerated under any circumstances. Poor Jay is all too aware of my double standards in this respect.

Suddenly at 8 p.m. it is all over, and our friends depart, leaving us alone in our new home. Too tired even to drive into the chip shop, and too hungry and brain-dead to tangle with the Rayburn, Jay lights the barbecue while I walk the dogs. We watch the sunset en famille, downing sausages and burgers with relish; not forgetting to take Piggy some sausage. She is not a happy cat, wedged behind her bed, prawns and litter tray untouched. She is so upset that she meows when she sees me. This melts my heart, so I gather her firmly in my arms and carry her into the house. For once she does not resist; I am obviously the devil she knows. While Jay glares threateningly at the dogs, I carry the cat round the house, crooning reassuringly, then risk letting her down to explore on her own. It is a novel experience to be actually wanted by the cat, but she does seem to appreciate me walking slowly round with her while she investigates the place. Much to our amazement, she settles down on the settee while we watch some television. Encouraged greatly by this response, I decide to try the *J cloth* trick. This is a technique used in dealing with cat behaviour problems and can be surprisingly effective, although the initial suggestion often produces baffled stares from owners. When cats rub their foreheads against people or furniture, they are in fact anointing the surface with scent from special scent glands on this area of their skin. Humans cannot smell anything, but it is crystal clear to cats. If you rub the cat's head with a clean *J cloth* then spread the scent on surfaces in the cat's surroundings with the cloth, the cat feels more confident and is less likely to carry out antisocial activities such as spraying urine. Piggy is a little startled when I mop her brow with the cloth but tolerates it well, although I do feel rather foolish polishing the furniture with the empty cloth . At the end of a very long day, we return Piggy to her kennel and enjoy the novelty of climbing the stairs to go to bed.

Chapter 21

The hot weather continues as we settle down in our new home. The surgery has been 'blooded' over the weekend – first a cat with an abscess, then a moribund young hedgehog suffering from the lack of food on the parched ground.

Never slow to come forward, Sheila has two cats for me to see this morning – one wets on the floor while the other has diarrhoea. It never takes long to get back in the old routine. I have tried to keep today quiet to deal with the numerous phone calls involved with moving house – insurance, poll tax, electricity and the rest. It is quite amazing how long it can take to make contact with a human voice, I think, listening to yet more canned music in a telephone queue.

There is some new wildlife up the hill this morning. Honky the stag and one of his harem managed to escape from the deer pen over the weekend, and are roaming free. I spot them on our walk; the hind is immediately noticeable – the bulky body moving tentatively between the trees unlike the roe deer who bound effortlessly away like wood sprites. Honky also looms into view, and we observe each other from a distance. He has always been quite a brave stag and is used to my chattering to him whenever we walk by the pen.

Piggy has been exploring in the garden after an initial sortie in my arms. I sit on the garden wall while she slinks through the bushes and sniffs at clumps of flowers. The garden is quite wild at the top of the banking and colourful with pink and white campion, bluebells and blossom. I suspect that gardening may need to take up more time than it did at the cottage – unless we can persuade someone to help out in return for my veterinary or Jay's design services. There is a long list of things which I would rather do than gardening. Luring the cat back into the house with yet more of her favourite prawns – I leave her in the sun room curled up on a comfy chair. Not such a terrible life, is it?

I leave early for evening surgery to allow time for another acupuncture session with Eeny. As Edith fishes her out of the cage, I can see immediately that she is much improved. 'She slept for hours after you saw her last, and has been better ever since,'reports her delighted owner. Just for good measure, we decide to give her another acupuncture session. Compared with the last time, there is very little resistance to the needles' progress, and they come out undamaged. I have noticed this phenomenon before, mangled needles and much drag when there is a major problem, fading to virtually nothing as the problem resolves. Perhaps this is an indication that the needles really do unblock obstructed energy channels, sacrificing themselves in the process.

During evening surgery, Solo, the cat nose job returns for a check-up. The wound has healed well and there is no expanse of raw tissue, only the thin suture line. Although the stitches will eventually disintegrate on their own, they are providing a focus for scab and hair material, so I decide to attempt removal. Solo is very good and sits quietly while I cut each stitch. Each stitch hole bleeds profusely as I remove the Vicryl. This is not a problem, as healthily healing tissue has a good blood supply, but it is ironic that the nose is bleeding more now than immediately after the op. Once again, I repeat the instructions to keep the cat in an easily – cleanable area of the house in case he shakes his head. Owner and vet alike are both pleased with the end result, and Solo is signed off. With luck, the tumour will not recur and he will live to a ripe, old age.

First operating day in the new surgery. Everything goes smoothly. I have only made one mistake with the positioning of equipment. I can watch the clock in the operating room – but Julie cannot as it is on the wall behind her. Jay will need to drill us another hole on the front wall. We begin to learn the characteristics of the new building. Being a stone structure for instance, we have a slight echo. As it becomes windier outside, the emergency door rattles slightly, but otherwise the surgery is very quiet. When it was windy along the road, you really felt as if you were in the middle of the storm – windows and door rattled furiously and the linoleum billowed off the floor. Our old extraction fan sounded as if a cat was being strangled whereas it is all too easy to forget to switch off the new ones.

As at the old surgery, we have observers while we work – the cows in the field are fascinated and frequently congregate to stare through the windows. The new surgery is larger then the old one, and both Julie and I notice this after a day's work. We seem to continually be trekking from one end of the building to the other to fetch some necessary equipment. This mirrors the situation in the house which is three times as large as the cottage. At least we will all be fit.

We have visitors while we work. The escaped stag and hind have wandered down the track above the house, and watch the comings and goings at the surgery. They listen intently while I shout a greeting to them. I frequently talk to them on walks past the deer pen, and they have become accustomed to me. This does not extend to all humans however; even if a friend accompanies me on a walk, the deer keep their distance. It is quite an honour to be accepted by them. By staying close to the pen, they are behaving the same as most animals do when released into new territory. They will initially explore a short distance from a familiar point (in this case, the pen; in Piggy's case, the house) but keep returning to the start. Once they are used to the area adjacent to the release site, they will gradually extend their range, becoming familiar with an ever-increasing area. Some years ago, I spent some time radio-tracking orphaned badgers and hedgehogs after their release to the wild, and they all followed the same behaviour pattern.

Knowing we were to be busy all day, Jay and I set to this morning before work, preparing vegetables and meat to be thrown into a casserole dish and left in the Rayburn all day. Tonight we reap the benefits – no messing with cooking when we come home tired, we just lift our meal out of the oven. Wonderful. Sheila visits us this evening to see the new house and to bring some house-warming presents – a book on Rayburn cookery and a device for making toast. As the Rayburn has no grill, this piece of equipment will be invaluable. It consists of two circular pieces of metal grid with a handle at one end and hinged at the other. The bread is sandwiched between the layers and placed on the cooker's hot plate. After Sheila has gone, I sit in my favourite spot next to the Rayburn, leafing through the cook book. As well as recipes, it is full of Rayburn lore and helpful tips, many dear to my heart: washing folded on the lid of the simmering plate will iron itself; boots hung by their laces on the rail will dry gently without damaging the leather; mugs sat on the side of the cooker will stay warm for ages. What a wonderful invention. As it thunders to life when the temperature falls, the throaty roar provides reassurance that we will stay warm and comfortable. I think Shergar is a very fitting title – and I can hardly wait until winter.

We have an 'eye' emphasis during morning surgery today. Every second patient seems to have an eye problem. First is Fiver, a dwarf rabbit owned by Shona, a regular visitor to the surgery. Shona's mother, who she lived with, died at Christmas time, and Shona has had a hard time coming to terms with her loss. The surgery became a regular port of call for her when she brought her mother's old cat for treatment for kidney failure. I think she enjoyed the company and was for ever popping in for no legitimate reason.

Most veterinary surgeries will have one or two folk like Shona on their books; lonely and not coping with life very well, they return to the place where they have been shown kindness and compassion.

When the cat died, Shona was distraught and thereafter would appear several times a week, perhaps bringing photos of the cat for our perusal, other times with plans for getting another pet. A dog was out of the question as Shona has arthritis and cannot walk far. Another cat was considered, but she felt too guilty at replacing the deceased cat. Finally, she acquired Fiver who has become the light of her life. He is a lovely little bunny who provides Shona with the affection and companionship that she craves. Not surprisingly, Alice and I dread the day if anything goes wrong with Fiver, and are understandably nervous when Shona comes through the door with Fiver in her arms, looking grim. 'He jumped up just as I was polishing the table,' she reports, holding the rabbit up for inspection. One eye is nearly closed and is watering profusely. It seems that he has had a face full of furniture polish.

The first step is to examine the eye with a pen torch – not easy to see anything as he clamps the lids shut. Next, I apply local anaesthetic drops and wait until they take effect and the eye opens. The conjunctiva is very red and he avoids the light of the torch. I continue the examination by putting fluorescein – a special dye – on to the anaesthetised surface of the eye. This dye will seep into any irregularities on the surface of the eye and outline the defect. It takes a few minutes to work so I busy myself by closing the heavy old shutters on the consulting room window. They cut out all the light leaving the room in complete darkness, perfect for eye examinations. Again shining my torch into Fiver's eye, it looks as if the dye is coating the surface of the cornea. For a better view, I use the blue light on the ophthalmoscope to outline the damaged area of eye more clearly. Poor Fiver, the polish has damaged almost the whole of the cornea (the clear front of the eye). The cornea contains no blood vessels; for healing to occur, blood vessels need to grow into the affected area bringing building materials to heal the defect, then regress once their job is done. Our job is to keep the eye in as good a state as possible while nature does its stuff. I give Shona some antibiotic drops to use and arrange to see Fiver again at the beginning of the week. Both Alice and I fervently pray that he heals uneventfully.

Bozo, the terrier is next, also with a sore eye. I follow the same procedure as before, scanning the eye carefully with the light after the dye has gone in. There is a suggestion of dye uptake in the middle of the cornea but it is not easy to see even with the blue light, so I try for an even better view using an ultra-violet lamp. The dye shows up really well using ultra-violet, and sure enough there is a small pinprick of damage in the middle of the eye. I suspect that Bozo has had another run-in with the family cat. Antibiotic cream for him, and an appointment for Tuesday.

The final eye case of the surgery is Florence, a middle-aged cocker spaniel with an eye thick with creamy discharge. This requires careful examination – bad eyes are not uncommon in spaniels and can be due to several structural reasons as well as trauma. Some have a tendency to grow extra eyelashes which rub on the surface of the eye causing irritation; in others, the eyelids themselves can turn inwards, also bringing lashes into contact with the eye surface. Another possibility is a condition known colloquially as dry eye. Its Sunday name is keratoconjunctivitis sicca, a title guaranteed to bamboozle most customers. This condition occurs when the eye produces less tears than it should. As tears lubricate and protect the eye, a reduction in quantity causes the eye to dry out and become uncomfortable and prone to infection.

Looking with my light, I can see no obvious damage on the cornea so the next step is to test the tear production in the eye. This is achieved by inserting a narrow strip into the corner of the eye and holding it in place for a minute. This is one of the longest minutes ever experienced in practice. The paper is uncomfortable for the patient who frequently struggles vigorously, but it defeats the object of the test to use local anaesthetic, as irritation of the eye is necessary to cause tears to be produced. Florence bears the discomfort stoically and soon we have a diagnosis. The tear production is measured by the distance which dampness spreads up the strip. Florence's production is well below normal. I routinely check the other eye which seems fine for now. I now need to explain the choice of treatments to the owner: Florence will need some antibiotic cream to clear the infection but this is only half the story. We can either replace the missing tears by using one of a variety of artificial tear products – basically lubricants which keep the eye moist and comfortable, or we can try to encourage the eye to produce more tears. This can sometimes be done using a drug known as Cyclosporin A. This is an immunosuppressive drug and works on the theory that the body is attacking its own tear glands and reducing production. The drug suppresses this destructive process and allows tears to be produced again. It is the drug of first choice for this condition and can be very effective, but it is very expensive, so it is up to the owner to decide if they want to give it a go. Luckily, this owner does, so we send him off with a tube of the product and arrange to see Florence next week.

All these eye examinations take up time, and I leave the surgery nearly an hour later than usual. Luckily, there is no need to dash home for more work. It feels quite odd to have a Saturday afternoon free, but there is one job which must be done. It is time for Kippen's annual haircut. He has an incredibly thick coat, and has been suffering from the heat both outside, and indoors, courtesy of the Rayburn. He is never particularly cooperative with me, so I steel myself for an hour or so chasing him round the consulting room with the clippers. The best tack is to stand astride him and shear whatever comes to hand. The floor fills up with clumps of tan fur and the clippers run hotter and hotter, making me alter my grip frequently. At times, Kippen looks as if he has been attacked by a demon barber, shorn furrows at all angles, until the job is finally finished and he actually looks quite presentable. All his fur has transferred to me, and I need to shower and even change my underwear to stop the itching of persistent bits of hair. To test the new Kippen, we go for a much-needed walk. Instead of trailing in my wake, the cool customer positively skips ahead with his 'sister'. It is me who brings up the rear, stiff after an hour spent hunched over the dog and finger tips stinging from overexposure to hot clippers. Thank goodness he only needs a full cut once a year.

A quick check on Eeny on the way home from morning surgery. I find Edith in the garden sitting on a low wall. At first I am concerned that she may have fallen and hurry towards her, only to be shushed by her touching her lips with a finger. I wait at the corner while she comes to me: 'I'm watching my house guests,' she says, 'Just wait for a minute.'

As we stand quietly, a swallow swoops under the lintel of the coalshed then reappears moments later and flies heavenwards jinking and twisting in the air. 'There's a brood of three and they're always hungry,' confides Edith. Eeny is fine, no need for more acupuncture. The poor dogs have to time their trips to the garden in between the swallow's trips to its nest. Edith waits until the coast is clear then ushers them out or in.

It is a beautiful day but Sheila is due in with some neuterings today so I put any thoughts of enjoying the weather out of my mind. My heart sinks as she unloads cage after cage into the surgery – *we'll be at it all day* – but a pleasant surprise is in store; out of ten cats, all but one are male, taking only a fraction of the time that females would. 'We'll no doubt pay for this later', I think as the last male is returned to his basket. Although numbers should even out at fifty – fifty, we do seem to get a preponderance of female neuterings.

I have a particular reason to be pleased at finishing early today – Jay has been going to see a Reiki practitioner regularly for treatment for a back injury. During the sessions, Jay has mentioned Kippen and the practitioner has volunteered to try her craft on him. They are both going for treatment this afternoon and Fintry will be left at home. She is not used to this and we are worried that she will resort to her old tricks of vandalising the house. This was the reason for her being re-homed when we first got her, and we had to endure several months of bed and carpet- ripping before she felt secure enough to stop. That she has turned out so well is largely due to the steadying influence of Kippen who has always been a relaxed, confident dog. I have to admit to a small thrill of anticipation at the thought of going on a walk with Fintry alone. The dogs and I used to go for miles together, but Kippen has slowed up tremendously over the last few months, and our walks have declined to sedate rambles with many stops for him to catch up. He has compensated for his arthritic limbs by developing an intense interest in every blade of grass or tree, and his progress is agonisingly slow. The day may come when he must stay behind, but he still enjoys his outings so much that it breaks my heart to even think of it. After I wave Kippen and Jay off, Fintry and I set off up the hill. She is not used to this, we usually ascend in the car. Revelling in a power-walk, I march the poor dog up the track, round the hill and down the other side. We come down the field by our old cottage then back along the road to the Laigher. I am sometimes quite shocked at our lack of homesickness for our old cottage, and feel something of a turncoat but, as Jay says, it is us and all our belongings that makes a house our home.

Fintry comes in with me to evening surgery where she stays behind the counter with Alice. She is very good except when she hears me reappear from the consulting room to call in the next client. Then she stands on her hind legs over the bar, observing all the comings and goings. She does not see many people at home so this is probably good for her. Shona and Fiver are in again. Fiver is more comfortable but the dye still shows a wide area of damage; in fact, it seeps under the top layer of cornea. Intact corneal surface should be watertight, this material is not healthy and needs removing. I instil more antibiotic into Fiver's eye and to Shona's horror, firmly rub the cornea with a sterile swab. Explaining that healthy cornea will not detach during this procedure, I tease the tags of loose tissue out of the eye. Shona looks even more anxious when I approach the eye with a hypodermic needle and actually begin to make multiple indentations in the cornea over the damaged area. This will encourage new growth into the defect. Reassured, Shona becomes chatty, 'I was talking to someone at the coffee morning yesterday,' she began, ' Big Jim overheard me saying I liked rabbits and asked me how I liked them. It seemed an odd question so I just said in their hutch – whereupon Jim said "och, no, I meant braised or in a pie."' Delivering the punchline, Shona's voice quivers with outrage, and we suspect that Big Jim will be crossed off her Christmas list forthwith.

I hurry home with anticipation after evening surgery, keen to hear how Kippen's therapy went. Jay says that he was very good, lying quietly on the floor while Karen's hands moved gently over his body. Like acupuncture, reiki works on the principle of correcting energy flow through the body, the practitioner having honed her senses to pick up imbalances. Karen detected a problem in his lower spine, and Jay said he squeaked when her hands remained over the area. We will just have to see what happens. He is returning next week.

We have our first setback with the Rayburn tonight – being clever or so I thought, I planned spaghetti for supper and put the sauce in the oven this afternoon. As we were both due in late, all that remained was to cook the pasta itself. As the cooker is on a low heat for summer, that took the best part of forty minutes. We must remember to turn it up in advance if we are likely to need food sooner than later. As our microwave oven has broken down, thinking ahead has become even more important if we are not to waste away.

The pleasant weather tempts me up the hill for an early walk. The dogs and I come across Honky and the hind lying in the undergrowth across the field. Honky's antlers are growing rapidly, sprouting like palm trees from the top of his head. The hind is putting her head down a lot, perhaps she is close to producing her youngster. With all the overgrown vegetation, there are certainly plenty of places to hide it from danger. The walk is a slow affair and I need to keep an eye on Kippen – one moment he is following, the next he is diverted into the undergrowth by an intriguing scent. He does not respond to my call (deaf or disobedient?) so I have to follow him, grab his collar and steer him back on the beaten track.

Unloading the dogs from the car, I notice that our pottery rabbit is missing from the line of creatures by the side of the surgery. I can hardly believe it and call Jay to make sure I haven't missed it. We are both mystified, what a strange thing to do. I wonder if it has been pinched for a joke and it will send us a postcard from somewhere. Perhaps it is the work of the phantom window-dresser from Clayfern surgery. Quite apart from arranging our furries in compromising positions, on more than one occasion, we found two or three of the toy rabbits with their heads stuck in the display sample of rabbit food. Alice and I racked_our brains to think who was in the waiting room before such changes occurred but could never pin down a culprit.

Morning surgery is quiet, probably as the electricity and telephone bills are out. This gives us time to do some paperwork. With the new surgery up and running, it is time to revamp the health and safety folder. More and more regulations make this area something of a minefield. In 1990 I think it was, the control of substances hazardous to health (COSHH) regulations burst onto the veterinary scene. In fact, they were probably one of the factors that influenced Jay and my decision to leave our bigger practice and start afresh on a smaller scale. These regulations require a practice owner to assess all substances held or used in the surgery for harmful potential. This even included materials such as Tippex and bleach. Following the letter of the law, if a nurse was washing the floor with bleach solution, she should be wearing rubber boots, plastic apron, gloves and a mask. Many points are of importance but, as usual, bureaucracy takes everything to ridiculous lengths. Together, Alice and I work our way through the file coming to the radiography section: 'Exclude pregnant women and adolescents under eighteen,' she reads ... 'So *that's* why you employ older staff.' 'No, it's mainly because they're grateful!' I respond, sniggering unpleasantly. You realise how many health and safety regulations there are when they land on top of your head.

The last of our run of eye cases turn up this morning. Florence, the spaniel with dry eye has improved well on her tube of Cyclosporin A, or liquid gold as we call it because of its price. She will probably need to stay on it for life but her owner is so pleased with the improvement that the expense will not bother him. Fiver is also in for a check- up. His eye is looking great, but we have another problem – a dreaded rabbit abscess on his chin. It seems close to the surface and is persuaded to drain without much difficulty but it is a worry. Abscesses are difficult to clear up, and if it is associated with the teeth in any way, then the outlook can be bleak. Shona is so pleased with the outcome of the eye that I have to let her down gently. I explain that abscesses can be a problem so we will monitor Fiver very carefully. I administer antibiotics and suggest we weigh him to keep an eye on his condition. Sometimes rabbits will show little sign of illness with abscesses but will gradually lose condition so it is handy to have an initial weight for comparison.

After our run of eyes, we are now in the midst (figuratively, not literally) of infected anal glands – in fact left anal glands to be exact. There is absolutely no logical reason why these should occur but I have seen two fresh cases this morning, and checked an on-going case from last week. Just one of life's strange coincidences. Eavesdroppers in the waiting room must think that I can only diagnose eye conditions or anal gland problems.

The rest of the surgery is rather pleasant, consisting mainly of animals I have known and liked since they were youngsters. There is Wolf, the German shepherd, in for his annual booster with his owner and her toddler whom he adores. I remember all the worry when she first found she was pregnant – would Wolf be okay with a baby? Then there is Suzie the retriever who came into the world by caesarean – performed by Jay, Julie and me; and Kim, the cat, who nearly died as a kitten with severe cat flu. We put an old terrier to sleep after seeing him over the years with trauma from a serious traffic accident, pneumonia and finally, a gradually failing heart. After he is dead, his owner and I discuss the options; 'You can bury him, or he can stay with me for cremation,' I say gently. After a moment's thought, the owner gives her decision 'Cremation – he always did like the heat.' '*Not 1000 degrees, he didn't*,' I think, trying not to smile. Inevitably, there is a particular kind of black humour associated with death which probably keeps us sane. A recurring gaffe which I try hard to avoid is the soothing of a fidgeting animal before his final, painless injection with the unfortunate words 'Oh, for goodness sake, you'd think you were being murdered.' Whoops. Another example of foot in mouth disease was delivered while sadly observing a particularly wasted patient lying at peace on the table – 'They turn into right little skeletons when they're dead.' Fortunately, folk seem to take such comments as they were intended, and bear no ill will.

Fintry has to join me during evening surgery as Kippen has gone for more Reiki. Earlier, Jay and I were discussing whether he was any better. It is in my make-up to be cautious at assessing cases. It is human nature to try to see improvement, and it is sometimes up to the vet to be the devil's advocate. Jay is convinced that the old dog has improved; he is certainly in good spirits and livelier than he has been, but I am not sure whether the Reiki is the only reason. Arthritis symptoms are notorious for waxing and waning for no apparent reason. Added to this, both dogs have been anxious with the build-up to the move, and Kippen has been suffering in the warmer house. It may just be that he is less upset and is feeling better after his haircut. It may even be that he enjoys the biscuits from Karen. However, for whatever reason, he has definitely improved, and it will be interesting to see how he does after a few more sessions with his therapist.

Chapter 24

Jay came home yesterday with exciting news. Jay's design firm does a lot of work for one particular builder, and the builder has just acquired a group of properties in Pitdreel, a small seaside town only an hour from home. The company wants Jay to do all the design work for them. The really exciting part is that one small flat is surplus to requirements, and we can have it for a greatly reduced price if we do it up ourselves. Jay has contacted our bankers, and we can add it on to our existing loan. This is craziness after all the expense involved with the move to the Laigher, but we both love the seaside, and it would be ideal for weekends and holidays. A locum is covering for me this weekend so we have come to see it. The car was full with dogs and bedding when we set off to the coast last night, and excitement was high. We may be heading like lemmings towards financial ruin, but we have convinced ourselves that it will be cheaper in the long run than paying for holidays anywhere else.

The little flat opens on to the main street in Pitdreel. This in itself is a novelty for us. It certainly is in a poor state and requires completely gutting, but Jay has good contacts for the necessary materials, and we will do all the work ourselves. After a chip-shop tea, I am all for exploring, but Jay is tired and settles to watch television while the dogs and I wend our way down a steep, narrow wynd to the harbour. Although a working fishing village, Pitdreel is extremely picturesque with its multi-coloured houses, pantiled roofs and bright fishing boats bobbing in the small harbour. I cannot believe our luck, and return full of high spirits to find Jay in ill humour; 'The TV isn't working properly,' is the dismal refrain, 'It will only receive Channel 4 ... of all the stations, *why* Channel 4?' Obviously not an intellectual.

So the next morning, after walking dogs and breakfast (rolls from the nearby baker's shop), we are heading into the neighbouring town to find someone who can repair aerials. We ask for a likely tradesman at a tea room tended by two elderly ladies. After much consideration and contradicting of each other, the leader does the talking 'Well, there's Dougie at the TV repair shop, he does aerials.' 'But he won't go up high,' pipes up the second-in-command triumphantly. Thanking them anyway with straight faces, we rush round the corner before collapsing with laughter – what kind of aerial repair man will not 'go up high'?

A trawl through the local antique shops, then back to take the dogs for a long, leisurely walk. We find a secluded spot by a shingly beach, and regress to our childhood days, investigating rock pools and scanning the beach for unusual stones. After finding some flint, Jay spends a happy if unproductive afternoon trying to light a fire by scraping two pieces of flint together, while I whittle an ornament from a piece of driftwood. After all the stresses of the last few months – with the inevitable arguments and grumpiness – it is wonderful to spend such a relaxing day, but it is definitely a good thing that we were not born in the Stone Age.

The following day, the weather has turned nasty, so we have a lazy start to the morning, beginning to plan the flat's revamp: painting here, tiling there, perhaps a new carpet for the living area. We warm to our theme, beginning to think of colours and designs. Our train of thought is only interrupted by one essential trip. On our arrival on Friday, we were thrilled to find that the property has a small, paved yard, perfect, we thought for the dogs' late night and early morning toilet requirements. However, an unforeseen snag has arisen – neither dog will 'go' on the paving stones. If let out when they must be bursting to do something, they merely walk round the perimeter then stand like lemons until allowed to re-enter the flat. This morning's long-lie was punctuated by the necessity to struggle into some clothes and take the pair of them for a morning wee. Luckily, there is a patch of waste ground not far away, and the beach is only a five-minute walk, so this is not a major inconvenience. Whether we will be quite so happy about it in the depths of winter remains to be seen, but for now, it is not really a hardship to amble slowly through such a picturesque environment.

After a leisurely lunch in the local cafe, we don waterproofs and head for the beach. In the wind and rain, we have the place to ourselves. White horses abound as waves argue to and from the shore. The grassy path on the headland is colourful with campion, poppies, bluebells and the last of the cowslips, and swallows fly below us on the beach, almost skimming the sand in their quest for insects. Mid-way through our walk, we come upon a strange sight – seven oystercatchers are standing by the water's edge, all facing in the same direction. 'Oh, look!' I point out to Jay, 'That one has only got one leg ... and so has that one ... and that one ...' Of the seven birds, only one has two legs. The dual circumstances of the birds' anatomy and orientation fascinate us, and we spend the rest of the walk thinking up increasingly bizarre reasons for them. Is it a disabled group with their teacher? Moslem oystercatchers facing Mecca (which explains the direction but not the leg)? An oystercatcher theatre group auditioning for Long John Silver? An oystercatcher yoga class? Oystercatchers having eaten too many radioactive oysters from the nearby power station ... and so on, the suggestions become more and more outrageous. Laughing fit to burst, we struggle back home against the hurricane-force wind, then jump in the car in search of high tea in the neighbouring village. High tea is a uniquely Scottish repast. It begins with a cooked meal served with tea and toast.

Once this is demolished, the waitress returns with plates piled high with scones, pancakes and cakes galore. It needs staying power to get through a high tea. Returning much later to the car after an excellent feast, Jay points to the windscreen which is liberally spotted with white bird droppings and howls with laughter – 'The revenge of the oystercatchers!'

Back home again and amazingly still relaxed after our first weekend off for months, I brace myself for a heavy day's operating. In addition to our 'owned' ops, we have neutering ops from the local charity. We are expecting ten puppies altogether but have no idea what sex they are. Yet again, all but one of them are males. This is very unusual. Julie and I can hardly enjoy the light workload for anticipating the inevitable payback. 'We'll probably get about fifty females next week,' Julie summarises what we are both thinking. Just as well that they are all males, as the appearance of two extra cases today has tipped a comfortably busy ops day into a long haul. Coincidentally, both are rabbits, and both are dental cases.

The first is a quiet little beast. He has suddenly gone off his food, and has the wet, slobbery chin characteristic of bunnies with sore mouths. He also has a watery eye. When associated with dental conditions, the latter symptom can be rather worrying. With rabbit bad mouths, it is possible for the tooth roots to grow in abnormal directions, and obstruct the tear drainage duct which carries excess tears from the eye to the nasal cavity, resulting in tear overflow. Sure enough, once the rabbit is anaesthetised, and I can examine inside his mouth, the extent of his problems becomes clear. His incisor teeth (those at the front of the mouth) are markedly overgrown and askew, growing into the side of his mouth. Even worse, the cheek teeth are in such abnormal positions that the bottom teeth have grown towards each other, forming an arch which completely entraps the rabbit's tongue. This is end-stage dental disease, and there is no satisfactory treatment – the most humane course is to put the rabbit to sleep while he is still under anaesthetic.

The next rabbit is a force to be reckoned with. He is also not eating and sporting the soggy chin suggestive of dental problems. Unlike rabbit number one, he is not a friendly individual and an initial attempt at examination has left me covered in hair, with long scratches on both forearms as if I have repeatedly attempted to slash my wrists. With difficulty, Julie subdues him in a towel while I gingerly inject the anaesthetic solution. He is treatable, only requiring some trimming and filing of his cheek teeth. As is often the case, it is the sweet wee thing who doesn't make it, while the unpleasant so-and-so lives to fight another day. Mr Nasty recovers quickly from his anaesthetic, and spends the rest of the day glaring malevolently from the corner of his kennel, daring us to make any moves in his direction.

We are now behind time to finish the next cases before their owner telephones for a progress report. I always like to have any operations finished before the owner rings in – I have a bee in my bonnet about it – as they often have to steel themselves to make the call, and it is a tremendous anti-climax if we merely tell them to ring again in an hour. Both Julie and I are slightly anxious about the final three dogs who have come in for routine dental work. They all belong to the same owner who positively dotes on them. The nightmare scenario of having to break the news of a death while under anaesthetic thankfully seldom occurs, but is an ever-present spectre. The prospect of holding such a conversation with Danielle is just too horrible to contemplate, and a malevolent little voice in the back of my head persists in saying '*Three* opportunities to see off one of Danielle's pets.' Other surgeons might play soothing music to keep them relaxed and focused, but, as always when under stress, we ease the tension by joking – 'Think of the first rabbit as a sacrificial offering to keep the fates at bay,' offers Julie. 'Extend her leg,' I order; poised to inject anaesthetic. 'It *is* extended,' 'That's not a leg, its a flipper!'

Once in action, everything goes smoothly, and the last dog is being moved into his kennel when Danielle telephones. After a clearing-up session, it is time for a much-needed lunch break. My hands have been inside some disgusting mouths today; '*You* make the sandwiches,' I suggest to Julie. 'I'll cut them into bite-sized portions that you can eat with a fork,' she offers helpfully. After much hand-washing a la Lady MacBeth, I return for my snack. Unfortunately, I have neglected to tell Julie that our electric kettle has finally given up the ghost. Our water here comes straight from a spring in the hills and is beautifully pure, but is death to kettles, causing elements to seize up and plastic sides to spring leaks. By sad coincidence our microwave oven has also chosen this week to cease functioning; so we are depending entirely on the Rayburn for all cooking and water boiling. As its output is turned down low for summer, it does take some time for a kettle to boil, and when I return from my ritual hand-washing, I find that Julie has given up attempting to make tea, and is instead pouring us both long, cool glasses of fruit juice. This is no hardship today, but perhaps I had better invest in a new electric kettle for those days when we really do need a strong, reviving cup of tea.

A mixed bag for evening surgery – the first patient is depressing. Skippy is a little dog who has always been extremely nervous, especially when coming to the surgery. We have all put in a lot of effort to ease her anxiety, starting with her attendance at the puppy classes run by Cath. During the classes, Cath gives the new owners basic information on training and socialising their pups, and the pups usually have a great time running around the surgery with their contemporaries ... and usually a few children thrown in for good measure. Not only do such evenings educate the owners, but they help to show the puppies that visits to the surgery can be fun. As is our way with all nervous pets, we have encouraged Skippy's owners to pop into the waiting room if they are passing, and either Alice or I finds time to talk to Skippy and give her some biscuits. All this effort has paid off and although Skippy will probably never enjoy visiting the surgery, at least she tolerates it. Unfortunately, I suspect her new confidence is about to be dealt a harsh blow.

The family is going on holiday soon, and Skippy has to go into kennels. The kennels have requested that all their inmates first receive a kennel cough vaccine. Some protection is conferred by the routine annual booster vaccination, but the vaccine which the kennels require is that against the bacterium *bordetella*, the vaccine that is administered intra-nasally. Extracting the vial from my pocket after warming, I fill the syringe, trying to appear nonchalant, and gently hook my free arm round Skippy's head, holding her nose steady for injection. Sometimes a casual low-key approach works well and the vaccine is in before the patient knows it, but Skippy reacts instantaneously to any attempt to steady her head and I know that our relationship is going to take a nose-dive (no pun intended). An undignified struggle ensues until several moments later, we are left with a distressed, panting, vaccinated dog, a dishevelled, hairy, scratched owner and an upset, but untouched vet. A prime example, incidentally, of veterinary self-preservation in action. Sometimes, I hate this vaccine – all our hard work gone to waste. Reconciliation attempts with biscuits are spurned by the dog; her one aim in life is to get out of the surgery A.S.A.P. As I dust off her owner, we both agree that we will not put her through that again. Most dogs can be done with only a little trouble, but there is always an exception.

My spirits are lowered even more when Shona and Fiver return for a check-up. Fiver's abscess is still on the go, and another can be felt near the side of his mouth. He is still bright, but when we weigh him, he has shed a small amount of weight 'Mind you,' says Shona in all seriousness, 'He's lifting his foot up.' If only that worked for all of us. It seems inevitable that Fiver must come in for surgery. The best way to deal with rabbit abscesses is to carefully remove them in their entirety. Unfortunately, they can crop up anywhere again, so repeated surgery can be necessary; and, if they have any connection with bad teeth or jaw infection, then the patient's outlook is truly dire.After imparting this gloomy information to a crestfallen Shona, I make an appointment for Fiver's operation on Monday. At least she has the weekend to spoil him and come to terms with his problem in case things do not go well.

Our last case is a racing pigeon which has been damaged by a sharp obstacle, perhaps a protruding nail or even a rat bite. The wound does not look too bad but the bird is very subdued. Stitching is not necessary, but antibiotic is definitely desirable. 'What weight is he?' I ask, knowing that many bird people keep tabs on their bird's weight. 'He's about a pound ... that's about ...eh ... five hundred kilograms,' says Effie, trying to help by converting to metric measures. What she means is five hundred grams, and her husband quickly corrects her, but the damage is done, the vision of a five hundred kilogram pigeon is indelibly etched on our brains, and smirks of mirth cross everyone's faces as the consultation continues. Now *that* is something I hope we never encounter.

Jay and I are both suffering from post-move after-effects. Neither of us can quite get used to the reduction in our daily tasks and, even when our jobs are running smoothly, we cannot relax for expecting some problem to rear its ugly head. I am just beginning to enjoy the extra time for dog walking and other leisure pursuits, but find it hard to shake off the guilty feeling that there is some work waiting to be done while I am enjoying myself.

However, the full ops day has completely banished all such thoughts from my mind, and even the dogs' walk has had to wait until after evening surgery. Passing the top of the deer pen, I see the first deer calf of the year, a small dappled creature tottering round its mother on shaky, stick-like legs. I have been lucky enough to catch a glimpse of a newborn calf almost every year. This is quite a coup as the baby calves are normally hidden away by their mothers for their first three weeks. They stay put, camouflaged by tall vegetation when mum goes grazing. Every year, I endeavour to carry the camera when calves are due – and every year, it is never with me when I sight the new baby. Typical. For weeks now, I will faithfully carry the camera and will never see another calf as young as today's.

The long grass in the fields across the valley is being stirred up by the brisk wind, and whirling trails are spreading up the slope, converging at the top like an invisible herd stampeding away from us. Quite an unusual effect. Standing in the barley fields by the woods is Honky. There is no sign of the escaped hind, perhaps she has had her baby and is holed up somewhere amongst the dense undergrowth. I must watch that the dogs do not disturb her.

Chapter 25

Fiver is in for his abscess removal operation this morning. Luckily his leg seems improved – I was worried that there might be infection in the joint which could have proved difficult to treat. He is anaesthetised with an injection of two combined anaesthetic agents, and placed on his back on a support bag. This plastic-covered bag is full of polystyrene beads and moulds itself to the patient's shape, holding them firmly in the desired position. It has the added advantage of conserving body heat, an important factor for all anaesthetised patients but especially for little ones.

Trimming up Fiver's chin with the clippers is not easy. As well as the discharging abscess, the area is disfigured with four other suspicious lumps. Luckily, all of the abscesses are discrete lumps just below the skin, and none connects with either teeth or jaw bone. After some careful dissection, I am able to remove them in their entirety, so am confident that no infection is left in the area. There is however the risk that others may crop up again, and more surgery will be required to remove them. It is unclear why some rabbits develop abscesses – it is known that they do harbour certain bacteria in their bodies, and it may be that affected rabbits have less efficient immune systems than their healthy comrades. There was no sign of any abscesses in Fiver before his trouble with his eye, and I wonder whether the pain and upset involved with that episode may have played a part in their development. We will never know. Extensive stitching is required to piece Fiver's chin together again – he does look as if he has been attacked by the mad axeman. I will need to warn Shona beforehand in case she gets a shock. He will stay on antibiotics for two weeks in an attempt to deter more abscess formation.

After the windy weather at the weekend, today is sunny and still.

Perhaps this is summer? I decide to take the dogs for a different walk, through the woods to the shingle beach at Peeswit Point. Ambling along the road, the smell of freshly cut grass fills my nostrils. Our neighbouring farmer is cutting a field for silage production. The harvested grass is packed into a silage pit and the low oxygen conditions within the pit converts the grass into a kind of pickled grass which is used for cattle feed over the winter months. There is an old farming joke regarding a layer of browned grass which could be seen on the side of silage pits throughout Scotland. It was said to occur when all the farm workers downed tools to attend the Royal Highland Show, thus allowing the grass on the top to burn, and was dubbed the Royal Highland Showtime Band. The show starts later this month, but I don't think we will be going this year.

Passing through the woods towards the river, leaves and small branches are strewn across the path- the legacy of the high winds – and the sharp, 'green' smell of bruised vegetation fills the air. As usual, the dogs sense our proximity to the river and bustle ahead, straight into the water. Fintry gallops clumsily through the waves while Kippen is content to stand with water lapping gently against his legs. It might ease his arthritic joints, but I must remember to give him some extra anti-arthritic tablets when we get home otherwise he will be stiff later.

Heading back along the road between fields of barley turning a pallid lemon-green and hedgerows dotted with pink and white dog roses, we come upon a distressing sight, a dead baby badger by the side of the road, still warm but beyond any veterinary help. She has been run over since we passed this way an hour ago. This is quite a turn up for the books. In the past, we have found evidence of badgers passing through this area – footprints and temporarily occupied holes – but there have never been resident ones on this side of the hill. The presence of a badger cub means that things have changed, but a baby out in the middle of the day does tend to signify that something is amiss. I divert into the strip of woodland close to the little corpse (which I gently move on to the grass verge) in an attempt to see if I can locate a sett. If the adult badgers have been injured or killed, there may be more cubs in need of help. However, the woods are so overgrown that it is impossible to see anything; all that I can do is to inform the folk who live next to the woods and ask them to keep their eyes open for any stray creatures. In my last practice, both Jay and I were involved in dealing with orphan badger cubs, so at least we have the experience should any appear. Making a mental note to return as soon as the summer vegetation begins to die back, I return home with my exhausted dogs.

The rest of the day remains quiet, so, contrary to my nature, I indulge in a spot of gardening. I weed amongst the fruit trees which are beginning to bear miniature fruits – I can't tell whether they are apples, pears or plums but inspect them every day in the hope that some recognisable features will appear. Our cherries are nearly ripe, but our predecessor did warn that it is a challenge to get at them before the birds have decimated the crop. I expect we will be buying them at the supermarket as usual. Any surplus apples or pears will be useful for the red deer. After half an hour's weeding, I have picked up thorns in both my hand and foot, and decide to call it a day – gardens seem to be dangerous places, I'm better off with savage cats and Rottweillers.

I am just beginning to get ready for the return to Clayfern for evening surgery when the telephone rings. The lady caller is in an intriguing dilemma: driving over a remote track near Drumdurn, she stopped and got out to admire the view. Returning to the car, she spotted a small brown dog under the vehicle. Any approaches were greeted by snarling, and any attempts to entice it out were ignored.

'I don't want to drive off and maybe squash him,' she says anxiously. The reason that she is ringing the surgery on her mobile phone is that she can see the surgery's name and telephone number on the dog's name disc. This is standard policy with the company who supply identity tags for our clients – client's name and phone number on one side; vet's on the other. With relief, I can see the solution to the problem 'Just see if you can get him to turn his head,' I instruct cheerfully. 'I've tried that,' she replies, 'But he snaps if I go any closer; I can only just make out your number.' Since the story has unfolded, my brain had been frantically searching its memory banks for the identity of a small brown dog from Drumdurn or thereabouts. Finally, the light dawns – perhaps it is Frankie Ewan. The snag is, Frankie's record card is at the Clayfern surgery. 'Let me check the phone book to see if I can find the number, I'll call you right back.'

Typical, not listed. Brain frantically trying to solve the problem, I come up with another idea. Alice lives in Drumdurn. She will be heading back to work soon, so she could leave a little earlier and call at the Ewans' house in the village en route. If it really is Frankie, then attempting to lasso him and drag him from under the car is not a good idea. He really is a little sod, but he also has a bad heart – so an undignified struggle could kill him. Best to locate his owners first.

Once Alice and the stranded lady are contacted, I set off for Clayfern hoping that all goes well – and it does, as Alice tells me when she arrives. Frankie wandered off this morning and the family have been distraught. Once they appeared on the scene, Frankie gave himself up gladly and the unfortunate lady could continue on her journey. Pondering the chain of events, it strikes me that there are two morals to this story – firstly, always carry a mobile phone; and secondly, if you must get stranded with a dog under your car, then do it in a small community where the vet has a sporting chance of being able to identify the stray.

Evening surgery is relaxed and peaceful. I could get used to this, I think as I water the garden before supper. Jay uses the hosepipe, but I prefer to trip to and fro with the watering can. I have an accomplice who follows me back and forth – Piggy the cat. She has settled here wonderfully well, spending her days in a day bed of ferns high in the banking then allowing herself to be enticed indoors overnight. On wet days, she has a cosy spot under the green shed from which she watches the comings and goings in the yard. It has become a routine for her to join me on my nightly waterings. I suspect I may be regarded as a bodyguard, allowing her to inspect the front of the property in safety.

The peaceful scene is unfortunately shattered by the shrilling of the telephone, closely followed by a summons from Jay – my services are required, a cat is having kittens but appears to have ground to a halt. After questioning the owner over the phone, it seems likely that a caesarean is going to be necessary, so I fall into the usual routine – locate Julie, prepare the operating room, put kettle on for hot water bottle etc. The small cat is only young herself, and is very disgruntled about the whole business. Luckily, she is a gentle creature, allowing us to administer an intravenous anaesthetic without struggling or complaint. One by one, I pass the kittens to Julie who moves into kitten revival mode, clearing secretions from mouths and nostrils, and rubbing each with a towel to encourage breathing. Two are fine and soon begin to squeak in protest, but the third is struggling for breath, the small body jerking with each attempt to inhale. Julie repeatedly clears mouth and nose of secretions and uses another technique to clear the airways. This involves cradling the kitten in a towel, supporting its head and body firmly while making a downward sweeping movement with the arms, the object being to dislodge fluid from the kitten's respiratory system.

Busily stitching up the abdominal wound, I am dimly aware that Julie has frozen in position at the bottom of her downward stroke, and is staring raptly at something on the floor. Seconds later, she resumes her movements, giggling to herself. 'Just look over there,' she says, when I ask what is so amusing. Staring downwards, her actions become clear – on the floor is a clumped dollop of fur, a stray lock from when the cat was trimmed up. It is exactly the same colour and size as the kitten's head, and for an instant before logic came into play, poor Julie thought that she had somehow shaken off the kitten's head. For hours after the event, this vivid mental picture will return occasionally, causing both of us to grin uncontrollably.

After the mother cat is finished and returned to a kennel, we continue to work on the poorly kitten, suctioning any stray fluid out of its mouth, directing a low flow of oxygen over its face and insistently rubbing its tiny chest. 'There she goes!' cries a triumphant Julie, hearing a series of anguished squeaks. 'Sorry, false alarm, that's just my stomach wanting its tea,' I have to reply. Luckily, after another fifteen minutes, we hear the real thing. An hour later, mother and three kittens are borne home by Mary, their relieved owner. The third kitten is still not one hundred per cent so Mary will have a long night ahead, but is well used to this type of situation, and in the past, has positively revelled in nursing poorly kittens back to life. This is lucky for us as it means that, after tidying up, we can both finally have our supper.

Chapter 26

On an early walk up the hill, the dogs and I disturb Honky in the long grass. What I initially mistake for a fallen tree branch is in fact his antlers. Far from taking off in a panic, he merely stands up and stares at us over the twenty yards between us, keeping us in sight until we disappear round the corner. Looking back, I see a strange sight – Honky has decided to follow us by ascending the small hill next to the track. All that is visible atop the hummock are his antlers, like two candelabras being carried unsteadily above the overgrown vegetation. It is quite flattering to be accepted by the stag, but I will be very cautious in autumn when the breeding season begins, and will keep my distance.

It is when wild creatures lose their fear of humans that trouble often begins. The cases occasionally reported in newspapers of owls or crows 'attacking' people are almost always perpetrated by birds which have been tamed by humans. Perhaps they were hand-reared before being released into the wild. They are only responding to a half-forgotten urge to be close to humans, and mean no harm, but it can be very frightening to be swooped upon by a large feathered creature. On the other hand, it can be serious if potentially dangerous creatures lose their fear of man. A friend of ours hand-reared a family of orphan badger cubs and rehabilitated them into a remote wood. During a night-time visit to the site several months later, one male badger attempted to attack our friend and he had to spend the night in a tree to avoid serious injury.

Alice and I cannot believe it during morning surgery but Shona and Fiver appear with yet another problem. A dog from the next street escaped from home early this morning and attempted to dig Fiver out of his hutch. Fiver escaped when the hutch tipped up, and was rescued by Shona's neighbour from under his garden shed. The little chap is covered in earth ... and is shutting his eye, the opposite one to that which was damaged a few weeks ago. Once again, the ritual of the local anaesthetic drops and dye solution show damage to the cornea. Off he goes again with more eye drops and an appointment for later today. 'That rabbit is doing his best to shuffle off his mortal coil,' Alice comments. Certainly if he was a cat, then several of his nine lives would be gone by now.

This has been a wonderful week – gorgeous weather coinciding with a quiet period ops-wise. Clayfern surgeries have been busy so money has been coming in, but much of the time between surgeries has been free for me to do as I please. The in-tray got sorted out on Tuesday, so the last three days have had a holiday feel to them.

To try to cool down in the heat, the dogs have spent considerable time in the river. This morning, Fintry is suffering for her enthusiasm in the water. Her tail has taken on the configuration of a shepherd's crook, jutting straight out for four inches from its base, then bending vertically towards the floor. It is obviously uncomfortable, and she has a very hang-dog expression. This is a condition known as *frozen tail* or *limber tail*. It occurs quite frequently, especially in Labradors who have been in water, and may be a kind of rheumatism. It usually lasts for two or three days then wears off whether treatment is given or not. Because she is in discomfort, I give Fintry a pain-killing tablet and much reassurance. Unlike her 'brother' Kippen, she is not used to pain and reacts very badly if anything is wrong with her.

Jay and Andy went to Pitdreel with Andy's trailer yesterday, and cleared the flat of all the old kitchen units and carpets. Next on the agenda is for us to chose some paint and blitz the place. As I can only venture to Pitdreel when I am off duty, I suspect that I will be doing less than my fair share of the work. It can be frustrating to be restricted to places within half an hour's drive from home. However, painting is not my strong point, so I will just concentrate on preparing appetising meals for when Jay comes home after a hard day's painting.

Knowing that few operations are booked in for today, I have volunteered to bath Edith's three dachshunds. Our former nurse, Gillian, used to run a small grooming service and regularly washed the girls. They are short-coated dogs who do not really need washing, but Edith has a bee in her bonnet about their summer bath, so I decided to get them done while we are quiet.

They are all set when I arrive at the cottage, smartly togged up in their posh red collars and leads, and squeaking excitedly at the prospect of a trip. Without more ado, we load them into the back of the Tundra, and I set off for Fern. Not long into the journey, an unpleasant smell hits my nostrils ... someone has had an accident. I accelerate and arrive at home just as Julie is parking. Poised to field any escapees, we open the tailgate. What a horrendous sight ... and smell, greets us. Dog dirt has been paddled all round the carpet, the dogs and their leads are covered, and worse, they have jumped up at the windows, managing to smear excrement over virtually every available surface. None the wiser, the little dogs are balanced at the very edge, desperate to fling themselves into our arms. 'I *don't* think so,' exclaims Julie, smartly shutting the tailgate again until we can don disposable gowns and gloves.

One by one, we carry the stinking, squirming creatures into the surgery and attempt to deposit them into a kennel, but they are having far too much fun for that, twisting free and padding all over the kennel room floor, leaving mucky footprints in their wake. Once they are finally corralled, we attempt to clean the car. Julie holds a large refuse bag open while I bin all the soiled carpet, then we mop everywhere else with disinfectant and odour eliminator.

Next, we turn our attention to the girls. One by one, they are bathed in our wonderful new Belfast sink, then hairdried and returned to a clean kennel. Lastly, we soak their filthy collars and leads. The idea was to take them home on the way to evening surgery, but I decide on a change of plan – get them home before they can do it again. A third clean Vet-bed is loaded into the car, dogs are lifted in and I set off again, leaving Julie to clear up the mess. Unbelievably, a hundred yards from Edith's, a familiar smell pervades the car -'Not *again*, girls,' I moan, accelerating up the hill. Luckily, they have too little time to become quite as filthy, and are smartly unloaded for their loving mum. 'Next time, Edith,' I say, somewhat heatedly, 'we'll come here and do them in your shower.'

Julie has cleared up by the time I return, and determinedly walks into the house where she has made us mugs of tea. Although there is another operation, I sense that mutiny is likely if we do not have our tea and bun first. 'How much did you charge her?' she queries through a mouthful of Danish pastry. 'Five pounds each,' I reply sheepishly. *'Fifteen pounds?* She shrieks in disbelief. I have to agree with her. Fifteen pounds for three baths, a car valet, two washing-machine loads plus mileage and time, not our most financially successful day.

Our next operation is quite a sad case. Mrs Cassidy's hamster (yes, she has one of them too) got caught in the wire of her cage wall and managed to break her leg. Bandaging hamster legs is rather a waste of time if the break involves the upper part of the leg. They have cone-shaped legs and any strapping simply slips downwards. Keeping the creature confined to a small area is often all that is necessary to allow the break to heal.

At first we thought all would be well, but the fracture ends have moved and one is protruding through the skin. Mrs Cassidy did not notice this for a day or so, and the whole leg is nastily infected. Amputation is the only answer. She knows that the risks are significant, but is fond of her wee Charlie. An injectable anaesthetic cocktail puts Charlie to sleep, then we place her on a heated pad and prepare for surgery. Trimming the area is risky – one false move and you have a bald hamster – but completed successfully, then the area is scrubbed with surgical antiseptic and draped with sterile cloths by a similarly scrubbed vet. The operation proceeds exactly the same as in a larger animal, but in miniature. Painkiller and antibiotic is administered before the sleeping hamster is returned to a toasty warm recovery box. Within fifteen minutes, she is fully awake and trundling round the box. The first hurdle is over.

A cat in some distress is brought in as an emergency. His breathing actions are exaggerated, and each breath is accompanied by a shrill squeaking sound, rather like a child's squeaky toy. Animals in respiratory distress need to be handled very carefully as they are inclined to panic, so a mild sedative is called for before we attempt to x-ray him. I think that he is unlikely to have a foreign body stuck in his windpipe but it is best to check. The x-ray shows considerable reaction round the airways in the lungs, but no sign of any foreign obstacles. This reinforces my theory that this is a case of asthma, and I medicate him accordingly with anti-inflammatory drugs along with some antibiotic. I am resigned to having an inpatient overnight, but by 4 p.m., he has responded so well that he can go home. It is the wife that picks the cat up during evening surgery. She tells us that the cat was playing with the duster as she polished the living room yesterday afternoon. It appears that the respiratory signs showed up shortly afterwards. This is quite reassuring, and helps to lend strength to a diagnosis of asthma. As she says, she now has two choices – either keep the cat out of the room being cleaned, or don't dust at all. 'It will depend how I feel at the time,' she remarks cheerfully.

Fiver is in again tonight for an eye check. It was so severe that I wanted to keep a close watch on him. His eye is looking better, but Shona has yet another complaint; 'His urine looks as if it has blood in it,' she reports. Not *another* problem – this rabbit really is doing his best to leave this world forever. Fiver himself seems absolutely fine, but I suppose I'd better follow it up. 'Bring me in a sample tomorrow and I'll check it', I suggest. 'I thought you'd say that so I've got one here,' she answers, triumphantly fishing a small vial from her bag. Sure enough the sample is a reddy-brown colour, but further questioning discovers that the rabbit has no trouble passing urine, and is eating and drinking as usual. There is no pain when palpating over his bladder, and no blood shows on the urine dip stick. I explain to Shona that rabbit urine can show wide variation in its colour, so it is best just to monitor the situation over the next few days. Knowing that she worries, I remind her that Fiver is still on his antibiotics for his abscesses so should be covered for any urinary infections.

Unbelievably, Shona appears yet again at the end of surgery with another sample. This time it is khaki-coloured. 'I don't think you need to rush down every time he goes,' I suggest gently, 'Perhaps just keep a note on a piece of paper and report later in the week.' Deprived of a project, Shona is momentarily crestfallen, then brightens as an idea dawns – 'I know, I've got my paints, I can chart it for you.' 'That sounds like an excellent idea, Shona,' I enthuse, wondering what works of art will pass through these doors in the next week or so.

Chapter 27

After a rainy few days, bright sunshine wakens us early this morning. We decide to take advantage of the extra time this gives us, and take the dogs for a lengthy walk. Despite the sun, wellington boots are required for forging through the overgrown vegetation which will take several days to dry out. There is plenty wildlife about – we disturb most of it on our travels.

Honky is lying in a woodland glade, an idyllic spot carpeted with tiny blue, white and yellow flowers, and fragrant with the scent of pine resin. As he watches us pass, supremely unconcerned, he is framed by purple foxgloves – what a photo that would be, but, as usual, no camera. Overhead, a buzzard silently takes off from the top of a tall pine. This is in complete contrast to the disturbed wood pigeons who noisily and ineffectually flap around until they finally fly free of their leafy prison.

Skirting the barley field, it is clear to see why there is such an ambivalent attitude to rabbits amongst our clients and friends. Up to twenty feet into the field, there is no crop, only one to two inches of stubble, kept short by the continual nibbling of the local rabbit population. They can be equally devastating amongst prized garden plants. A friend thinks she may have found the answer – an old countryman has suggested she applies a solution of Epsom salts around her plants. Such a simple solution would be tremendous, otherwise people tend to take matters into their own hands with air guns or even snares.

The other day, a cat was brought to the surgery, having been freed from a snare intended for rabbits. Luckily, his cries had alerted a neighbour and he was released without serious damage, although his midriff will be tender for a day or so. The barley heads are formed now, but are still green. We need more sun to ripen all the crops. I show Jay a trick which my friends and I performed as kids. If you nip off a head of barley, and place it between your sleeve and skin – filaments first – it will crawl up your arm. At least it seemed to when we were children, but today's demonstration goes like a damp squib and Jay is singularly unimpressed. Perhaps you need to wait until the barley is ripe?

Coming down through the trees, the advance guard of dogs disturbs two squirrels prospecting on the forest floor. One shoots up a tree trunk with much chattering and swearing, and the occasional slip. The other only climbs to a height of about five feet on the opposite side of the tree to the dogs, and freezes stock-still like a statue. Is it hiding? I wonder, and, to test my theory, move slowly towards its side of the tree. Sure enough, it scuttles round to the far side. Moving towards it again, the same thing happens. I am actually playing hide and seek with a squirrel. After three goes, it loses patience and sets off up the trunk again with much swearing. We suspect that the first squirrel was a youngster, as yet lacking in experience and guile.

This revives fond memories for us – several years ago, a client brought a baby squirrel to the surgery. Its mother was found dead, so we became the guardians of the baby, and brought her up. When we first got her, she was about three weeks old; her eyes were still closed and she was totally dependant on us for feeding. She would clutch the milk-containing syringe with both hands and suck greedily. Rationing was necessary as she would readily over-eat, then suffer from indigestion, groaning and rocking miserably from side to side, both hands clutching her taut little belly. She slept in one of my furry slippers in between feeds. Watching her rapid development was fascinating. Over the next week, she became more vocal, and once her eyes opened, there was no stopping her. New behaviours appeared from one day to the next – self-grooming, play fighting and anger responses. She started eating solid foods, soaked cornflakes and brambles initially, then her first grape at five weeks, before moving on to nuts, and developing the skill to gnaw through the toughest of shells. Gradually she began to explore her surroundings.

One of our biggest surprises was how bad her balance was to begin with. Placed on the back of the settee, she would teeter and sway alarmingly, causing both of us to hover anxiously nearby, hands cupped to catch her if she fell. Before long however, she was skilled at leaping from surface to surface, and we transferred her into a shed bedecked with branches to perfect her technique. Her bed was in a wooden hutch in the shed, and she was dining exclusively on fruit and nuts. From a furry baby – all head and spindly legs – she was now streamlined and looked like a small adult. In the wild, young squirrels are fully developed by ten weeks of age, and by this time, our Elsa had learned all we could teach her. It was time for her release.

The hutch was carefully wedged between the branches of a tree near our home, and after some hours of acclimatisation, the door was left open. We kept a close eye on her hutch, keeping it topped up with her favourite foods so it remained a secure base from which she could gradually return to the wild. For many weeks, we were privileged to be greeted by our handsome foster squirrel whenever we came bearing gifts. It was a wonderful feeling to shout for Elsa, and, after a few minutes, witness her speeding across branches and down the tree trunk on to our hands, scoffing the proffered nuts and lifting her foreleg for her armpit to be tickled, her favourite treat. Unfortunately, after a month, she no longer came to our calls. We hoped fervently that she had successfully become independent, but could never know for certain. Like any children, you can only do your best for them while they are young, then once they have fled the nest it is up to them. The one skill lacking from Elsa's repertoire was the ability to interact with other squirrels, and we could only pray that this had not led to her downfall.

My car needs to go in to the garage this morning, another slow puncture courtesy of the assorted nails filling in the trenches in our yard. The sooner Julie's friend appears with some tarmac the better.

Being car-less can be a real problem with four miles between surgeries, but the garage attempt to make life easier for me. If I drop the car off on the way to morning surgery, then they endeavour to have it ready for collection after surgery is finished. The walk up the village is a pleasant start to the day with much greeting and exchanging of pleasantries. Retrieving the car after a couple of hours, the mechanic comments yet again on how clean its undercarriage is. This is thanks to the long grass between the tracks en route up the hill.

A mixed bag for morning surgery. Unfortunately, the first patient is Charlie, Mrs Cassidy's hamster. She seemed to have recovered well from her leg amputation last week, but this morning she is dull and lifeless. The wound looks fine, but the hamster is obviously in dire straits, I cannot tell exactly why.

'The cat chased her the other day, and she hasn't been right since,' says Mrs Cassidy, 'I think that its time for me to part with her.'

Looking at the huddled little creature, I am inclined to agree, and the deed is done. 'At least she had a good week,' remarks Mrs Cassidy as she departs. *That's true,* I think, then start to doodle with figures on a piece of paper as a thought strikes me – the average hamster life span is around two years; the average human is seventy years. Therefore, a week to a hamster is worth approximately thirty five weeks to a human. Looked at that way, the outcome of the surgery does not seem such a disappointment. She was not a young hamster, but all the same, it is a pity that she had not lasted for longer.

Our next customer is Leo, the Labrador. Leo is a spry fourteen year old, and trots happily into the consulting room. He does not look at all ill, but his owner reports that his drinking has increased alarmingly recently, and he has also become very greedy, grabbing scraps off the floor as well as polishing off two big meals a day. An examination reveals no obvious abnormalities, but I suggest a blood test to investigate further. As Leo's owner says, it is not the drinking that she objects to, but the getting up at all hours to allow him to part with the results of the drinking. Alice steadies him gently while I trim up his foreleg then apply a dollop of local anaesthetic cream. Once reserved for the most cowardly of our patients, I tend to use this cream most times that we need to take blood nowadays. It cuts down the involuntary jerking of the leg when the needle makes contact, and makes our job easier. At my age, I'm all for anything that makes the job easier, and it is more pleasant for the patient.

The blood is divided into two small tubes and parcelled up for transport to the laboratory. I have asked for routine biochemistry and haematology to be carried out. The biochemistry screen measures levels of certain substances in the blood. If these differ from normal levels, then certain inferences can be made. For example, the substances *urea* and *creatinine* are increased in the event of kidney malfunction; *ALT* and *bile acids* will be raised if there is a problem with the liver. Haematology examines the different constituents of the blood – mainly red blood cells and the several types of white blood cells. Variations in the numbers and percentages of the cells present also helps towards reaching a diagnosis. For a simple example, if a lab result showed increased urea and creatinine, coupled with an increased *neutrophil* (type of white cell) count, a reasonable interpretation would be that an infectious process is affecting the working of the kidneys (as the neutrophil count increases when infection is present). It is not always possible to come to a diagnosis after one single blood test, but it is often one step closer, and often provides useful information about what the condition *isn't*. Leo's results will be through tonight. I also ask Leo's owner to drop in a sample of his urine this afternoon. I will check that here and take that information into account when reading the lab results.

At Fern surgery, we have another day of dentals. This has been our lot on Fridays, and it does make sense to do such 'dirty' procedures at one time. We are presently awaiting the delivery of a new dental machine – an air-driven machine similar to those used in human dental surgeries. All the tools will be conveniently arranged on a bar at the front of the machine which is itself on a mobile stand. There will be an ultrasonic scaler and polisher similar to that we already use, but the biggest improvement is in the drill which is high-powered and operates at approximately three hundred and fifty thousand revs per minute, a great improvement on our present drill which only makes thirty thousand revs per minute, and generates much heat into the bargain, making sectioning of teeth or bone something of a marathon. And yet, only a few years ago, our present set-up was regarded as state-of-the-art. It is increasingly hard (and expensive) to keep up with advances in technology.

After the dentals are recovering in their kennels with their shining choppers, there is one last job to be done, two blood samples for the Pet Travel Scheme, the scheme whereby animals travelling to certain countries can return to the UK without having to go through quarantine. The whole procedure is quite a palaver – not for the faint-hearted.

The animal first needs microchipping so it can be uniquely identified, then it has a rabies vaccination, then a month after that, a blood sample to ensure that the rabies protection levels are adequate. One health check later, its certificate can be signed, but it is not valid until six months later (as it is impossible to tell whether the raised rabies levels are due to the vaccination or infection with the disease, the animal effectively undergoes its six months quarantine *before* it travels abroad). Quite apart from these requirements, the animal also needs an import certificate for the country it is visiting. Each country varies in their requirements; some require the certificate to be signed within forty eight hours of the animal's arrival in the country. This can be a hassle for our Scottish clients as they have to travel the length of the UK before they can cross to the Continent, and there is little room for delays. Within forty eight hours of returning to the UK, the animal must be treated for parasites at a veterinary surgery in the foreign country, and obtain a signed statement confirming this.

British vets are watching the scheme with considerable interest as there is a real chance that we will begin to encounter illness due to parasites not found here; several cases have already been reported.

Today's challenge for Julie and me is to extract two ml of blood from two miniature Papillion's – small, excitable dogs belonging to a small, excitable owner. A previous attempt to collect the blood during a routine consultation failed dismally, so today the plan is – detach dogs from owner for an hour (probably the most useful part of the exercise), mildly sedate them, apply local anaesthetic cream and collect blood. The first dog goes remarkably smoothly, but the second is like getting blood from a stone. The sedative has dampened the worst of her wriggling but she keeps up a constant squirming which makes life exceedingly difficult as I desperately try to coax blood from her vein. Drip by drip it lands in the collection tube while Julie employs heroic manoeuvres to keep the limb outstretched. At last, the two ml line is reached, and I withdraw the needle with considerable relief. Irritatingly, for someone with seemingly no blood a minute ago, the dog's leg drips enthusiastically all over the floor on the way back to the kennel. Handling the precious samples with extreme care, we parcel them up and hand them over to Pete the postie with all possible speed.

Rest and recreation time. The dogs are bored with our trips up the hill, limited as we are to the tracks, so I set off to pastures new. Our neighbouring farmer has just mowed his clover field, the very spot for a gentle ramble. This field appears to be something of a thoroughfare for foxes and roe deer, and the dogs are in heaven investigating the novel scents. The river stretches away from the bottom of the next field; today it is as calm as a millpond. At first glance, I think that one small boat is about to ram another, then realise that it is merely a reflection in the water. The river reflects perfect images of clouds and nearby trees, even a heron at the water's edge. Gazing at the inverted images almost gives me vertigo.

The barley next door is subtly changing from green to tan, and looks luxuriantly bushy, almost like fur in appearance. The malty smell of ripening grain is so evocative of this time of year. Kippen reappears from a forage in the overgrown verge, the unmistakable smell of fox on his head. I wipe his face with a hanky then discover that the smell has transferred to my fingers. It proves indelible for most of the rest of the day. A flock of sheep are clustered together in the next field, one lies at the centre of the semi-circle, perhaps they are being briefed. Shortly afterwards, they disperse to graze – now what was that about?

Leo's urine sample is delivered during evening surgery – apart from being dilute, there is nothing of interest to be seen. One step forward, we know now that he is not diabetic, and there are no clues of any abnormalities in the urinary tract. It is sometimes quite exciting to be poised at the beginning of the diagnostic trail. I am looking forward to receiving Leo's results. Preliminary suspicions are forming in my mind, but I will say nothing until the information is at hand.

Keeping the ball rolling nicely, Leo's blood results have been faxed through while I am at Clayfern surgery, and I peruse them on my return to Fern. As is often the case, they do not clinch the diagnosis, but move things along by allowing certain conditions to be discounted. Several levels are raised or altered, lending strength to a suspicion which has been forming in my mind. I wonder whether Leo could be a case of *Cushing's Disease* or, to give it its official name, *Hyperadrenocorticism.*

I telephone to explain the results to Leo's owner, Lynn. A small physiology lesson is in order first to help her understand what *Cushing's Disease* is. *Cortisol,* the body's own corticosteroid, is produced by two glands called the *adrenal glands.* There is one on each side of the body, next to the kidneys. The production of cortisol in the glands is controlled by a hormone produced from a 'master' gland in the brain – the *pituitary gland.* If there is a tumour of either the pituitary or adrenal glands, then excess cortisol is produced, causing deleterious side-effects. The most common symptoms are – drinking and eating a lot, hair loss, reduction in muscle tone leading to a pot belly, poor wound healing, thinning of the skin and a plethora of other effects. The most usual victims of this disease tend to be middle-aged or elderly, small, female dogs which Leo certainly is not, but everything else seems to fit, so I suggest a second round of tests. There is a treatment for Cushing's disease which involves using a drug which destroys adrenal tissue; it can be incredibly effective, but if used in a patient who does not have the condition, it is likely to be fatal. Thus it is essential for us to reach a definite diagnosis. The next test is called an *ACTH stimulation test* and requires two blood samples – one is taken to measure the patient's basal cortisol level; then a synthetic version of the hormone manufactured by the pituitary (ACTH) to stimulate the adrenal gland is injected into the blood stream and another sample is then taken in one to two hours' time. A greatly increased cortisol level in the second sample points to Cushing's disease. Some clients tend to give up at this point, unwilling to spend more money on an elderly dog whose life expectancy is not great in any case, but luckily Lynn is keen to prolong Leo's life as much as she can, and is game to carry on. I order the synthetic ACTH from our supplier, and book Leo in to undergo the test on Monday.

On our evening walk up the hill, we fleetingly see Honky and the hind. I have a romantic notion of the happy couple living peacefully together, but suspect that all will change during the breeding season: she will be dropped like a hot brick in Honky's attempts to get back in with the rest of the hinds. Stags are not into monogamy. It is easy to see where they have been – the long grass is flattened, and steaming heaps of deer dung anoint the ground, not at all like the delicate pellet-like droppings of the roe deer. Unfortunately, Fintry has seen them too and rolls ecstatically in the 'deer pats'. We drive down the hill with all the windows open, and bath the dog the minute we arrive home.

Chapter 28

Before morning surgery, a new walk in the freshly baled hayfield only yards from the house. The dogs are thrilled at having novel territory to explore, and snuffle eagerly round the bales and the verges. The smell of new-mown hay is wonderful, and I relax, sitting up on a bale listening to a flock of tits in the dog rose bushes, observing the view. The neighbouring fields are varying shades between green and tan; the oilseed rape is dishevelled and tousled, a waste of space as far as walks are concerned. The tide is nearly out and horse-shoe shaped sandbanks are visible on the river, each left with silvery zigzags of water reflecting the sky. Clumps of reeds are growing on the distant banks, from a distance like dark, oblong boxes. Pastures new should gradually appear later this month as fields are harvested or mowed, and each will be as diligently explored as we have today.

The main event this morning is the next step in Leo's diagnostic trail. The synthetic pituitary hormone arrived in Saturday's post, and he is due in first thing. At 9 a.m., we take a sample of blood for measurement of his body's cortisol, then inject synthetic ACTH into the vein. At 10 a.m. he returns for more blood to be taken. If the second blood sample shows a large increase in cortisol, this is strongly suggestive of Cushing's disease. As is usual before blood sampling, Leo has been starved for several hours beforehand. As a treat after his final sample, Alice offers some biscuits from the treat jar and nearly loses fingers in the process. Leo falls on the treats as if he has not eaten for days. This gives us some idea of how difficult life is for Leo's owner at the moment. He is drinking sixteen pints of water per day as well, and she has to get up at all hours of the night to let him out. If we do not diagnose Cushing's, then I suspect Leo's outlook will be bleak as the poor woman just cannot cope.

After morning surgery, there is an hour to spare before further work, so I decide to visit an elderly friend. Mrs Gladys Cross has been a client for years, but last year it was necessary to put her old dog to sleep. Gladys decided not to get another pet as she was getting older herself, but we have still kept in touch, and I visit when the opportunity arises. Jay and I went to her ninetieth birthday party two years ago and thoroughly enjoyed it ... as did Gladys who was seldom off the dance floor. An impressive array of friends and family were present including children, grandchildren and great-grandchildren. Although old age is catching up a little with her physically, mentally she remains as sharp as ever and is a witty, amusing companion. I have not seen her since the purchase of the Laigher so there is plenty to talk about. Born and bred in this area, she tells fascinating tales of life in days gone by.

One concerns the lady of the manor whose bathchair was towed round the neighbourhood by a Shetland pony. The local children were expected to curtsey as she passed, otherwise a week's notice might be given to any parent unfortunate enough to be a tenant of the 'Big House.'

'What are you doing with all your spare time now you've moved?' Gladys enquires.

'I've started to paint with watercolours again,' I reply, a little embarrassed, 'I'll not be giving up the day job, but it is very relaxing ... in fact, if you don't mind, I'd like to try doing your house.'

Gladys' house is very picturesque, thatched, with a colourful cottage garden full of wild flowers which attract multitudes of butterflies.

'Feel free,' she says, so I whip out my camera from the glove compartment and set about taking photos. I would be useless let loose in the countryside with an easel, as my favoured modus operandi is to photograph a likely subject and paint it in the comfort of my own home. As I am thus occupied, Jim the local grocer arrives with supplies for Gladys.

'I'm going to paint her cottage,' I explain, in response to his enquiring glance.

'When?' he asks,

'Probably Monday or Tuesday evening,' I reply, thinking, *What an odd question. Is he interested in the result?* Distracted by Gladys making coffee, I think no more of it, and spend another half an hour discussing Rayburns with my friend. She has an ancient solid-fuel Rayburn, and is skilled at using it. 'These hot days I only light it two hours before I need it,' she volunteers – 'Just give it time, that's all you need to know'.

On the way home, I drop off some worming tablets for Edith's brood. She is pottering in the greenhouse: 'These are my passionflowers,' she shows me proudly, 'They only flower for one day every year – just one day then they are gone.'

'What are they like?' I ask, intrigued.

'Well, I have blue ones and red ones ... if you want I'll give you a ring when the next one flowers and you can come to have a look if you're not too busy.' *Anything for a new experience*, I think as I take my leave. Let's hope they don't flower on of our madly hectic days.

Up at the farm, there is the usual collection of cats to attend to for Sheila. Pete the postie brings a parcel into the surgery. It is a stout cardboard box containing the incinerated remains of Sid, a particularly unpleasant old cat who thankfully passed away in his sleep last week. He has had innumerable ailments over the years, many of which would have been the end of cats half his age, but the lovely Sid always managed to recover. Treatment always involved much slight of hand and avoidance tactics, even for something so innocuous as a simple injection, and for anything more major, sedation was always necessary. Julie, Alice and I have all had our share of scratches and punctures from Sid, who was known to everyone as Hissing Sid, or Sid Vicious. Despite his faults, his owner loved him dearly and requested his ashes for scattering in his favourite spot in the garden – apparently a bush from which he used to rush out and terrorise the neighbour's dog.

'There's some bits leaking from the box,' observes Pete as I sign his delivery form. Sure enough, some dusty material lies on the consulting table. I had planned to hand over the unopened box to Sid's family, but decide to check inside. They would not be best pleased if half of Sid's ashes have leaked away. The container is intact however, the particles are seeds from the discrete little posy of dried flowers which the cremation firm attach to the jar of ashes. 'You could plant them in the garden,' says Sheila, scooping them into her open palm.

'As long as we don't have a crop of lots of little Sids,' I return, quaking at the very thought.

Leo's results come through just before evening surgery – negative, not quite what we expected. This is not the end of the line, as this test can occasionally be negative in cases of Cushing's disease. The plot thickens – we now have to perform yet another test, known even more grandly as a *low dose dexamethasone suppression test*. Poor Lynn, Leo's owner, is struggling with all these names. I let her into a secret – it takes me all my time to get all the words in the right order. With a sigh, I ring our suppliers and place an order for the required drug. The next test will take place on Thursday. Sid's owner comes to collect her sad cargo. It is the first time that I have seen this lady since she brought the deceased Sid in last week. The most striking thing about her is that she does not have Sid's trademark scratches on any exposed skin surfaces – the poor woman used to look like she habitually slashed her wrists, but we all knew it was just Sid.

Up the hill with the dogs later, I finish the camera's film on some shots of Honky in the long grass. He doesn't bother to move as I frame his magnificent head in the lens. There is a rook family in the woods behind the thinking stones, and unusually gentle, intimate cawing can be heard as we pass by. There is little point in stopping to sit, the flies are out in force and we each have our own little flock in attendance. They are driving poor Honky and the other creatures mad. Like a scene from a Hitchcock film, flies surround the car when we get in again.

The telephone is ringing as I return home, and I grab it suspecting it might be Jay. Instead it is Gladys, laughing like a drain. Answering her door a few minutes ago, she was met by Jim resplendent in a white boiler suit. 'I can't come in the evenings,' he said, 'But if you show me where the paint is, I'll make a start, and Kate can finish it later.' The misunderstanding has made Gladys' day.

After giving the dogs their tea, I drive into Stramar to meet Jay who has been at work. Jay has spent every spare evening recently painting at Pitdreel (perhaps we should divert Jim over there), and this evening it is time to choose a new carpet for the living room. 'Nothing fancy, just cheap and cheerful,' we agree. I am very taken with a smart tartan rug, and keep coming back for a second look. 'Aye, the Scottish genes will out,' says Jay, 'It'll be baffies [boot-like slippers, usually also tartan] and the *Sunday Post* next.' I heard recently from a mutual client that our local doctor has a cottage in the village next to Pitdreel. 'Why there?' asked our client. 'Because its not Clayfern', came the dour reply.

Enjoying an evening play with the dogs in the garden, I smile fondly at my partner – 'Just listen to the burn trickling away, isn't that peaceful.' 'Actually,' says Jay, 'Its a cow having a wee.' A look over the fence confirms this, but it seems sad to have one's illusions so cruelly shattered.

Two days later, Leo and Lynn are waiting for me at 9 a.m. The area of poor Leo's front leg where the last blood sample was taken is more bruised than normally expected – another sign suggestive of Cushing's disease. I liberally anoint the target area on both legs with local anaesthetic cream before gathering all the necesssary paraphenalia for the test. For accurate results in this test, it is important that the patient is unstressed as otherwise his cortisol levels will be elevated anyway. For this reason, we decided to forego the usual period of starving. Like a shrew, Leo is looking for food every couple of hours, and starving him does make him very stressed. He is very good while I take the blood and inject the corticosteroid *dexamethasone* into his vein. The rationale of the procedure is that a feedback mechanism will normally reduce the body's production of cortisol for approximately seventy two hours. Leo will come out to Fern surgery for another sample in four hours, then back to Clayfern for a final one at eight hours post dexamethasone. Lynn is sent off with a tube of local anaesthetic cream to apply before each sampling.

Working through a consignment of neuterings for Sheila, we chat about topical news. It is a shock for all the locals to hear that Pete the postie is due to retire soon. What will we do without him? 'Nothing much today, Kate,' he will say, passing over the mail, or 'It's only your car's tax reminder.' He suffers with us through agonising waits for big bills or tax rebates, and announces their appearance with triumph. It will seem strange not to have one's post personally vetted before one gets it. Misdirected letters never occur with Pete – we have received mail with glaringly incomplete addresses such as 'The vet in the cottage by the river' or 'Sheila the cat lady,' and little else.

'We should get him a retirement present,' says Sheila, and together we mull over likely items. I have recently taken delivery of a magnificent painting of our locality, specially commissioned by Jay for hanging in Clayfern surgery. It shows our river and hills, and many of the creatures that inhabit them. The 'muriel' has been a great talking point amongst clients. 'What about a picture like yours?' she suddenly suggests. This strikes me as a good idea, but to be sure, I telephone a sample of neighbours. 'Go for it!' is the unanimous response, so, after the operations are finished, I telephone the artist with our ideas – 'The same familiar scenery with perhaps a red post van and a little figure in a postie's cap.' To my relief, the artist will be able to finish the piece before Pete is due to go. Between us, Sheila and I will contact as many locals as we can and try to extract a donation. Pete is very popular so this should not be hard. Many folk are clients of the surgery so if they don't cough up, I can always add a little extra on to their bills.

Up the hill with the dogs, I happen upon the runaway hind. Instead of running away, she takes a step or two towards us, and stares fixedly at the dogs. This is unusual behaviour, and may mean that she has a calf. When protecting their young, the normally shy hinds can be quite aggressive – we have frequently watched them in the pen, chasing a passing fox into the distance. There is nothing to see nearby but I shall be watching very closely in future.

Fintry comes in with me to evening surgery as Jay is taking Kippen for his Reiki session. He has been going for several weeks now, and it is hard to say how much it is helping. We do think that he is more cheerful after a session – although this may be due purely to the therapist's biscuits and a snuffle round her interesting garden, but whatever the reason, he is now included whenever Jay has an appointment. Fintry is not used to being left on her own, and in case her previous house-wrecking tendencies re-surface, it is safer to bring her into Clayfern and allow her to stay with Alice behind the counter. She too has lots of treats and a short, brisk walk with me on the way home.

Just before I leave, Edith rings to herald the flowering of a passionflower. With Fintry loaded in the rear, I drive to Edith's home. Poor Fintry, when I reverse into the drive, she is spotted and screamed at by the three dachshunds. What an incredible noise from such small animals. Edith drags them into the house before escorting me to the greenhouse. There a blue passionflower is blooming in all its glory. It is really quite a complex flower: outer mauve petals encircle a cluster of thin filaments which begin in the centre of the flower as purple then change to white, and finally royal blue. Inside the filament circle is a cruciate arrangement with four knobbly bits. 'It is supposed to tell the story of the crucifixion, but I can't remember exactly how,' says Edith vaguely. I think I get the rough idea.

Unfortunately, my intended walk in the hayfield is stymied – the farmer has moved all the bales back to the barn and has put the cattle in to graze. Poor Fintry has to make do with yet another run up the hill. At home, both dogs greet each other with great excitement, partly I suspect, because Jay has been to the chip shop on the way home.

Leo's results come through overnight. We have hit paydirt with this latest test. The results confrm that he _is_ in fact suffering from Cushing's disease. I telephone the supplier of the treatment drug to be told that we need a *Special Treatment Authorisation* from a department of the Ministry of Agriculture. The drug is not manufactured in the UK, and must be imported from Canada. The helpful receptionist explains that an application form can be acquired from the ministry's internet web-site and gives me its address (or *u.r.l.* for the technically minded). Feeling very pleased with myself for achieving this unscathed, I carefully fill in the form and send it to the relevant department. Hopefully we will have Leo on medication before long – Lynn is approaching the end of her tether.

Mrs Cassidy brings her old cat into morning surgery for her 'G and T', as she calls it. The cat suffers from chronic renal failure and looks dreadful, although she remains surprisingly cheerful – the typical creaking gate. Every three weeks or so, she comes in for injections of vitamins and anabolic steroid which seem to pep her up. Mrs Cassidy is worrying about the next trip in three weeks time as she will be on holiday, and the cat will be staying with her niece in Drumdurn. I know that the niece is a mobile hairdresser and suggests that she brings the cat in. 'But she's only got a bike,' wails Mrs C., 'She doesn't go very far.' Trying not to concentrate too much on a vision of a hairdresser on a bike – curlers and scissors protruding from every direction, Alice and I endeavour to solve the dilemma. 'If she does stop eating, I'll pop in, in the passing, if your niece lets us know,' I reassure her the worried old lady. Drumdurn is not that far, and I can take the dogs to the nearby woods and make an outing of it.

One of today's operations is an investigation of an elderly cat who has stopped eating. She is somewhat stroppy and needs a mild sedative before she can even be examined. A gentle palpation of her abdomen suggests a mass which also shows up on x-ray. Her owner is phoned and we prepare for an exploratory operation. 'I put an old dog with an intestinal tumour to sleep last night,' I comment as we clip up the cat's abdomen, 'I bet this is the same.' Uncannily it is. At first I think the growth might be removable, but a closer inspection reveals that it has spread to other areas, and the only option is to put her to sleep. I've heard of the animals going in two by two, but the illnesses ... ?

The weather is unseasonally cold with a north wind blowing, but it is bright, so I take the dogs on a fresh walk up the hill behind Duncraig. The scenery is different here, more reminiscent of the Highlands than the gentler grass-covered hill behind the house. Bare rock platforms cover the summit, surrounded by purple bell heather. I see a white version and gather a sprig for luck. The wind rustles through the marsh grass, and the rowan berries are already darkening. Even this early in the year, flowers are gradually turning to fruits. There are waxy green cones on the larch trees, and green beech mast and ash keys. In a small valley, honeysuckle all but obscures a stand of larch, the smell is heavenly.

Waiting for Kippen to make it up the last slope, I sit on a rock contemplating the scene. Bees flit from plant to plant, and I watch fascinated as a skylark mobs a hovering kestrel. The skylark is tiny beside the bird of prey but approaches it again and again, trying desperately to deter it from descending on its young. The kestrel is determined, and veers away repeatedly, only to return to hovering mode. Unable to watch the slaughter, I stand, wave my arms and shout ... and succeed where the skylark has failed. To be sure, I stand guard for a few minutes. A grasshopper 'cricks' away in the grass, and I try to spot it. Hearing them is easy but they can be hard to locate. Not so today, there are several including some little ones – a grasshopper family perhaps? They really are well named as they spring acrobatically from one blade of grass to another.

Driving back past the farm, I notice that the combine harvester is in the yard. It will be getting its once-over before the harvest. The prospect of some new walks is quite exciting. To ring the changes yesterday, I attempted to take a short-cut through the woods only to find nettles and sticky willy (cleavers or goose grass) performing a double act – the sticky willy clung to my clothes and pulled the nettles perilously close to any naked flesh. The dogs did not enjoy the experience either.

Arriving home mid-afternoon, I contemplate my options – shall I cook tonight's tea at a low heat for hours, or shall I turn the oven up before evening surgery and cook it at a higher heat for half an hour. Decisions, decisions. While I dither, the phone rings, it is friend and client Alison. Alison belongs to the local miniaturist group. These skilled individuals both make and kit out dolls' houses in astonishing detail. Knowing the affection with which I regarded the first surgery – the green shed – Jay asked Alison if she could make a scale model for my birthday. That was almost two years ago, but Alison has been ill and we have all been busy so the project has rather lapsed. It sounds as if Alison has taken up the reins again. She is coming into Clayfern surgery to take some photos of our posters to be scaled down, and wonders if I could take a photograph of some bones. The reason for this puzzling request is that her camera does not produce negatives. Negatives are ideal to use as x-ray films on the viewer. I'm not sure if it is a compliment that she assumes that I might have some bones knocking about the place. As it happens, I have just been sorting some old slides which include various x-rays of broken bones. That should be the very dab.

We are on the verge of going to bed when the telephone shrills. Sighing with resignation at the

prospect of an emergency, I am pleasantly surprised to hear Sheila's voice instead. Coming home late, she has just seen a young badger foraging at the roadside not far from where the other one was found dead. At least some are alive after all.

Chapter 29

A much needed day off. On our morning walk, I collect Sheila's dog Jonno before heading up the hill. He is even older and stiffer than Kippen, so our progress is slow. Kippen is deaf, and Jonno is nearly blind as well, so the trip is not particularly relaxing. No sooner has one been fielded, than the other disappears behind some undergrowth. It is like an outing of the geriatric dogs' society. Packing them into the car is also quite a procedure – Kippen attempts to leap but occasionally needs a quick grab round the middle to prevent him falling back. Jonno knows his limitations – he puts his front legs on the tailgate and waits patiently for his hind end to be lifted in. Fintry watches the loading procedure with fascination having hopped in with no effort at all.

With everyone exercised, we set off bright and early for a painting session at Pitdreel. Jay has done brilliantly; there is not very much still to do and after a morning's work, the whole flat has been completed. After exhausting the dogs on the beach, we drive farther along the coast to a village which is staging an exhibition about the doomed liner, *Titanic*. Listening to me planning this outing, Julie brought us an interesting item to show to the *Titanic* enthusiasts – a copy of the *Daily Mirror* dated Tuesday April 16th, 1912, found lining a drawer in one of her antiques. The truly remarkable thing is the reporting of the sinking – *Everyone Safe!* blares the headlines, *Helpless giant being towed to port by Allan liner.* Oops. Sitting in the inevitable cafe after viewing the exhibition, and showing off the paper, we read the rest of it. What interesting snippets there are – *Covent Garden porters demand a minimum wage of 22s a week; Rome tour £14.14s; Death from injured nose* – this concerns an unfortunate man who slipped on orange peel in the street and injured his nose, which subsequently caused lockjaw and death.

And finally, *The New Storm Queen, waterproof weather veil – its so simple and it cannot slip.* The latter is accompanied by a picture of a happy lady sitting in her open- topped car (as I suppose they all were then) with her weather veil tied in a large bow round her throat. As we return home, the heavens open and we are everlastingly grateful that our car was manufactured in 1998, not in 1912.

Next, we go shopping for kitchen units for Pitdreel. Choosing a sink called '*Alicia*' which is decorated with flecks of grey, I appreciate that this will be an ideal opportunity for teasing Alice ('It will always remind us of you etc ...). While we indulge in a businessman's lunch, Jay recognises some business acquaintances at an adjoining table, and we chat rather stiltedly until the model of the Green Shed comes up in the conversation. The obviously very well-heeled couple thaw noticeably, 'Oh for goodness sake!' says the wife, recognising kindred spirits, '*We* started out in a chicken shed.' From that moment, we all get on like a house on fire.

When we arrive home, there is a message on the answering machine from Lynn, Leo's owner – 'Any sign of his drug? He is getting me up every hour of the night.' Right enough, I have heard nothing so give the ministry department a ring. 'You filled in an old-style form, and the information is incomplete, so we have sent it back,' says the chap on the line. 'Well, it was from your web site,' I retaliate, thinking *Good grief, it's not even on its way.* What other information *do* you need.' 'The dog's name and type.' Taking a deep breath, and resisting the temptation to explode 'Well why could you not ring me? – Or even make it up,' I explain the situation in full detail. To give the man his due, once he realises the urgency of the case, he is helpfulness itself. If I fax through these details, he will fax the special authorisation back by Monday. I suspect that sitting behind a desk examining forms may dull folks' critical judgement, and make it easy to lose sight of the fact that we are dealing with a real flesh-and-blood patient here. The drug can be dangerous, but I can think of cheaper ways of poisoning the neighbourhood than going to the trouble of obtaining it under false pretences. Bureaucracy! I know it is for good reasons, but I never can get on with it.

In the evening, the beautiful weather lures us outdoors. Kippen has really had enough exercise for one day so we compromise and the whole family goes for a peaceful walk in the garden. It has all sorts of interesting nooks and crannies which are intriguing to dogs and humans alike. Up the slope is a tangle of bushes and trees, festooned with curtains of honeysuckle. This is home to several families of birds and their hungry offspring. As a result, I suspect we will not see many of our cherries when they ripen. At the moment, they are turning red but are still hard and bitter. The miniature fruits on the other trees are becoming recognisable as apples, plums and pears. We should be very healthy later in the year.

On the way to morning surgery next day, I spot the tractor mowing in the set-aside field. This is the earliest date that this can be done, allowing ground-nesting birds to fledge at least one clutch first. The sweet smell of freshly cut grass wafts through the open car window, raising anticipation of a new walk soon.

True to his word, the man from the ministry has faxed through Leo's special treatment authorisation (STA) so I telephone the suppliers – yes, I can finally get the drug ... but first, can I just fill in a new account form and an order form, and also send the STA. All this form-filling is becoming a pain; the dog will be dead of old age before we even begin treatment.

Morning surgery is fairly busy, the hot, still weather is tough on arthritic and chesty patients. These usually elderly animals cope quite well normally, but are pushed to the edge by extremes of temperature. We also have two requests for 'emergency' dentals as soon as possible, the reason being that our clients have a house full of guests attending the Open golf championship, and the guests have commented on the ripe odours emanating from the resident dogs' mouths. They will be fitted in tomorrow, a good opportunity for the new dental machine to do its stuff.

The heat is also affecting my beloved Kippen. Our horizons have narrowed so much in such a short time. Only last year, we would walk for miles, but now we are reduced to short rambles, taking half an hour to cover what we used to do in ten minutes. To keep them cool, I take both dogs into the woods. Down the track we go, Fintry skipping ahead pretending to flush and chase squirrels, while Kippen strolls gingerly as if on eggshells – a gait all too familiar to owners of elderly, arthritic dogs. Thank goodness he paces himself now, stopping frequently to investigate intriguing scents. We head uphill to intersect with another path leading back to the car. Protective of my old friend, I bring up the rear. On slopes, his legs sometimes give, landing him in an undignified heap and, although he is an independent devil, he will tolerate a hand cupped round each thigh for support if he falters. Once on the track, we stop for a breather, and even Fintry checks that her brother is rested before we continue slowly long the sun-dappled grassy path.

I watch Kippen ambling along – big hairy feet and body the colour of sun-dried grass, dark head and dark V-neck which becomes more pronounced in winter (we call it his cricket pullover) – and a lump forms in my throat. He is heading down the all-too-familiar slope that many old dogs take. Being a vet, I cannot pull the wool over my own eyes – his legs will get gradually worse and one day, we will have to make a decision. I see the same scenario every day – but not with my Kippen. It sounds trite but he is such a *nice* dog, gentle, intelligent and happy with a sharp sense of fun. The thought of losing him seems suddenly unbearable. I know what Jay would say – 'He's got plenty of time yet,' but I know his time will come before too long. We were watching a television programme recently where a guest stated their most hated thing was the fact that dogs' lives are so much shorter than humans. You may think that you have your life-time's companion, then they are gone in a mere twelve or so years.

Lost in thought, I have lagged behind, and I suddenly notice that Kippen has stopped. He is looking over his shoulder as if to say *Come on,* Mum. When I hasten, he wags his tail and continues en route.

Banishing my maudlin thoughts, I look to see what he has found – a deep hole dug by a forest resident. That looks like old wasp byke material in the depths, I think, investigating with a stick. *Bad* move, some disgruntled wasps are still in residence. Kippen and I leg it briskly along the track, watched from a safe distance by a bemused Fintry. Just like old times. As if to prove he is not due for burial yet, the old dog has a dust bath under an up-rooted tree, coming out black and stiff with grit. Clouds of dirt billow from him after a pat, a carpet beater might be necessary when we finally get home.

The hot weather has continued all week, and everyone feels like wee greasy spots. As we begin another run of dentals, the tractor and trailer pass along the road. That can only mean one thing – the harvest is about to begin. Sure enough, the combine harvester lumbers past in the field between the Laigher and the river. Excellent! This is a particularly pleasant field in which to walk. Unfortunately, there are no other fields ready for harvesting, so there is a risk that the farmer will plough this one soon after it is done. We must make sure that we have a few trips down to the river first.

Outdoors, the buzzards continually scream overhead, probably adults teaching youngsters to fly and hunt, and flies make all animals' lives a misery. To combat this, two horses by Abbeygate Farm have fringed veils on their foreheads – full of eastern promise, but probably very practical. Indoors, both surgeries feel warm and muggy, and clients seem more awkward than usual. The schoolchildren are on holiday so we either get groups of five or six in with their minder of the day, or cancelled or last minute appointments as the families forget their sick pet and head for the coast, only to realise out of hours that their animal really is ill and needs attention. Nerves are frayed and we all feel as if we could do with a holiday. Due to a small inheritance, Jay and I have achieved the near-impossible and have booked a locum for two weeks next month. We are going to Pitdreel, and can hardly wait. I cannot remember when we last had two weeks off – it must be at least ten years ago.

The new dental machine is definitely going to earn its keep. It has been invaluable. The drill is wonderful, cutting through teeth like a knife through butter, making extractions so quick and easy. Unfortunately, it sounds exactly like a human dentist's drill causing us several queasy moments. Another boon is the compressed air and water spray which clears blood and debris miraculously, keeping the operative field crystal clear. Already I don't know how we managed without it.

Leo's drug appears sooner than expected, not in the post but by courier late in the afternoon. I go into Clayfern early to have time to work out his dosage, and to write out instructions for Lynn. I am responsible for *pharmacovigilance* (a wonderful term), and must ensure that the drug is used responsibly and safely. Leo will be on daily dosage until his eating and drinking subside, and/or side effects develop. Lynn must wear gloves to administer the tablets, and wash her hands carefully after use. We do not want *her* adrenal gland to be affected.

Late in the evening, it is finally cool enough to take the dogs out for a stroll, not far, just a wander round the farm, accompanied as always by the shrieking of the buzzards. I am pleased to find that the wild raspberries in the hedgerows have ripened and are as sweet as I remember them. The dogs and I spend a happy five minutes eating them straight from the cane. I notice that Fintry, like Kippen, has learnt to pick the berry gently off the husk. Before eating them, I inspect the berries carefully for insects, although, as Julie says, they will be full of raspberry as well.

The dogs appreciate the novel smells and we enjoy the sights, especially in the barn which is a veritable nursery at this time of year. Several swallows' nests are glued to the girders, cup-like affairs often with little black and white faces peering out. Parent birds swoop in regularly with yet more food then return to their aerial gymnastics gathering more insects. Pigeons and starlings also nest in the roof. The pigeons give themselves away with their soft cooing, followed by wild whirring of wings when they are disturbed. Large piles of bird dirt are a real give-away for locating nests. Sheila's cats are intrigued but the birds are safe in their lofty perches.

Chapter 30

It is cooler today than of late, and we are not wakened at crack of dawn by the morning sun streaming through the windows. The farm cockerel's crowing is muted too – Sheila has obviously not let the birds out yet, so we manage to have a Sunday long lie – only until 8 a.m., but luxurious all the same. In the past, turning in bed or even a mere sigh would rouse Kippen who would be up and raring to go immediately – his deafness has its advantages.

The whole family piles into the Tundra, and we set off down the newly harvested field. At the bottom is one of my favourite corners on Fern – all the more alluring because we can only visit there for a short time between harvest and re-seeding. An old barn nestles into the hillside, the ground coming to within the top three feet of the back wall. It is unlikely that it was built like this, it must be due to the gradual movement of earth over the years. Quite amazing. Swallows swoop in and out through the skylight with their usual precision. Close to the barn, a stream runs down the boundary of the field cutting a deep crevice from which sprout alder, ash and wild cherry trees, many covered in impenetrable creepers of ivy. Ox-eye daisies, poppies and bindweed cover the banking in profusion. Waiting for Kippen to catch up, we spy a striking insect flitting from flower to flower. It is a *six-spot Burnet*, a day-flying moth with irridescent green wings blotched with red spots. At different angles, the wing colour appears black or even blue. I count the spots on the moths nearby and discover that they really do have six spots. Our knowledge of entymology is increasing daily as a result of waiting for Kippen.

Although slow, there is nothing wrong with Kippen's memory. He heads straight for the pool of muddy water where the stream disappears into the reeds. This has always been his wallow, and he emerges after several moments of happy splashing – coated in tenacious mud. Before we can stop her, Fintry follows suit. Luckily, we are heading for the river so they can have a good clean. The broken fence is still there allowing us easy access to the overgrown strip of rough grass before the river's edge. Avoiding dog rose thorns and brambles, we emerge on the shingly beach. Fintry heads straight for the water while Kippen disappears into a stand of reeds, reappearing with a football clamped between his jaws. He *always* finds a ball at the beach and had amassed quite a collection at our old cottage. This is the first for the Laigher. We make our way slowly along the shingle, Jay throwing sticks in the river for Fintry as we go. When we first got Fintry, she was afraid of water but followed Kippen's lead. Now she swims like a seal, and even drops her stick in the shallows for throwing – just like Kippen. She must have got water in her ear as she is shaking her head violently while swimming to shore, still hanging firmly on to her stick. Even Kippen hears this and looks up to see what the commotion is.

We beachcomb as we go, examining weird shapes of bleached wood and interesting stones. Jay has been given a worry stone by the Reiki practitioner and thinks I should have one too. The search is on, and, much to Jay's disgust, I discard many proffered offerings before settling eventually on a smooth, semi-circular piece of flint. Whether it will stop me worrying remains to be seen. We collect two stones too intriguing to be left. One is mottled giving the appearance of snakeskin – this seems to be a result of tiny cracks filling with earth; the other is a pinkish-blue wedge of stone with a top layer of white quartz, rather like an iced slice of cake. These may be the solution to a bone of contention between Jay and I. There is a barren patch of garden at home which Jay wants to fill with colourful shrubs, but I am unwilling to obscure the magnificent view. In a mutual brainwave, we decide to build a rock garden, collecting weird and wonderful stones from the river's edge and beach. This is the perfect time of year for such a scheme as we will soon have easy access through all the harvested fields.

Flushed with success, we make our way home for a late breakfast. Sitting in the kitchen, we notice a baby blackbird is on the ground, closely attended by its anxious parents. Unfortunately, the trees are so thick that we have no idea where the nest is, but the adults seem to be doing a sterling job of keeping the youngster fed and sheltered in small nooks and crannies. Our job for the day will be to remain in the garden, poised to chase off marauding cats. As the sun has burst forth, this will not be an onerous task. While Jay goes for the Sunday papers, I mend my sunglasses. A missing screw is replaced admirably with some fine orthopaedic wire, twisted into place with orthopaedic wire twisters. Sometimes being a vet has its advantages.

No sooner are we settled into deckchairs with papers and lemonade to hand than the telephone rings, someone has found a badly injured wild rabbit. 'Just bring it along to the surgery and I'll do what is necessary,' I say ... but that would be too easy; the people have no transport, and no one who can bring them along. There is no alternative but for me to collect it.

I do hate such calls – there is a fine line between helping folk out and being taken for a soft touch. Many prospective clients would be all too happy to never lift a finger but to have the vet turn out, attend to their pet and leave with only the vague promise of payment sometime in the future – which never materialises, and it can be impossible to distinguish between genuine cases and those just 'trying it on'. Vets are in the difficult position of being a caring profession, but on the other hand, having to charge their clients to make their living. However, this is a wild rabbit, and at least the people have taken the responsibility of putting it in a box and calling for help. I will not be charging them anything.

Muttering a little to myself and feeling hard done to, I clamber into the car and set off for Strathdhu, a small hamlet fifteen minutes away. Approaching the village sign, I spot the family at the side of the road, cradling the rabbit in their arms. It is badly smashed up, and humanely putting him to sleep is the only course of action. As is frequently the case, I warm to the people more in person than on the phone when they came across with the '*We've got this problem and it's up to you to fix it, and we're not going to put ourselves out at all*' type of attitude. I load the small corpse into the car, and we part amicably. Driving home, I feel quite guilty about my irritation at having the day disturbed – after all, the rabbit wasn't having such a great day either.

That evening, curious to know how Leo is doing on his new treatment, I ring his owner Lynn for a progress report. After three days of treatment, his drinking has dropped from sixteen pints per day to thirteen, but he is still as ravenous as ever. Still, that's a start, and I reassure Lynn that it is early days yet.

I start the next day tired, courtesy of several emergencies over the evening. The last weeks have been really hectic, producing the feeling of being relentlessly worn down. There has been a surge of challenging and difficult cases, and my brain has been especially taxed diagnosing, then explaining, reassuring and empathising with clients and patients. I feel almost bled dry. Even the much-needed holiday is adding to our stress levels, as both businesses have required more work to prepare for our absence. I have ordered large quantities of drugs so that the locum does not run short, extra oxygen for the anaesthetic machine; written clinical notes up more comprehensively than usual when I am the only one who reads them; compiled large lists explaining quirky parts of the surgery's running, contact numbers for Alice and Julie and instructions for equipment in the house (as the locum will be staying) and care of Piggy. My brain is so over-active that it resembles a wasp in a jamjar. Jay is much the same, on the go from dawn till dusk, making sure that everything will run smoothly, if only for just two weeks.

Still no rain. Queuing in the post office after morning surgery, I meet the man who lived in the Laigher before our predecessors. 'Is your water supply still okay?' he asks. 'Do you know something we don't?' I reply. Unfortunately, both counter assistants choose that moment to serve each of us so I never hear the reply. Watering the flowers before my first appointment is due at Fern, I find myself grudging every full watering can. It will be awful if these plants have our last gallon. Luckily, rain is forecast so, hopefully, the dilemma of 'to water or not to water' will not arise.

We have some pups to neuter for the charity today, and a school boy observing to see if a career as a vet is for him. The puppies are wet and sticky – they have been car-sick en route and have been sick over their fellows. Our student has gelled hair and looks quite similar 'Has anyone thrown up over you this morning?' jokes the irrepressible Julie. The student might as well make an early start in getting used to the peculiar brand of humour common to most veterinary surgeries. These work-experience days can be a trial for us, but are invaluable for the young folk. They can see whether the real job comes up to their expectations. Some will decide that veterinary life is not for them, but for others, it strengthens their resolve to work hard at school and try to be accepted for the veterinary course. This young chap seems interested and keen, and is not put off by my rude assistant.

As usual, we chat easily while anaesthetising and preparing our first patient. Rob asks intelligent questions and watches everything closely – until a short distance into a spay when I notice he has gone quiet, and is shuffling around. I raise my eyes from the op site just in the time to see him slump against the wall, and begin to slide gracefully down. This happens in seconds and Julie – who is listening intently to the pup's heart – has not picked up that there is a problem. Descending to a sitting position, Rob now lists to one side and looks in imminent danger of crashing on to the floor. With a shock, I suddenly realise that the tile floor is unlikely to be as forgiving as the wooden one in the old surgery, and lunge round the side of the table, hands outstretched to cradle Rob's head before it makes contact. In my mind, I hear the sickening thud and imagine the consequences – possible resuscitation, the ambulance, the phone call to parents etc. It is quite amazing how much can go through your mind in an instant. Luckily, I catch him in the nick of time, and am gently propping him in a safer position when Julie comes to lend a hand. 'Look at his hair,' she mutters as he begins to stir, asking drowsily 'Did I faint?' 'You did indeed,' answers Julie, surrepticously mopping gobbets of blood from his elegant tonsure while I scrub up swiftly and return to my charge. Perhaps a judo mat might be in order if we continue having students. After his initial embarrassment, which we dispel by mentioning casualties from the past – including one hulking lad with a reputation around the school as a *hard man*, and several who have gone on to become vets – Rob relaxes and thoroughly enjoys the remainder of the day.

The afternoon passes quickly, working through a batch of cat neuterings for Sheila. This is her busy time of year, as cats are having kittens by the dozen. There is also a cat demat to be done. One carrier-bag full of fur later, the cat looks like a skinned rat but will be a lot more comfortable. A good spraying with insecticide is necessary as fleas scuttle away from the approaching clipper blades. There are loads of fleas around at present; they are always at their worst in the summer, but can survive all year round, especially in centrally heated houses. They add to the annual influx of seasonal itchers which veterinary surgeries always have at this time of year. Some of these animals are reacting to fleas, others to the various pollens present in the environment. Life can be most miserable for them without treatment.

As I work, I keep an eye on the movements of the farm vehicles, worried that they will plough our field before we have the chance of more trips to the barn by the river. The oil-seed rape is being swathed – the stalks being chopped down by a special tractor. The oil-seed will dry on the ground for a while before the combine harvests it. The farm tractor is out spreading fertiliser on a grass field, and the deep thundering of the grain dryer tells me what Colin the farmer is up to. Good, everyone is otherwise occupied, for today at least.

I arrive home late after a busy evening surgery. Incredibly, we appear to have another potential Cushing's disease in the pipeline. No cases for years, then two on the trot. Susie has had an initial blood sample taken this evening. If she proves to have Cushing's disease, it would be very convenient if she could share Leo's drug supply – the medication is extremely expensive – but I suspect that might be too easy. No doubt, we will find out in due course. 'Where are the microchips?' Jay asks as I walk through the door. 'At Clayfern surgery,' I respond, before realising that we are talking about the chips which cook in microwave ovens, not the ones which identify animals. A sure sign that a holiday is sorely needed.

It would have been nice to spend the remainder of the evening relaxing, but an emergency traffic accident puts paid to that. The dog does not look promising. He was lifted off the road after the accident and has not stood or walked since. He screams whenever his back is touched, and his hind legs are limp and unresponsive. Unable to watch their dog in pain, the owners are desperate to leave. Taking the owners' telephone number, I send them home while Jay and I prepare for a busy evening.

'I'll phone you whenever there is any news,' are my last words before they leave, and we carry the stricken creature into the operating room to get to work. After setting up a drip and administering strong painkillers and a mild sedative, we manage to take an x-ray of the relevant area. The news is not good. The dog's back is broken and the fragments widely separated. His spinal cord will be damaged beyond any chance of recovery. He has to be put to sleep. I try to telephone the owners, and am concerned that the phone rings unanswered. I look them up in the telephone directory and try again – still no answer. I ask the operator to check the line – it is functioning normally. Now I am in a quandary – there is no doubt that the dog must be put to sleep, but some owners like to be with their pet when they go. Should I go ahead anyway, or give them more time? The dog is comfortable now, so waiting a little longer is feasible.

Banishing thoughts of my yet-uneaten supper, I settle down on a cushion by the dog's side, stroking his head and crooning gently to him. Jay brings me a cup of tea. Every ten minutes, I try again to reach his owners. Eventually, after forty minutes, the phone is answered. I break the news and mention rather pointedly that I have been trying to reach them for nearly an hour.

'Oh,' says the male owner, 'My wife was really shaken, so we went to the pub for a drink to steady her nerves.'

They give their permission and an overdose of anaesthetic is added to the dog's drip allowing him to sleep painlessly away. This situation can occur surprisingly frequently, and, for the life of me, I cannot fathom the owners' thoughts. Last month we kept a dog under anaesthetic for thirty minutes while trying to contact an owner to tell him that his pet had an incurable cancer. He had been told exactly the same as tonight's people – 'We are going to do X and will let you know as soon as we have some news.' If *my* dog was being treated somewhere and I was told I would be telephoned, I would be sitting within two feet of the phone all day.

Another client special is when the vet attempts to telephone the number given on the emergency pager, only to find it engaged. This is equally baffling – the answering machine message clearly states '*Please leave your name and telephone number, and the vet will ring you back within ten minutes.*' In such cases, I usually explain to the operator that I have received an emergency call and ask them to check the line. Flustered people will sometimes fail to hang up properly, although sometimes it transpires that the owner decides to fill in time before the vet calls by ringing a friend or relative to tell them what has happened. One client thoughtfully decided to keep the phone off the hook so that the vet could get straight through. Sometimes the workings of clients' minds can be truly baffling, and is probably best not dwelled upon. When their little foibles become irritating rather than amusing, it is a good sign that we need a break.

In the cool of the evening, dogs and I amble slowly along the track. Beside us is a raised banking which amazes me with its resilience. Each year, the farmer cuts it back to allow the combine to pass, yet it recovers within weeks and once again bristles with wild flowers – sky-blue scabious; purple, yellow and mauve-white vetch; yellow hawkbit; purple knapweed and thistle; creamy yarrow and cow parsley. It fairly teems with insects, and I linger to inspect more six spot Burnets, grasshoppers and ladybirds. My pace is so slow that Kippen overtakes – a first these days.

We have not seen Honky or the hind for days, but rounding the corner, I spot the hind in the long grass. I peer to see if a baby is with her, but can see nothing. If she has one, it should surely be old enough to be with her by now. All the youngsters in the pen have joined the main herd and are clearly visible on the hillside. From above the deer pen, our 'walking' field is visible, and I can see that the plough has gone over the tram lines – the hard tracks left by the tractor. The tractor usually loosens these up first before continuing over the rest of the field. We must try to get down there again before it is sealed off for another year.

Chapter 31

There is a nice surprise regarding our possible second case of Cushing's disease – the ACTH test has produced a positive diagnosis. No need to proceed to a third test. It would be so handy if Susie could share Leo's pot of drugs – the drug is expensive and there is all the paperwork involved with applying for a special treatment authorisation – but this may be too easy for the Ministry. I cannot delay any longer, the phone call has to be made ... again, I have a pleasant surprise, it seems that this is not a problem. Brilliant!

Leo has been on his treatment for almost two weeks now, and is down to drinking eleven pints of water per day, still high but better than the original sixteen pints. Lynn reports he is possibly showing signs of slight weakness, so I add some *prednisolone* – a manufactured corticosteroid to his daily medication. It may be that his body is missing the sudden reduction in cortisol, so we will temporarily add a little back.

Alice is on holiday this week. She has been looking forward to it for weeks, but on Saturday was actually quite reluctant to go. I feel exactly the same about Jay and my impending break. Alice and I are used to each other's *little ways*, and are quite proprietorial about our respective files and patients. The thought of someone else gaining access to our little niches causes a degree of trepidation. However, like I will, she managed to overcome the urge to stay, and is no doubt having a wonderful time and barely giving the surgery a thought. I am coping well with Julie, Jay and Cath's help, but quite miss my usual Clayfern sidekick. As Jay and I are due to go on holiday next, Alice and I will not see each other for three weeks – how will we keep up with all the gossip?

After morning surgery, poor Julie exchanges her medical hat for her more usual surgical one, and follows me to the farm surgery for the day's operations. When she goes on holiday, Alice in turn fills in at Fern. They enjoy the change, but are secretly glad to revert to their normal duties. Both are slightly apprehensive about working with another vet. Neither of the nurses are qualified – that is, they have not gone through the formal training and sat the examinations which entitles them to use the initials V.N. (veterinary nurse) after their names, and worry that they may not be good enough for the locum. Having said that, all the locums and part-time vets who have worked in the practice before have been impressed with their work, and one mentioned that they were better than some qualified nurses with whom she had worked.

Today's agenda consists of yet another set of two similar cases. The patients – both dogs – are suspected of having a problem with a foreign body, but not one in the gut as is more usual. The first dog – a springer spaniel – has a soft swelling on her foreleg, just below the knee. The owner reported that two weeks ago, there was a blister-like lump between the dog's toes on the same leg. The circumstances are very suggestive of penetration by a grass seed or similar. During exploratory surgery, the leg swelling consists of an area of fibrous tissue in the centre of which nestles a one-inch-long grass awn. Removing this foreign object should prove curative. Such seeds can travel widely in the body. My most unusual example concerned Chloe, a crazy Afghan hound belonging to Alison, the maker of the miniature surgery. I first met Chloe when Alison brought her to the surgery (the original green shed) with a cough and high temperature. Antibiotics settled down what we thought was an infection, but we were concerned to find that the same symptoms recurred in a couple of weeks. More antibiotics did their stuff, but Chloe next appeared several weeks later with a large swelling by her breast bone. By now, I suspected that the symptoms might be caused by a wandering foreign body. Such objects often attempt to 'find their way out' of the body (in fact, the body tries to expel them). Operating on the swelling, I traced a track leading towards the chest wall, but it petered out after a few inches. Once again, Chloe was discharged, and I hoped that the troublesome foreign body remained somewhere in the fibrous mass removed.

After several months, both Alison and I thought we were home and dry, but another lump appeared on the opposite side of the dog's chest. Suspecting that sophisticated techniques might be needed for the search, I endeavoured to refer Chloe to the nearest veterinary school for specialist attention. Unfortunately, the earliest appointment available was in three weeks time. Before this time, the lump increased to massive proportions and burst spectacularly, discharging its contents in a mess of blood and gore. As the appointment came closer, the wound was receding nicely, but I persuaded Alison not to cancel. So, Chloe duly went to the vet school where the specialist thought he saw a suspicious shadow in her lungs. Her chest was opened and many fibrous tracts were found, evidence that a foreign obstacle had passed that way – but nothing was ever found. Chloe returned home and recovered uneventfully. I am convinced that the foreign body exited when the second lump burst. It probably gained access to the lungs when she galloped through a field of grass with her mouth open, and, in hindsight, her various symptoms could be explained as the grass seed's wanderings in the tissues.

Our second case, a Labrador, is also suspected of having symptoms caused by a foreign body. A large swelling has appeared on the top of his head. There are no skin wounds, but I have already managed to withdraw some pus in the surgery through a hypodermic needle. As is often the case, no impressive foreign body is to found, just a mess of pus and fibrous tissue. No doubt the FB may be within this lot, but finding it would be harder than a needle in a haystack. I content myself with removing the abnormal tissue, syringing the cavity with saline, securing two drains in place and closing the wound. Shaven-headed, with the drains sticking out on either side, the poor dog looks as if he has been involved in some Frankenstein's monster-like experiment.

Just time for a quick walk up the hill before returning to Clayfern

– and what a triumph, a glimpse of hind ... and youngster, a stocky white creature reaching almost to her shoulder. Both take fright and bolt into the woods, but my day has been made.

Coincidentally, after reminiscing about Chloe and Alison, there is a message on the answering machine from the same lady when we return from our walk – the model surgery is finished, would we like to collect it? After checking that Jay is free, I call her back and arrange to go after evening surgery.

Still trying to clear the decks as much as possible for our locum, I deliver dog food and medicine to Edith McNaughton on my way to evening surgery in Clayfern. On my way out, we have our usual tour of the greenhouse, no passionflowers today, but *green* carnation flowers. Where does this woman get those things? 'I see you're wearing red socks,' she comments as I flash some ankle while climbing into the car. 'They're my *Winnie the pooh* socks,' I reply, theatrically displaying the socks in question. Edith laughs, and delivers one of her famous one-liners which can be taken either as compliment or insult 'Och well. At least you're young at heart!'

During surgery these days, there is the usual procession of seasonal ailments produced by the hot weather: hirpling and panting old dogs, victims of strokes, and maggot-struck creatures. If infested for less than twenty four hours, then the latter animals only harbour maggot eggs which can be relatively easily removed, but if left for longer, the maggots hatch and burrow into the tissues causing severe pain and damage, leading to shock which is often irreversible. In hot weather, it is especially important for owners of small pets such as rabbits and guinea pigs to inspect them at least once daily for any wounds or soiled areas which will attract blowflies. Interestingly, I read an article recently describing the use of specially produced sterile maggots in actually treating many types of infected or necrotic wounds in humans and donkeys. Apparently, in these species, healthy tissue will inactivate the digestive enzymes produced by the maggots thus limiting their action once they have removed the abnormal tissue.

Unfortunately, neither rabbit, guinea pig nor sheep tissue can do this, so the maggots can continue to wreak havoc.

And of course, there are the seasonal itchers – hardly surprising given the multitudes of corn lice, daddy-long-legs, moths, flies, bluebottles, bees and wasps around. In the surgery after dark last night, when I opened the outside door, a veritable army of insects of all shapes and sizes swarmed into the lit up room. I shall not be sorry to temporarily relinguish this mish-mash of ailments to Emma, our locum. Susie, our latest Cushing's dog, is responding well to her medicine, and Leo is down to eight pints per day. I ask Lynn to stop giving the drug daily, and move him on to once-weekly therapy. This will last for the rest of his life. The prednisolone seems to be doing the trick and he no longer appears weak. It is good to leave things on an optimistic note. The final client is in for some worming tablets and brings a smile to our faces. Already the owner of a rather grumpy miniature poodle, our client also took on a standard poodle pup earlier in the year. The poor pup's life has been made a misery by old Grumpy – but now the worm has turned, the standard poodle towers over the miniature, and is no longer putting up with his unpleasantness. For the last month, the nasty character has been receiving his just desserts and has had to reform to save his skin.

Jay is waiting outside the surgery, and we head straight for Alison's house. Whenever we enter her work room, I know that we will not be disappointed. On the table stands an exact replica of my beloved shed, even down to the windowsill with the missing chunk of wood and the brass plate with my qualifications. Alison demonstrates how the front and roof open to display the inside. The detail is truly amazing, it is like a trip down memory lane. All the kennels, table and x-ray machine are there, in exactly the right place. There is a vet in a green overall with hair just like mine. Alison told me over the phone that this caused her much difficulty as most dolls for dolls' houses come with ringlets. I had thought of arriving in a wig just to fox her. Just like the original surgery, there are miniature posters, a day book, clinical record cards in a box, a towel rail holding a towel and even working lights – a strip light overhead, an x-ray viewer complete with x-ray and an examination spotlight. 'Watch the spotlight doesn't burn the vet's hair,' warns Alison. Uncannily, this occasionally happens in real life too.

Every moment, we spot another detail – there is a pigeon on the roof which reminds us of the one that stuck around for a while – he loved that roof – and a frog on the steps (how did she know?). For a while, we just stare in wonder while Alison looks anxiously on. She had been concerned that we would not like it. She need not have worried, it is absolutely perfect, and I will treasure it forever. Jay promises to make a case so that it can be displayed at the surgery without the danger of children's prying hands.

Although both shattered after a week of planning and preparing for our absences, Jay and I are lured out later in the evening to a barbecue with friends. It just goes to show that a change is better than a rest, as we feel more relaxed afterwards than we would have been after a night draped over the settee. As we cross from the car to our back door, a crescent moon floats high above the river, and a warm wind rustles the leaves. A bat laps the house repeatedly. Over the hills, layers of colour rise – pink to parchment to cream to light blue, blending into inky dark sky peppered with stars. The wheaty harvest smell pervades the air. In the garden with the dogs for their bedtime outing, we watch a lone car working its way along the road, lights coming and going, flashing between trees and bushes before finally sweeping past. The thicket in front of the field is silhouetted against the sky, the different leaves making intricate patterns. The navigation buoy flashes reassuringly in the river. For some reason, catching sight of it always makes me feel safely at home. Strange to think that in less than twenty four hours, we will be watching the sky and the flashing of the lighthouses at the seaside.

We both awake with feelings of nervous anticipation. Going through the day before a holiday is difficult as we are both mentally beginning to shut off from work, and are terrified that some emergency will prevent our escape. Jay goes to work to finish paying bills and finalising work for Jack, the second-in-command. I have a reasonable morning surgery, followed by a visit. My next job is to go shopping for the locum (lots of microwave meals to save her from battling with the Rayburn), then I pack, load the car, water the garden (still no rain) and exercise the dogs. We catch a quick glimpse of the hind and her youngster which I have begun to think of as her son, he is so big and stocky. Much splashing attracts me to a water trough where a large insect is in danger of drowning. Grasping a stick, I fish it out of the water and lay it on a branch. It is really large – it must be over an inch long, yellow and black with a yellow syringe-like rear. I could hear the splashing noises from at least ten feet away. Intrigued enough to look the strange creature up in a reference book later, I learn that this is a *horntail*, one of the sawfly family. The strange nether portion is an ovipositor with which the fly lays eggs in pine trunks. I have never seen one before.

Jay arrives home at 5 p.m., and the locum arrives at 6. We spend nearly an hour going over my carefully prepared list, then, at last, we are off en route to Pitdreel. Once there, we settle for a Chinese takeaway and a bottle of wine. Jay laughs at my description – my brain feels like a *brillo pad* – but, to me, this describes aptly the tight, clenched feeling when the brain is so overloaded it will not relax. I ease it away with more alcohol than I have had in quite a while.

Chapter 32

We still waken at 7 a.m., but after a blissful night's sleep. The dogs need their first outing so we head to the beach. It is going to be a glorious day: sun shining, gentle breeze and waves breaking softly on the shore rattling piles of shells like wind-chimes. The heady realisation that we have nearly two weeks of this begins to dawn. Both of us need to resist the temptation to plan. Our lives revolve round timetables – for me: *9-10 a.m. surgery;10.45 a.m. appointment at Fern; finish ops by 2 p.m.; dogs out till 2.45 p.m.* ... and so on. I tend to do the same on holiday and it drives Jay mad – 'If we go for a walk till 10 a.m., then we can get to town by 11; spend an hour shopping then lunch between 1 and 2 p.m.' Arriving home for breakfast, we run suddenly and totally out of steam. It might have been the preservatives in the Chinese meal the night before, or the wine, but we end up toasting the holiday with fizzing glasses of A*lka Seltzer*.

The two weeks flash by at the speed of light, and all too soon, it is our last day on holiday. We have to get home this afternoon to allow Emma, the locum, to travel to another job. We have had a marvellous holiday, and, for the very first time, we are both reluctant to go home. The weather has been kind to us, and we have spent the majority of our time on the beach, beachcombing, having barbecues and even swimming. On sunny days, we set off to 'our' beach, loaded like pack ponies with food, drinks, towels and a variety of other paraphernalia. Descending on to the sand, it was traditional to dump our loads and follow the dogs to the sea. Kippen was rejuvenated. He loves the sea and spent hours standing chest-deep, allowing the water to lap over his legs. Another trick was to actually lie down in the shallows. Fintry meanwhile, charged around like a dervish, raising great sprays of salty water. The water was crystal-clear, and we humans were tempted in several times. It was very cold but worth it once you got going. The dogs were comical when we swam – there was a film whose title I forget, but involved children who were possessed by aliens. They spent much of the film walking hand-in-hand like robots to vantage points and staring blank-faced at adults in trouble. Our dogs were very similar. With Kippen a head in front, they walked together to the edge of the rocks and watched us with baleful expressions. A few minutes later, they would move off to a fresh position and resume their vigil.

Once out of the water, we cooked sausages and marshmallows either on disposable barbecues or on 'homemade' fires. Again the staring dogs were in constant attendance, but this time showing considerably more emotion. The fire required near-constant sorties along the beach in a quest for more driftwood, and an excuse to beachcomb. Beachcombing at the seaside yields a very different haul from that by the river. Rubber gloves featured most frequently, closely followed by rope, fragments of net and the inevitable assortment of plastic, wood and bones. While we relaxed after our meal, watching terns and kittiwakes dive spectacularly for fish in the distance, Kippen would retreat with his bone to an eyrie in the dune grass, but Fintry was a nuisance. She obviously disliked lying on sand, and constantly vied for the lion's share of our beach towels. Any move from the centre of the towel was immediately followed by the invasion of a wet, sandy Labrador. Other days, we went to an isolated rocky cove and dabbled happily in the rock pools, remembering holidays spent as children carrying out the same activities.

For a little variety, we attended several events at the sea festival in the nearby village. The ceilidh, as always, went down well. A particularly rowdy *Strip the willow* reminded me of the day I qualified as a vet. The class had a celebratory ceilidh which continued nearly all night. Much alcohol was drunk and much stress let off after the tension of final exams, and, during a wild *Strip the willow*, my partner let me go as we birled madly out of control. I sailed up the floor on my face, luckily somewhat anaesthetised after an evening's celebrating.

The only after-effect (apart from a splitting headache which could not honestly be blamed on the fall) was an impressive bruise covering the entire side of my face. Each day, I thought it could get no worse but it did, changing from black and blue to maroon, and finally to a rather jaundiced yellow and grey. At each job interview, a hurried explanation was necessary to justify my lurid appearance. Telling this tale to Jay probably explained why my grip was more vice-like than usual during our present-day dance.

One day, the harbour area filled with a variety of stalls – food, crafts, information on local attractions to name but a few. One stall explained a research project at the local marine institute. Seals were being radio-tracked to provide a wide range of data. One glance at the equipment showed how technology has moved on since my badger radio-tracking days. While I spent hours on dark hill sides, loaded down with heavy radio receiver and three – foot aerial, searching for signals from our target, the seal researchers sit at a computer, plotting their subject's course. The signal is picked up by satellite and relayed to base. That's the way to do it! – but secretly, I think my way was probably more fun.

Even walking round the picturesque villages has been pleasant, the whitewashed cottages and pantiled roofs clinging to the steep coastline. I have told Jay that I wish a pantiled gravestone, inscribed *At least she was young at heart.'*

I suspect that the biggest reason why the holiday has been so successful has been the total lack of responsibility – no patients or customers to worry about, no bills or repairs, not even house-cleaning or gardening. The flat is so small that ten minutes tidy is all that it needs. No wonder the thought of returning to our busy lives does not appeal. I feel myself tensing as we approach home, and Jay is the same. In minutes, Emma will brief me on any problems or glitches that have occurred while we have been away. Jay gets a stay of execution until tomorrow, but will be flung back into the swing of daily life again then.

Remarkably, there are no glitches or problems – Emma has been amazingly efficient and everything seems in order. She has kept a list of cases to be discussed so that I am up to speed when she leaves. She seems to have had a busy, but enjoyable fortnight and has appreciated the pleasant lifestyle. Sad to say, she is moving to another part of the country with her husband soon, as otherwise we might have happily shared the practice together.

Once the washing machine has done its stuff several times over, and we have unpacked and eaten, we wander into the garden with the dogs. This is a wonderful place, but, just for tonight, our hearts have been left behind in Pitdreel, remembering the moonlight on the water and the lighthouse flashing on the horizon, while fishing boats leave the harbour for a night's fishing out at sea.

Although we have not been sleeping late on holiday, it is still a shock *having* to get up in time for work the next day. A quick walk with the dogs before breakfast alerts us to changes to our territory. As expected, the stubble field by the barn has been ploughed and re-sown. Already, the new crop is one inch high and looks like patchy grass. The vegetation in the verges and up the hill has peaked, and is now past its best, showing signs of dying back. Some leaves on the trees have begun to shrivel, the beech mast is brown and toadstools are flourishing. In the garden, the fruit trees are ripening and the rowan berries are pillar-box red. Autumn is not far away.

Emma told us that she was late home two nights ago as the farmer at Abbeygate Farm was burning stubble, and a thick pall of smoke totally obscured the road. Several cars eventually went through in convoy. The farmer has got his just deserts for obstructing the highway – several fence posts have also burnt through, and the wires are hanging limply today, swaying in the breeze.

Starting work again reminds me of swimming at Pitdreel – after the initial shock, you quickly acclimatise. It is quite pleasant to see friends and acquaintances again, and after an hour, I feel as if we had never been away. Alice has enjoyed working with Emma – who kept her supplied with ice lollies during quiet moments. The fortnight has gone smoothly, the only difficulty has been for my nurses who had to get used to working for a right-handed vet (I am left-handed). For most procedures, Emma was taken aback by the nurses positioning equipment – and themselves, in the way that works for me. They have had to adapt, and I have spent morning surgery re-arranging my bits and pieces as I like them. It does feel odd to have one's anonymity gone again – back to being a vet rather than just a person. All my life, I have been a vet before anything else and now I find I want some time without it. This is the first time I have not been keen to come back to work, and I am not used to the feeling; it is somewhat unsettling. Perhaps it is just the reaction to a particularly hectic year and an idyllic holiday.

Talking this over later, I find Jay feels the same. Working all hours to build up the design business has not been easy either. We both resolve to try to win more time off. I have just read an article about high-flyers in New York who spend Monday to Friday lunchtime in the city, then the long weekend at beach houses. That would suit us fine, all we need is a similar salary to pull it off.

Another, more leisurely, trip up the hill the following morning results in an excellent sighting of the red deer family – Mum, Honky and baby – now nicknamed Gray. Another exciting find is that our badger sett – in the past only occupied occasionally – now appears to have permanent residents. All the signs are there: the well-worn trail from the sett, the scratched tree bases and the latrines – holes dug and used as toilets.

In the past, both Jay and I have spent hours watching badgers overnight, and look forward to doing the same here. One particular sett we visited had an impressive tree platform built above it by members of the local badger group. One had to be in position well before dark, and stay very still for what seemed like hours before any badgers appeared. When they did, it was magical – they are such comical creatures to observe. One night, we watched them changing their bedding. This involved a badger exiting backwards from the sett, hauling an armful of straw and dried grass. This was dragged slowly and deliberately for almost fifty yards before it was dumped and the badger came back for more, carrying out the same procedure several times.

In summer, one can often watch cubs at play. When a few months old, they are smaller and lighter in colour than the adults, and full of fun, ragging each other unmercifully.

One badger group member had badger-watching at her local sett down to a fine art. We went with her one evening. Arriving at her house in good time, we found her making up a pile of jam sandwiches (badgers are very sweet-toothed). She then grabbed a rucksack and lantern, and we walked briskly towards the sett. Scrambling down a steep banking, we recognised the tell-tale trodden-down earth by the sett. Our friend hung her lantern – fitted with a red filter to minimise disturbance – to a nail protruding from the tree trunk, then handed each of us a thick mat from her bag and indicated a levelled area of banking where we were to sit. What followed was one of our best ever badger watches. Mum ventured forth first, followed by three cubs. All tucked in to the sandwiches then indulged in a spot of mutual grooming, followed by a cub rough and tumble, refereed occasionally by mum who intervened when things got too heated. I am sure that they knew we were there, but had been gradually habituated to non-threatening human presence. This is what I intend to do with 'our' badgers.

To this end, the afternoon sees me back up the hill, laying a trail of jam butties from sett to nearby stubble field. Badgers are omnivorous, although their staple diet is earthworms, they will eat almost anything else too. The rationale behind the jam sandwiches is that they are less likely to be eaten by other forest residents. Laying the trail up the sheer slope from the sett to the field, I realise too late that Fintry is following close behind, eating the jammy pieces as she goes. Still, some remain to tempt our badgers. I have also brought some windfall apples for the deer family. Our nephew Tom and family are coming to stay next week, and my optimistic plan is to train the wildlife to put in an appearance. Sure enough, the deer are grazing not far from the thinking stones. 'Come on,' I yell to get their attention, ostentatiously opening the bag and lobbing apples towards them. To their credit, they remain alert and watch my antics closely, but do not bolt away. They are half-used to the dogs and me already. Quite a decent day's work, I think as I gather empty bags and bemused dogs, and head back home.

Driving into the yard, I find Jay purposefully rescuing our bicycles from the back of the shed. In a fit of enthusiasm, we have decided to try cycling to maintain the improved level of fitness we attained on holiday. Much dusting off of cobwebs and pumping up tyres later, we have a test run to the farm. I had forgotten how uncomfortable the saddles were. After trying unsuccessfully to work out what the gears actually do, I settle on one and give up further changing up or down. My next project is to use the bike to collect donations and signatures for Pete the postie's retirement. I suspect Jay's is mainly to show off in front of Tom. After the wailing and moaning which follows the stiffening-up of muscles in the evening, there is every chance that the bikes will end up thrown back into the depths of the shed where they will remain undisturbed for another ten years.

Chapter 33

A fairly light working day allows me to move on with my various non-veterinary projects. An early trip up the hill to deliver more butties – carefully supervising both dogs this time – yields more evidence that badgers are in permanent residence.

A large wasp byke has been dug out of the banking. It must have been almost the size of a football, but all that is left is an inner shell moulded to the earth. Ripped-out pieces of honeycomb walls lie on the ground with dazed or dying wasps crawling over them. What a rude shock the poor things must have had. There are even some pupae still to be seen within the hexagonal cells. This is typical badger handiwork. They have powerful feet with long sharp claws capable of considerable damage. When we had badger in-patients at our last surgery, they were housed in specially constructed cement kennels with doors reinforced with steel plates, as they have been known to dig their way out of wooden sheds.

Leaving the dogs at home, I get on my bike once again and sally forth on a collecting round. Swallows are swooping overhead, making more noise than normal. I suspect that, as with the buzzards, this means that the youngsters are learning to fly. Watching carefully, I think I detect a few smaller and less skilful than their adult counterparts. Up the road, I pant, carrier bag containing Pete the postie's retirement card banging annoyingly at my legs, pleased with myself for finally making a start. It is rather nice to realise that we actually know everyone within several miles radius of home. As Pete goes next week, I cannot delay any longer. Four miles and ten houses later, I freewheel disconsolately home. Out of the ten homes, only one person was in. I am totally knackered with nothing to show for my trouble. Perhaps this bike thing is not such a good idea.

A second fairly quiet day allows me to have another bash at collecting for Pete's retirement. This time I take the car. Largely by default, I have become the organiser of both the gift-ordering and the official presentation for our local area which coincides roughly with the parish of Claybraes – or the Water-side as we are known to the neighbouring parish of Duncraig. The 'do' is to take place at the farm surgery next Friday. After calling at the Laigher, Pete has only to deliver to the farm along the road before his round is finished. He passes us again on his way back to base, a circumstance which will be used to our advantage next week.

As well as collecting signatures and money, participants need to be informed of these arrangements. In contrast to yesterday, most folk are at home today, so my progress is satisfactory but slow. In fact, so slow that I wonder whether I will complete the four-mile circuit in time for evening surgery. Several people need to be found first – this involves expeditions into their gardens or outbuildings, tentatively calling their names. Once located, everyone wants to chat and I am offered innumerable cups of tea. It seems that our modest effort is in competition with Duncraig's grander affair, and one or two folk have been unfortunate enough to be nobbled by both 'sides.' My status as organiser is unwittingly ratified when I receive an invitation to bring all the Water-side faction to Duncraig's evening bash on Saturday. Of course, I make the same offer in return. A twinge of anxiety strikes me – this affair is growing legs.

Having missed out on an afternoon walk, I load the dogs into the Tundra and shoot up the hill after evening surgery. A sick dog is being brought to the surgery at 7 p.m. but there should be time for a quick stroll before then. I leave the dogs rootling in the stubble field while I clamber down towards the badger sett, clutching my bag of butties, but when I emerge on to the field, there is no sign of Kippen. He has totally vanished. Not particularly worried, but with an eye on the time, I head across the field with Fintry. Any exhortations to 'Find Kippen' are met with a stoney stare, so I continue to bellow his name and scan the horizon for any movement. Ten minutes later, I am becoming anxious. It is now 6.40 p.m. and we should be heading downhill soon. Arriving back at the car, I load Fintry and drive back across the field, shouting Kippen's name.

Jay is not home yet, and neither is Sheila apparently as my mobile phone calls remain unanswered. From its description, the sick dog may need hospitalising and connecting to a drip so I am unlikely to be free to recommence the search quickly. I am in a quandary – reluctant to leave my missing geriatric, but aware as usual of the call of duty. Still not sure what I am ultimately going to do, I drive back to my original parking spot, but, before I get there, I spot my tired old dog, walking wearily up the track. He stops uncertainly when he sees the car, looking anxious and lost, obviously not recognising the car. I am out of the door like a bullet, calling his name, and in an instant, his demeanour changes – the ears prick, the tail wags furiously and he heads towards me at a lurching run. The poor old fella looked so lost and confused; he must have been really scared. I must make sure that I *never* lose sight of him on a walk from now on. After much cuddling (from me) and squeaking (from him), he is loaded into the car and we pelt down the hill, arriving in the yard at 6.58 p.m.

No sign of any clients. In fact, there is no sign of anyone until the phone rings twenty minutes later. They have had a puncture, but are on their way now; they should be here in fifteen minutes. Half an hour later, another call – they are lost. Thinking uncharitably that the dog will be dead of old age never mind illness by the time they get here, I give directions. They finally arrive at 8.30 p.m. Luckily, the dog is not as poorly as described on the initial message, and I finally sit down for supper at 9.15 p.m. Vets know all too well how just one call can completely scupper your night, but this is usually *after* you have at least seen the animal.

Despite a light working day, I go early to bed, exhausted. All the mental angst has completely worn me out!

Nephew Tom and family arrive next day, and immediately, Tom

and I get into a huddle. There is so much to do during his stay. One year, he and I exhumed a deer skeleton which he endeavoured to fit together again. On this visit, We shall probably continue in much the same vein. On walks, I casually note the position of any dead animals, and will probably return months later to see if any bones remain. This is frequently disappointing, as the forest residents seem determined to spread such remains far and wide. However, during the last week, I have located some bones for Tom to 'discover,' and have ordered a book from the Internet to spur his interest. The book is called *The Bone Detectives* and explains the many facets of a forensic anthropologist's work. As I thought, Tom is fascinated by the section on facial reconstruction and is raring to reconstruct the faces of the crow and rabbit skulls which we bear home from our walk. 'So they will be John Crow and Jane Doe!' jokes Jay. Already this gives Tom a purpose – we need to go into Clayfern to find some plasticine for the task, but beforehand, I try to teach him the rudiments of identification. He gets the crow skull easily due to the beak, and the rabbit skull by the teeth.

'But which leg bones are which?' I ask, before beginning to explain my train of deduction. Both are similar sized, and both rabbit and crow bones are light. The crow's front limb bone has a large crest at the top where the massive flight muscles attach. 'What we need now is a picture of a bird's skeleton,' I say, getting really carried away by now, beginning to delve into our extensive book collection. Sometimes I forget that he is only ten, and has limited powers of deduction and concentration. He wanders off to play with his *Pokemon* cards (the latest children's craze) while I spend the next twenty minutes researching in the office. I enjoy these visits as much as he does.

Tom comes in with me for morning surgery – not so much for the surgery's sake as to buy his plasticine. It is a pleasant morning during which I vaccinate the kittens which Julie and I delivered by caesarian several weeks ago. It is funny to think that we were responsible for bringing them into the world. There is an anxious phone call from Hector, Lena's owner. 'She's been injured,' he pronounces dramatically. 'Where?' asks Alice. 'In the garden,' is the reply. Once he comes in, we discover that the wound is actually on her lip. It might be an old cut, but it looks rather odd. I suggest that we remove the affected area tomorrow, and send a biopsy to the lab for analysis.

Tomorrow is going to be busy as we also have another twosome of similar conditions – two dogs with ulcerated left elbows. These are elderly, heavy dogs who have a habit of thumping down on hard surfaces. In the warm weather, they seem to actively seek out cool surfaces like concrete or tiles, and eventually develop a thickened area of skin over the boney elbow. This callus can fissure and develop infection which in severe cases can cause a raw depression to appear in the centre. Both dogs have been treated with antibiotics and surface cleansers, but the skin refuses to heal so tomorrow's plan is to remove the unhealthy tissue and stitch the healthy skin edges together. We also have several routine neuterings booked in, but at least today is only lightly booked so I can keep Tom amused.

On the way homewards, we visit the post office for plasticine. Unfortunately, there is no rabbit- or crow- coloured material available – our reconstructions are going to be multi-coloured. Next, we call in on Edith and her girls. Tom has met them before, and wants to see everyone. He is taken on the tour of the greenhouse with three flowering passion-flowers, and chatters excitedly about all and sundry. It is lovely to see the young lad and elderly lady so obviously enjoying each other's company.

When we arrive home, our mission for the day has a tinge of urgency about it. Racking my brains, I have remembered seeing a sheep's skull wedged in the river banking. The problem is that the field is being ploughed at this very moment. I know that it will take John about two full days to complete the full field, but Tom has no idea of the ploughing timescale ... no time for lunch, we need to load the dogs and set off immediately. Luckily, after all the hype, the skull is still there, complete with horns: 'That would be great for Halloween with a candle inside it,' I muse, no doubt earning yet another schoolboy brownie point. Inside this supposedly mature woman, a child continually tries to get out – and a gruesome one at that.

Evening surgery is carried out minus Tom – probably just as well as it becomes rather sombre. The owner of Susie, our second Cushing's disease dog, drops a bombshell – she was hit by a car on Sunday and was killed immediately. What a shame – it shows only too clearly that no matter how old they are, dogs *never* get any better with cars. 'I'll be back with another one,' says her distraught owner as he returns her medication, 'The wife and I can't stand the house being so quiet.'

Our next case does not bode well either. Corrie, an eight-year-old cat looks alert as he is carried awkwardly into the surgery, but once placed on the table, his hind legs flop limply to one side, and he can only prop himself into an uncomfortable crouch.

'He was fine this morning, but I've just come home and found him like this,' explains his owner. I start an examination at the front end, looking first for signs of shock or trauma, my brain sifting through possibilities – spinal injury or pelvic damage could cause such symptoms. Corrie's colour is fine and he seems alert enough, with no obvious pain. His chest sounds clear although I detect a mild heart murmur on listening to his heart. This might or might not have any bearing on the case so is noted as I move on. There are no cuts or abrasions on the cat's body; nothing to indicate a traumatic incident, but once I reach the rear end, the diagnosis suddenly becomes obvious. Corrie's hind feet are ice-cold, the quicks of the nails showing a bluish tinge and I can feel no pulses in the femoral veins – the large veins which run down the inside of the thigh. The cat has an *aortic thromboembolism*. A thrombus (plug of material – largely blood clot) has lodged at the bottom of the aorta, the main artery supplying the back end of the body, just as it splits into two to supply the hind legs, and the blood supply to both hind legs has been cut off. The heart murmur might suggest that the thrombus material has come from there. Because of the clot's position, this condition is also known as a *saddle-thrombus.*

The lack of blood supply has left the cat with hind limb paralysis. Such cases occur occasionally, perhaps about one per year, and I have never had much success in treating them – almost inevitably the cat ends up being put to sleep. The most unusual aspect of Corrie's case is that he appears to be in no pain. Usually these patients are in agony and can sometimes be heard yowling along the road before even entering the surgery. Reducing the pain becomes the most pressing action, and can be hard to achieve. Despite pain relief and treatment, most have gone from bad to worse and have had to be put out of their misery. It may be that Corrie was in pain while the family were at work, but he seems remarkably cheerful now. Largely because of this, the owner and I decide to attempt treatment.

I start with an injection of *heparin* – an anticoagulant – to hopefully start dissolution of the clot, and follow it with a low dose of sedative to calm the cat and to utilise the drug's side-effect of dilating peripheral blood vessels. The aim of treatment is to dissolve the thrombus, but the hope is also that the body attempts to restore circulation to the hind limbs by re-routing blood through smaller blood vessels. The *vasodilator* effect of the sedative may help this process. Having explained this to Corrie's owner, I ask her to begin to give Corrie a quarter of an *aspirin* tablet every two days. As her husband has a circulatory condition which necessitates the same treatment, she understands my drift, but asks why the cat should only get his *aspirin* every second day. This is a typical example of why knowledge and caution is necessary before using any drugs in a veterinary context – different species often deal with drugs in very different ways. Cats lack some of the enzymes necessary to break down *aspirin*, and it lasts longer in their bodies than in humans or dogs. More frequent dosage would allow the drug to build up in the system and cause toxic side-effects.

Booking Corrie in to be seen tomorrow, I warn his owner to get in touch if he deteriorates in any way. I am not very optimistic, but as the cat is not in any distress, treatment is certainly worth a try. After they have gone, I reminisce with Alice about my last thrombo-embolism case, which was truly dramatic. Finding their cat dragging her hind legs and yelling when touched, the distraught owners telephoned to say that their cat had been run over. Performing my usual front-to-back examination, I noted that Fyllys's chest sounded a little harsh and initially suspected lung bruising due to the accident. It was only when I discovered the lack of pulses in the hind limbs that the owners admitted that they only suspected a traffic accident. As pain control was going to be of vital importance, I admitted the cat after some initial treatment, asking them to phone in an hour for a progress report.

Again I was rather pessimistic about Fyllys's prospects, but had no idea how swiftly her condition would deteriorate. Literally minutes after her owners departure, I thought that Fyllys's breathing was slightly worse and set about providing her with some oxygen by mask. Within fifteen minutes, her breathing was laboured and she was gasping for breath. Nothing I did was of any help. Less than half an hour after they had gone, I rang the owners explaining her deterioration and requesting permission to put her to sleep. In addition to an aortic thrombo-embolism, it appeared that Fyllys had also suffered from thrombus material entering her lungs – *pulmonary thrombo-embolism.* Her distress was so great that putting her to sleep was the only humane option. The speed with which her symptoms worsened was truly terrifying. I was powerless to do anything to help.

Well immersed in work again, I need to change gear when I get home to see what Tom has been up to in my absence. I don't find this easy when my head is full of just-seen patients, so plead for five minutes peace in the office to look up aortic thrombo-embolism on the current feline medicine CD-rom. When a condition is only seen infrequently, it is worthwhile doing a little research to make sure your knowledge of treatment is still up-to-date. The CD-rom service which provides me with dog, cat and rabbit information is up-dated every two months, so the suggested treatment regimes are sure to include any new developments. I am reassured to find that my treatment choices appear sound, and discover that, according to the expert authors, for a decent outlook, we should be expecting the circulation to the hind feet to begin to improve within twenty four to forty eight hours. Corrie is booked in to be seen tomorrow – all we can do is wait and hope.

Satisfied that there is nothing more to be added to Corrie's treatment, I can 'switch off' now and pay attention to Tom, who has been waiting patiently. This rather uncompromising attitude to work can be somewhat unpopular with family and friends, but Jay has learnt over the years that it is better to leave me to sort out my concerns and end up with a relaxed Kate, than to insist on my immediate attention and know that my mind keeps wandering off elsewhere. There is no doubt that being attached to a vet is not an easy option, and many relationships fall by the wayside. Luckily, Jay and I have always been quite good at give and take, and with the design business, it is quite often me that is left twiddling my thumbs these days, while Jay attends to some vital last minute arrangements. Part of our long-term plans is to make sure we have plenty of time just to be together enjoying ourselves. We are very lucky that, after nearly fifteen years, we still look forward to and enjoy each other's company.

Tom has been waiting patiently to show me his handiwork. Psychedelic crow and rabbit heads are perched dramatically on the utility room draining board. I don't need to put on an act, I am truly impressed, they really look like the real thing (apart from the colours of course). I suspect such a task would have taken me hours and would be worse than these which apparently took about twenty minutes. The rabbit has perhaps a little too much teeth showing so I suggest an extra dollop of plasticine. 'Perhaps he has a hare lip,' comments Jay and we all collapse with laughter. Our miniaturist client Mavis has supplied some beads for eyes and they look really good in situ.

After tea, I make up more badger butties while Tom collects

windfall apples for the deer and we set off up the hill in the Tundra. The sandwiches left yesterday have been devoured – we have switched from jam to honey as the badgers are so fond of digging out wasp bykes. Some time this week, the plan is to attempt a badger watch so the bait has to be particularly appealing.

Next, we drive towards the thinking stones, park and walk over the rise to look down on the stubble field stretching to the woods. Our luck is in, the whole deer family are there and lift their heads suspiciously as we come into view. Honky has lost the last vestiges of velvet from his antlers and they look smooth and hard. 'I wouldn't like to be stabbed with them,' comments Tom a little uneasily. 'They are more scared of you than you are of them,' I reply confidently, noting all the same that the hind has taken a few steps forward, no doubt getting ready to protect her youngster if necessary. We empty the bag and retreat below the horizon, peeking out after a few minutes to catch sight of Honky making short work of an apple. Mum and Gray are more cautious but they may come round in time.

This will be our routine for the next few evenings. Meantime, I must make sure that we have all the necessary equipment for a successful badger watch. The torches will need new batteries, and I must try to get hold of some red cellophane to drape over the light. Badger eyesight is not particularly sensitive, and they do not appear to notice when they are caught in a beam of red light. Heading down the hill as dusk approaches, we notice that the tractor is still out ploughing. I really hope that he does not turn his attention to the field into which we are enticing the badgers – at least until after Tom goes home.

Chapter 34

All today's operations go according to plan. Hector's Lena has her lip lesion removed with as wide a safety margin as possible. This is important in case the lesion is cancerous, as some cancers spread readily into adjacent tissues even though it looks normal. A biopsy is taken and parcelled up to be sent to the lab. 'And the autopsy will tell you what it is?' queries an anxious Hector. 'It should do,' I reply, suppressing the urge to add on the facetious comment – 'But I don't expect things to go *that* badly.' Out of the corner of my eye, I see Julie smiling as she passes behind Hector to retrieve his dog. Clients getting words wrong frequently gives us amusing moments, but we would never draw attention to their mistakes, often made unwittingly in the heat of the moment. Last night, I had a *repressed* (instead of *depressed*) cat. Such a cowed creature is hard to imagine.

More chopping-out is required with the two elbow cases. The skin on one patient's elbow is so abnormal that I end up excising a doughnut-shaped – and sized – piece of tissue. This makes the skin available to suture over the wound rather sparse, so I employ two techniques to improve the chances of uneventful healing. First, I tack a biological material derived from pig intestine over the defect. This sterile material acts as a scaffold enabling healing cells to migrate easily into the area. Next, I undermine the skin above the elbow and gently pull it into position, then, to increase the surface area and thereby reduce tension on the wound edge, I make multiple small stabs into the loosened skin. This technique is known as *meshing*, and can be very helpful where spare tissue is hard to come by. If each small wound gapes by only three millimetres, it still covers an area significantly larger then the original skin would. The small circular defects heal quickly and easily. Many sophisticated reconstruction techniques are

220

available nowadays, including procedures originally only used in the realms of plastic surgery.

Specialist reconstructive surgeons are a joy to watch.

Once the ops are finished, there is still time to devote to Tom although we cannot stray too far from the recovering patients. I have been a little anxious about Pete's retirement presentation on Friday. Although everyone is due to arrive at 12 p.m., Pete is not particularly punctual and I have an uncomfortable vision of everyone standing waiting in an awkward silence. As most folks know each other, this is somewhat unlikely, but it has been the necessary spur to push me into finally commissioning the Green Shed into a museum for the ever-growing collection of old medical instruments which have been living in boxes in the office. With Tom and Julie's help, we evict countless spiders and creepy crawlies, before laying the exhibits out with explanatory texts. So much has accumulated over the years – there are interesting antiques from the veterinary, dental, medical and pharmaceutical professions of yesteryear. While Julie and Tom organise the sections, I consult my reference books and produce short paragraphs to guide any visitors. Blacksmiths were popular village residents in olden days – in addition to their regular work, they also did much of the early veterinary and dental work. At least if Pete is late on Friday, our guests can while away the time by inspecting the exhibits.

The whole family have planned to go out together in the afternoon, but an emergency scuppers our intentions. Perro Smith is an elderly collie/spaniel cross-breed. For months, a soft lump has been slowly growing next to the black tip of his nose, just above his nostril. His owners have been reluctant to opt for surgery, but suddenly the lump has either ruptured or been ripped, and has bled like a stuck pig. We have been calling him Pinnochio, but now he is more like Rudolph, the red-nosed reindeer. The decision has been made for us – surgery is now essential.

The surgery goes rather better than I had feared. There is little surplus skin in this site, and I suspected that leaving an open wound might be necessary, but there is enough mobility in the surrounding skin to cover the defect. Perro has had the opposite of a face-lift. Fine sutures complete the job, then we finish by fitting an Elizabethan collar round the semi-conscious dog's neck. This will be unpopular, but a good rub or scratch could cause major wound breakdown.

From admission to departure, Perro has taken up nearly three hours. Jay has also been delayed at the office, so it looks as if the family outing is off. To make it up to Tom, I invite him into the surgery while we clear up. In his *Bone Detective* book, the text mentions the technique of shining ultra-violet light on bone to obtain a rough estimation of age. If the whole bone reflects the UV light, it is probably less than a hundred years old. We just happen to have an ultra-violet lamp which is used as an aid in the diagnosis of ringworm. Approximately fifty percent of ringworm types will fluoresce under UV light – a welcome confirmation when dealing with the usual small bald, scaly patch which *might* be ringworm, but could be almost anything. So, we darken the room and run the light (known as a Wood's lamp) over our bone collection. No antique bones – all under a hundred years old. Nevertheless Tom is well impressed, obviously feeling that we are on the cutting edge of science.

We spend the remainder of the afternoon using the metal detector at the heap of stones by the beast of Fern's lair. The old road research is still tucked in the back of my mind, awaiting activation. Unfortunately, metal-detecting scores badly compared with bone-hunting; there is no instant gratification and Tom is bored. I should have hidden some treasure beforehand but did not think ahead enough. Still, I do have my work cut out, remembering where old bones are and feeding half the population of the woods. Jay now calls me the *bag lady* when I set off on feeding sorties. I think I will make more use of the metal detector when Tom goes home, it sets an ideal pace for Kippen. As Tom detects, I have a covert itch – *berrybugs* are driving me mad, and always in the most embarrassing places, not scratchable in polite company. For a minute, I wonder if Tom has taken my tip about rosehip seeds to heart. As children, we crushed the red hips and extracted the hairy seeds. Covertly placed down a victim's jumper, they were excruciatingly successful as itching powder.

Off to evening surgery where Corrie is first in. Still cold feet and no pulses, but bright and attempting to stand. He can just about prop up unaided for a few seconds although his hocks are nearly parallel to the ground. Any locomotion consists of the front legs doing the work with his hind legs being dragged behind him. However, he is not distressed so it is worth seeing what tomorrow will bring. 'Give him enough rope to hang himself,' is my rather gloomy private thought.

Evening surgery also brings a welcome visit from Leo, the Cushing's disease patient. Now on weekly medication, he is drinking a mere three pints per day, and sleeps through the entire night without wanting out. His owner is looking better than she has done for ages – the benefits of unbroken nights' sleep.

For our feeding expedition tonight, Tom and I change to peanuts – another badger favourite. Another dog favourite as well, judging from Kippen and Fintry's enthusiasm. They share some of the bag, but there are unfortunate side-effects -if they have the same effect on the badgers as on the dogs, then we should be able to *smell* them even if we cannot see them.

After supper, Tom and I head up the hill and park in the stubble field about a hundred and fifty yards from the pile of peanuts. It is going dark at around 8.30 p.m. these days so we need to be in position a good half an hour beforehand. We wind down the windows and sit quietly waiting.

Actually seeing badgers is really just the icing on the cake for me – I just love being outside at this time of night. There is an expectant feel as the light gradually fades; a blackbird alarms in the bushes and a car passes in the distance; a bat flits briefly round the car before careening further along the field; an owl starts to call in the woods and is answered by another in the east wood; and a gentle breeze rustles the leaves in the trees before fading to absolute stillness. As the daylight fades, our eyes begin to play tricks, seeing imaginary shapes in the distance which turn out to be tree stumps when checked through the binoculars. I had wondered beforehand whether it was possible for the garrulous Tom to stay quiet for any length of time, but he seems to be touched by the same magic and is as quiet as a mouse. Suddenly, there is movement at the edge of the woods. We sit alert and peer through the binoculars – one rabbit hops into the stubble closely followed by another. We watch them for a while as they gambol together – I suspect this might be a mating dance (the culmination of which would have caused much giggling from Tom) but nothing happens, the participants seeming suddenly to lose interest and turn their attention to foraging along the tramlines. Two or three more rabbits join them.

The night is rather cloudy, and we are having trouble seeing anything at all now, so decide to give up on our badgers and head for home. Rabbit eyes reflect pink in the headlights as the car starts, and we slowly trundle across the field, looking for an exit on to the track. Other eyes shine pale in the lights, and we leap out to sight three roe deer in the binoculars. They are not sure what to do, and stand stock-still in the powerful beam. I switch off the lights for an instant, then on again to catch the same three looking back as they head into the woods out of harm's way.

Slowly passing down through the woods, Tom points to a sudden movement on the track – a frog is crossing the road. We watch him scuttle over the tyre marks and into the undergrowth under the trees. It has been a productive evening, and despite not having seen badgers, we have thoroughly enjoyed our night-time safari. Listening to Tom regaling the family with all the excitement of the evening, I am sure that it has made up for the fruitless metal-detecting expedition.

Chapter 35

Pete's presentation day dawns dry and bright. Not earth-shattering in the scene of things, but exciting for us locals. Today has been kept clear of ops, and I hope for a quiet stretch – at least till after 1 p.m. No such luck!

As I walk through the door at Clayfern, Alice reports that a cat with a suspected broken leg is en route. Still, I think, it can be medicated, x-rayed and left until after the do to be fixed. Corrie, the thrombo-embolism cat is in for a check. He can just totter about, although his right foot still knuckles badly. Both hind feet are warmer but I cannot detect any femoral pulses – the blood must be finding its way by an alternative route. We discuss the use of small socks or pads to minimise damage to the top of the right foot, and to protect some raw areas between his toes which may be associated with self-trauma following returning circulation. Still, he has bucked the trend – the reference article says that, for success, circulation to the feet (as gauged by warmth) should return by twelve to twenty four hours, yet it has taken Corrie four days. I am guardedly pleased ('Typical cautious vetspeak,' as Jay would say) as my previous success rate with such cases has been truly dismal.

Next in is a puppy with a swollen face. The terrier's head is grotesquely enlarged, turning him into a bulldog look-alike – little eyes almost hidden in puffy cheeks and large thick floppy lips. The owner suspects something life-threatening; I suspect a bee or wasp sting. There are lots of such insects around, going slightly drowsy with the cooler weather but still capable of causing trouble. Sure enough, there is a tell-tale sting on the inside of the lower lip. The pup's breathing and circulation are not affected. Although dramatic, such reactions are rarely dangerous and will gradually deflate after an anti-inflammatory injection.

Next potential emergency – a dog whose suture line has partly broken down after suture removal. This occasionally occurs, hard to say why, but this is a very old dog whose healing potential may be less than ideal. Luckily, she is a quiet old thing and stands quietly while I instil local anaesthetic and staple the gap closed. I realise that time is nearly up and there is no sign yet of the cat with the broken leg. Alice fields a phone call which turns out to be the very person – she is having transport problems; someone is coming to pick her up, can they come out to Fern? I experience that familiar feeling of frustration with Murphy's Law – is it so much to ask to have just one quiet morning?

The stapling has made me late, so I thunder off to Fern. Luckily, I have help. Jay has bought cakes, biscuits and drinks, some wine but mostly soft drinks in view of the fact that everyone has to drive to get here. Tom has crayoned a Happy Retirement banner and is blowing up our supply of balloons (we could only get Happy Birthday but will hang them writing to the wall). My patient arrives promptly. It is only a kitten which has fallen off a chair, and is sporting a tender leg. I don't feel a break, but will sedate and x-ray him to be sure. No, no fracture, just badly bruised. I give him a painkiller and install him in a warm kennel to come round. His owner is to ring at 1 p.m. and can pick him up soon after.

With time in hand, we lay out food and drinks and decorate the consulting room. The decorously draped picture is on the table pushed up against the wall. Pete is due to deliver here before finishing his round, so the balloons will not go up until after he passes. The bush telegraph is up and running – Barbara rings from Dhu farm , 'He's just been here,' then Sheila 'He's leaving our yard now.'

I saunter casually out to the car as if to collect a forgotten item, and intercept Pete at the gate. 'Could you pop in on your way back,' I ask, 'I've got a sample for the lab.' 'Sure thing, Kate,' he replies, ever-helpful even on his last day.

I skulk until he goes, then the team swings into action, erecting the banner and tying balloons to the fence. With a punctuality frequently lacking in their normal visits to the surgery, folk begin to arrive. Never mind the soft drinks, our neighbours are not backward at having a celebratory dram, asserting that 'Jist a wee yin'll be okay.' Our thoughts of a bucolic evening with the surplus booze fade into the distance. A last minute arrival screeches into the last parking space – 'He's just behind me,' she gasps. The poor man is pounced upon as soon as he opens the van door. I *wondered* why no one stopped to chat today,' he exclaims, spying familiar faces, 'Barbara only waved from behind the window, and Sheila stayed in the garden.'

A worthy parishioner makes a short speech, the gift is unveiled, then the assembled party fall to chatting. 'Are you going on holiday, Pete?' one asks, then when he replies in the affirmative, 'Send us a postcard ... in fact, send one to your first call and your successor can bring it to everyone else!' This hints at Pete's willingness to transport provisions, borrowed books and the odd note from one neighbour to the next. The Post Office profits may well go up once he has left. 'Well, you know where the back door key is' ... 'And the coffee,' chirps another. 'You could start a new career as a burglar,' muses our neighbour. All in all, a good time is had by all, and the socialising continues for some time after Pete has left, trailing balloons tied to his bumper. The museum is opened for anyone interested and sparks some interesting reminiscences.

Finally, they all go and we set the surgery back to rights. As Pete is used to encountering me with blood-stained hands, and the others are mostly of farming stock, an emergency during the proceedings would not have been a total disaster, but all the same, I am relieved that all went smoothly. In this job, it is often something of an accomplishment to get through a social event unscathed, and the proceedings have left me surprisingly exhausted.

Next day, there has been a subtle change in the weather as befits the onset of autumn. There is a slight chill in the air, and there is condensation on the car windows this morning. Some swallows and martins are still flying about, but they are gradually beginning to leave for warmer climes. Some leaves are beginning to tan and fall.

Tom and family are leaving today, so he is up early to muster his collection. He has skulls of a crow, rabbit, sheep, deer and a fish (found on an outing to Pitdreel yesterday). The last is a strange light bone shaped like a platypus bill. We have scanned and printed pictures of skeletons and their live counterparts. His model of an archeological 'dig' bought by Jay has yielded a sabre-toothed cat from a lump of chalk, and he has chosen one of Honky's antlers. It has been quite a week – the museum is finished, the postie is retired, deer and badgers have been fed, metal been detected and the area denuded of skeletal remains. Tom is my little soulmate, sharing my interests and – like me – mixing his metaphors, talking of 'Bullets in china shops' as I talk of 'Carrots at the end of the tunnel' or 'Being hung for a sheep as a goat.' What will I find to do when he is gone?

Jay is taking the family home and returning tomorrow, so I have the place to myself – as usual, my on-call situation prevents my going too. After their whirlwind departure, I resist the temptation to lie down in a darkened room, instead making a strong cup of tea, and, in the time before morning surgery, settling to whittle down my in-tray which has reached epic proportions – payback for all the time off this week. For the next twenty four hours, I will free-base, eating junk food when hungry, watching television and going to bed when I feel like it. Tomorrow I will do the dishes and tidy the house before Jay's return.

Julie and I are going on a staff jaunt out today. One of our suppliers is holding an equipment fair in Stirling, and we are nipping down. A married vet with children has recently moved into our area and she has offered to cover for me for short periods of time. Today is her 'test run.'

As usual before any event out of the ordinary, I am like a hen on a hot girdle during morning surgery, anticipating the emergency which will necessitate cancelling the trip. As witnessed on Pete's retirement day, the requirement for a few quiet hours is like a magnet to emergencies. However, the morning passes uneventfully – very sociable, just not much money. Mavis comes in to order dog food and to enquire if the beads worked as crow eyes. I have saved her some plastic trimmed off an Elizabethan collar – knowing the miniaturists is very handy, it means never having to throw anything out. Mrs Cassidy comes in carrying a large suitcase. 'What on earth has she got in there?' ponders Alice. It transpires that she is going on holiday, and cannot take more than fifteen kilograms on the plane. She has brought the empty case today, and will return later with it filled. This seems rather pointless unless she is to fill it with a known weight of clothes, but *ours not to reason why*. As well as animals, our scales have been known to weigh local slimmers and prize vegetables heading to shows, but this is a first. Hector is next with Lena for a check-up. Her lip wound has healed well, and the lab report confirms that it was a benign growth.

Pager dropped off with the new locum, we head for the open road and arrive on the outskirts of Stirling sooner than expected, giving us just the excuse we need to visit a nearby antiques and craft warehouse. Julie is always on the lookout for items for her shop, and sorting the museum has whetted my appetite for old instruments. Luckily, there is nothing suitable so Julie contents herself by buying a slab of tablet (an extremely sweet Scottish form of fudge). 'Just a wee bit,' I say, but, as usual, scoff the entire half offered on the way to the equipment fair. Also as usual, we are both feeling sick as we draw up at the venue.

It is only really at conferences that we get the opportunity to view equipment and quiz manufacturers or reps, and such events are usually down south, requiring considerable effort and expense to attend. So this is a treat. 'Oh look!' I say at the first stand, picking up a steel splint-like object, 'One of those gadgets to keep the leg extended when on a drip.' '*Actually,*' counters the rep, 'It's a horse oral speculum.' Much hilarity all round – I am never exposed to large animal equipment these days, but can see that this is in fact the case. No doubt pinning me down as a harmless eccentric – and possibly an easy touch – the rep enthusiastically extols the virtues of the company's new pulse oximeter/carbon dioxide detector. It is useful to limit the build-up of the latter waste gas (produced when we breathe out) in an anaesthetic circuit, so a visual display of the percentage of the gas breathed out is an added safety feature. Perhaps he re-defines his opinion of me when Julie mentions that we already have a pulse oximeter, and I enquire pointedly about a potential trade-in – not so green after all, maybe! Pulled up short after being told that our device is now only worth a tenth of its purchase price when acquired a mere three years ago, I cool off slightly and set off round the other stands, promising to at least think about it. Knowing me well, Julie obviously suspects this is something of a token gesture 'When are you getting it?' she enquires innocently. I do like toys – possibly starting off in a shed has made me sensitive, but I do like to be well equipped with good quality equipment. I shall consider the matter over the next few days.

Apart from getting somewhat lost while leaving Stirling, we are on the motorway home in good time to take over from the locum before child-picking-up time. The fact-finding mission has been very successful and I am quite proud of my restraint in the face of such a concentration of goodies. Today has been good value – antiques, equipment ... and a tour round an historic city.

Chapter 36

The morning's big excitement occurs when, on an early walk up the hill, Jay and I find a badger's latrine hole – liberally seeded with roasted peanuts. This might not make everyone's day but it certainly gives us a thrill.

Yesterday's operations have been re-scheduled for today, with the result that we will be totally out of synch for the rest of the week. Luckily, we are not wildly busy and even have time to see a rep booked in by mistake. 'Order six packs of bandages and we give you a free set of underpants,' she announces, no doubt surprised at the sudden interest generated in her offer. However it was a mere slip of the tongue, underpants sound more exciting than underpads (the proper offer) and set the trend for the day's conversation. Julie remembers that when our locum Emma was here, her underwear came out of the washing machine a vivid pink after mixing with a new T-shirt, and, mortified, she hung them out of sight in the garden. 'The locals would just have assumed that we hadn't gone away,' I muse, strangely comforted that I am not the only one to do such things. Both Jay's and my undies change colour regularly depending on what they have been washed with. At present, they are all a rather fetching blue.

Life is too short to sort your washing into separate lots. Mrs Slob lives!

The ops are routine this morning with one exception – our own dog, Kippen. He has a small *haematoma* (collection of blood) in his ear which requires draining. I first noticed it a week ago, but ignored it in true vet-owner fashion. Like cobblers' kids being worst shod, vets' pets often fare badly in the scheme of things. Although incisive and detached with other people's pets; with our own we are reduced to indecisive jellies, unable to map out even the simplest treatment plans.

Only last week, I examined a neighbouring vet's cat for her. She is an excellent clinician, very experienced and highly competent, but loses all clinical judgement when faced with illness in her own pets. In turn, she operated on Kippen two years ago to remove a benign but annoying growth.

Anyway, Jay has nagged me incessantly about the ear, so I have at last turned my attention to our own dog.

Luckily, Kippen does not require a general anaesthetic today as I am planning to drain the haematoma through a small hypodermic needle. Several years ago, the only treatment for haematomas was to open them surgically under full anaesthesia, drain out all the collected blood then flatten both sides of the earflap together using large, staple-like stitches to prevent more fluid accumulation. Some surgeons even used small buttons under the knots to reduce the tension on the stitches. The end result looked quite bizarre, and the treatment was occasionally ruined by kindly folk undoing the stitches, thinking the buttons had been stitched on as a cruel joke by vandals. Anyone who has ever had any dealings with cats will immediately realise that such an act would be virtually impossible without benefit of efficient anaesthetics.

In recent years, new methods of dealing with haematomas have been experimented with, with varying degrees of success. As they are less invasive and do not require anaesthetic, they are always worth a try, and surgery can still be used as a last resort if they are not successful. My preferred technique is to give the patient a dose of anti-inflammatory drug three days before draining the blood by syringe, then injecting long-acting anti-inflammatory into the vacated cavity between the outer and inner sides of the earflap.

Before morning surgery today, I anointed Kippen's inner earflap with local anaesthetic cream, and re-apply some as soon as I return to the farm. I am using this cream more and more these days. Anyone who has had a blood sample taken will realise that *Just a little sting* is a total euphemism – being stabbed with a sharp object is damned sore, and I do believe that the adage *Do as you would be done to* is an admirable one to live up to.

Working with a relaxed, non-resisting patient also makes our job easier, so plastering on local anaesthetic cream makes sense. Kippen is surprisingly good when his haematoma is stabbed, and even stays still while I withdraw fifteen millilitres of blood then inject anti-inflammatory when drainage is complete. Julie and I distract him afterwards with a juicy chew. The fresh needle hole usually bleeds a little, and head-shaking at this stage can successfully pebbledash every surface within a two-metre radius.

The patient is recovered enough to come for a walk in the afternoon. I take the car along the road into another favourite field, negotiating a troop of young pheasants dithering by the verge. There are many around at this time of year making a country drive quite a hazardous venture.

Our field was harvested earlier this week, and I am horrified to see that ploughing has started already. The weather has been so poor lately that the harvest is far behind schedule, and all that is left for the farmers to get on with is to plough and re-seed finished fields. Our only hope is that some land is left fallow until spring barley is sown early in the new year, otherwise we will be relegated to hill walks again until winter frosts renders sown fields passable. I trudge down the field while both dogs forge ahead. The old chap is remarkably spry today. This may be partly because he had a Reiki session yesterday, but also because this is a new walk and, like his owner, he appreciates the novelty.

It is hard to believe that only three weeks ago I was living in shorts and T-shirts. Today I wear sweatshirt, waterproof and wellies. This field is quite exposed, and the wind rips across it bringing tears to my eyes, and shaking plump sloe berries and rosehips from the hedges. I sample brambles as we walk, savouring their rich fruity taste. The dogs prefer raspberries and strawberries, so I pick unhindered by hopeful sidekicks. I really must bring a bag next time and collect a batch to bake into a tasty bramble crumble, perfect for chilly autumn evenings.

Evening surgery is brisk, with yet another infected elbow callus, the product of large, heavy dogs lying on hard surfaces to keep cool. Sometimes the hardest part of treatment is enticing the patient to recline on a comfortable soft bed rather than tiles or concrete.

Corrie the thromboembolism cat appears for a check-up. He is doing well, and his owners are manfully attempting to dress his weaker foot so that the rubbed area does not get any worse. The inflamed areas between his toes are clearing up, and his outlook is looking excitingly hopeful. Cheered by this, I joke with the next client. 'The same old scabby thing,' she says, steering the cat basket through the door. 'But she's *your* scabby old thing,' I reply, light-heartedly. 'Actually,' she says, ' I was talking about the basket.' In fact, the basket holds a kitten with ringworm. Adopted from a cat home, she sports suspicious bald, scaly patches on her ears. These fluoresce gratifyingly when illuminated with the ultra-violet lamp. Before I return the lamp to its cupboard, I covertly check my own patch of ringworm – a small circular lesion on the back of my hand. There is a limit to how long I can pretend that this is a burn; I really must be diligent in applying anti-fungal cream twice daily.

For the cat, I dispense tablets and a shampoo to reduce environmental contamination. Although not particularly serious, ringworm can be a nuisance due to its ability to persist in the cat's surroundings. It forms spores which are virtually impossible to destroy. This is the reason why cats from sanctuaries occasionally come with the infection, once the ringworm is present in the environment in the form of spores, it can survive for years. Establishments with wooden cages are more likely to have problems in this respect, as at least plastic or fibreglass kennels can be wiped clean, and possess fewer nooks and crannies for spores to inhabit. I am sure there is more ringworm around than ever gets diagnosed – or even examined. The lesions are not particularly horrible, and will self-cure in time.

It is worth remembering that there are many species of ringworm, many of which are present in the soil, so the unfortunate family pet is not always the carrier when a human becomes infected. Handing out the printed instructions which go with the shampoo, I warn the owner that shampooing a cat is not always so easy as the manufacturers would have us believe. Give up if the going gets too tough, is my advice. Some cats are cooperative, but the cosy pictures of relaxed felines reclining in basins of water are too much of a fairy tale for my liking.

There is time for a walk up the hill before evening surgery. The wind is freshening, and branches flail to and fro as we walk through the woods, clumps of leaves shaking like hysterical hands before dislodging and spiralling to the ground. The noise is considerable, like the rush of a mighty waterfall. The track is muddy from the rain and, emerging from the trees, I look for clues as to who has been around.

There is the convict-suit arrowhead pattern of birds' prints, and the large cloven shapes of red deer hooves – three times the size of the smaller roe deer. A delicate, well-defined print which will belong to one of Sheila's cats – a petite but hardy creature who lives in the woods. She meets us occasionally on walks and is sociable for a while, purring and rubbing against my legs, but only accompanying us for a certain distance before returning to her territory. She has been seen nipping down to the farm so is obviously not lost, just enjoys the outdoor life. Looking carefully, I finally find what I hoped might be there – badger tracks, distinctively broad prints with the imprints of the creature's sharp, powerful claws. They cross the track from one field to the next, probably heading for the burn at the bottom of the slope. Badgers often travel on well-defined paths, and already there is a distinct trace through the field. As virtually no one else comes up this hill regularly, most of the tracks through wood or field are produced by the wild residents. When walking on one, we are following the footsteps of a deer, rabbit, badger or fox. I find this rather exciting, and try to imagine myself in the animal's shoes, so to speak, trundling under low hanging branches, diverting to investigate a rabbit hole or snack on some plump mushrooms perhaps before reaching a good spot to find earthworms and grubs, digging many shallow scrapes to winkle out prey.

I remember following radio-tagged badgers on many such expeditions, sometimes being able to watch from a distance; at other times, piecing together their activities from the noises they make. They could hardly be described as stealthy, and their energetic crashing through the undergrowth and snuffling out food could be heard over quite a distance.

Jay goes off to work early next day, so, being up and active with time to spare before morning surgery, I grab the metal detector and set off with the dogs down the as-yet-unploughed stubble field leading to the river. This type of activity is excellent for Kippen as he can rootle about while I do too.

There is a big signal from near the old bothy and I begin to dig with my trusty trowel. A cylindrical object nearly a foot long appears as the earth is moved. It crosses my mind that it could be a bomb, but curiosity overcomes caution and I continue to dig until I unearth – a piece of drain pipe. A quick glance at the bothy confirms that all its gutters and pipes are intact, so at least this is an *antique* drainpipe. It doesn't really matter what you find, the excitement is in the thrill of the chase. We squeeze through the fencing on to the beach, and move slowly along, partly metal-detecting and partly beachcombing.

The first find is a concave shield of bone with a spine down the centre, and indentations at each edge. This is a bird's breastbone – it provides a broad surface for the massive flight muscles to attach. It is over six inches long by three inches broad, and I suspect it may belong to the dead swan spotted farther along the coast last month. It will be a good project for Tom to decide what type of bone it is – no conventional presents ever from Auntie Kate. The metal detector also detects an ornate handle, of the type seen on cauldrons – or garden buckets as Jay disparagingly says later. It is quite addictive this metal detecting – the quickening of the pulse when a signal is heard, then the mounting excitement as you unearth the mystery object. Several coke cans and a sheet of lead flashing later, I gather my treasures, muster the dogs and head slowly back up the field. A very pleasant start to the day.

The petrol crisis is hotting up. Hauliers protesting against yet more increases in fuel prices are blockading refineries, and supplies to petrol stations are drying up. Panic-buying is making the situation worse, and cities like Edinburgh and Manchester are already out of fuel. Luckily both Jay and I filled up at the weekend so are not in imminent danger of running out, but the implications are worrying. Jay travels miles every day, giving estimates to customers, and so do the workmen. Deliveries of the necessary materials may have trouble getting through. It is sobering how dependent modern life is on fuel. On the surgery side, maintaining a service from four miles out of town could be a worry. I could get on my bike, but inevitably would end up with a sick animal to bring back to the farm surgery. We do have a client who brings her dog on the back of her moped, but I doubt if most would be so accommodating. I drive slowly into morning surgery to conserve petrol. Cycling in would not be so bad, but the hill on the way back is a killer.

As if to prove the point, I do end up bringing a dog back up to the farm surgery. Duke, a young Labrador was operated on earlier in the year after swallowing a rubber ball which lodged in his gut. For the last twenty four hours, he has been showing the same symptoms of vomiting and refusing food. The latter is a highly suspicious sign in a Labrador as, almost without exception, they are all gannets.

'We have been watching him so carefully, I can't understand what he might have got,' ponders Dave his owner. The x-ray is something of a puzzle – Duke's first dietary indiscretion – the ball – showed up as an object denser than the surrounding tissues. This is the normal picture for most foreign bodies, but a lighter oval shadow is visible on today's radiograph. As I begin the surgery to retrieve the obstacle, Julie and I try to guess what it could be, but fall far short of the answer – a boiled new potato still in its skin. This is a most unusual finding, as one would expect such a thing to be digested in the stomach with no trouble. Both our dogs will eat such potatoes left over from our meals, as I'm sure do many others. However, this potato has somehow bypassed the stomach and is tightly wedged in the small intestine causing damming back of fluid in front of the blockage: there is no doubt that it is causing a problem. As last time, the operation is uneventful and Duke is soon recovering in his kennel.

After the operation, time out again for Kippen and Fintry. Clutching a bag of peanuts, I lay a trail from near the sett on to the stubble field, intercepting a hopeful Kippen en route and guiding him back along by the collar. No peanuts for him today. Fortunately his ear has healed well so there has been no need to ask my vet friend to perform any surgery. Everywhere I tread, there are clusters of ladybirds, there does seem to be a glut of them just now. Avoiding them while leading the dog is not easy, but I do my best.

A large drug order arrives this afternoon – more than I would normally order, but a safeguard in case the fuel situation worsens. The driver has been told that he is a priority case, but, even so, finding an open petrol station has not been easy. After several days of supplying cars from out of town as well as locals, our local garage is now closed, although the doctor told me that the garage had kept secret supplies for emergency vehicles. 'Does that include vets?' I enquire over the phone, 'Yes, but don't tell anyone else,' is the furtive reply.

Evening surgery is brisker than anticipated, clients seem to be getting in so far. We have two diabetics on the go at present – a dog and a cat – and both are in this evening. They are still at the stage of coming in daily while we edge up the dose of insulin to control the disease, and both are doing quite well. I am still trying to train one owner *not* to bring the daily urine sample in a *Tupperware* container – I seem incapable of opening these without getting soaked. The diabetic dog's owner has only enough petrol left to make the trip tomorrow – I do hope that the petrol crisis is not going to cause such problems. While discussing the situation with Mrs Cassidy (who has come in to weigh her full suitcase), she makes a generous offer 'In my shed, there is half a gallon of unleaded petrol from the war. If you are short, just help yourself when I am away.' 'That was kind of her,' I comment as she heads off with suitcase in tow –' but I didn't know they had unleaded petrol during the war.' 'She said from the *mower* not the war!' corrects Alice before we succumb to a fit of the giggles.

Secure in the knowledge that further petrol supplies are obtainable, I set off to Stramar to view the articles due to be sold at the auction on Friday. Not very conservation-conscious, I'm afraid, but I have been looking forward to this trip for over a week. The auction is selling off the entire contents of an old chemist's shop, and I hope there may be many interesting things to be found. I can't make the auction itself, but leaving bids is the next best thing. Doing my bit to save petrol, I trundle in at a leisurely rate. There are fewer cars on the roads than usual, and the trip is really rather pleasant. I think I may endeavour to drive more slowly in future.

As expected, the auction hall is an Aladdin's cave of intriguing finds. After half an hour of enthusiastic rooting in boxes and sacks, I leave bids for several lots of old chemist's jars; a rocking chair for Andy's Christmas as he always hogs ours by the Rayburn – this one needs some refurbishment but might fit the bill; two brass cauldrons for re-sale; and a rusting implement on a stand which I cleverly deduce (because the old label says Halls clippers) is an old hand-driven shearing device. Jay will kill me if I get that.

Home after evening surgery, I scan the paper to see what is on the television. Ah good, *Vets in Practice,* interesting viewing for most UK vets. As Jay might settle down with drinks and snacks to watch football, I ready myself for the start of the programme showing young vets at their daily work. It is probably a national sport amongst the profession to criticise and heckle the participants – again similar to Jay's football-watching antics – but in reality, I have a great deal of respect for the stars managing to carry on their daily routine under the constant scrutiny of a TV camera. I have been filmed only once and found it a most unnerving experience. The number of TV programmes featuring vets and animals has multiplied recently, and public demand to see us in action seems limitless.

Chapter 37

We wake to the comforting sound of the roaring Rayburn. A quick look out the window confirms that it has gone colder. Both cars' windows are obscured by condensation, and a jacket is necessary for our morning walk. The first V of geese honks high overhead, but they carry on heading northwards, ignoring our fields. There are still the occasional swallow and house martin to be seen, but not many, most will be now flying over Europe en route to Africa.

In Clayfern, Alice confides that she has donned her winter vest, and is in mourning for summer, but I am in happy anticipation of the pleasures of the second half of the year – walks on stubble fields on crisp mellow days; autumn clothes – warm fleeces, bright jumpers; moleskin trousers and comfy old fell boots; curling up in front of glowing fires; comforting winter stews and puddings; perhaps loads of snow. I am definitely a winter girl at heart.

Mrs Cassidy is in again this morning – this time to weigh a full carrier bag. 'They're not restricting the weight of your hand luggage as well?' Alice enquires, puzzled. 'Och no, this is just my tartan skirt and top. I want to see if they can fit in my case.' As she is six kilograms under her limit, I shouldn't think there will be a problem. She is certainly getting some mileage out of this holiday. We are nearly as excited as she is.

Duke comes in for a check-up after yesterday's surgery. He is very bright, and I remove his intravenous canula (left in place in case he required more fluids) and dispense some cans of recovery diet. 'After that, gradually move him on to light foods such as egg, fish or chicken with boiled rice or potatoes for a few days,' I parrot off my usual advice. 'That'll be *mashed* potato, I take it,' says Dave wryly. Duke's last episode ate into the family's summer holiday fund; this time it is the Christmas stash that suffers. We make the usual joke about fitting a zip before he departs.

Our next client brings in a cat with an abscess, a routine case. 'He ate a whole rabbit the other day,' she mentions, 'Beforehand, he was standing over it growling, and afterwards, when he walked, his stomach swayed from side to side – he just looked like a small lion; it was quite frightening.'

I tell her the tale of a road traffic accident cat which was rushed to the surgery one day. Many cats will attack humans if something unpleasant is done to them, or if they are cornered, but this cat was actually stalking us. It had obviously had a bang on the head which had affected its temperament, and it was completely unnerving to watch the small but fierce creature coming at you from across the room, slowly and deliberately, with murder in its heart. Ordering the owners from the room, I backed into the corner and loaded a syringe with tranquilliser while my nurse grabbed a large bath towel. Acting in concert, we threw the towel over the cat and injected the drug. There was much screaming and struggling (mostly the cat) but at last, silence. After being admitted for some treatment to reduce the effects of brain bruising, and attention to her other wounds, that cat was absolutely fine. Scary however, to see how wild they can be under the thin veneer of domestication.

Being an out-of-towner, the client has a question 'Is there anywhere in Clayfern that I could buy some turps?' 'At the electrician's,' we answer in chorus. That is all part of the quirky appeal of small towns – the Clayfern undertaker is also the taxi driver – and painter and decorator, while in Pitdreel, the Sunday papers and morning rolls are to be found in the fish and chip shop which opens specially.

Corrie the thromboembolism cat returns for a check up. He is doing very well but the top of his right hind foot has become abraded from dragging on the ground. I bandage it up, and request his presence again in a week, or before if the bandage is dislodged. Some cats are expert at removing bandages so a week may be somewhat optimistic.

With a 'Hello, stranger,' I welcome the next patient into the consulting room. It is none other than Don, the gentle old Labrador who caused such trouble with his non-healing leg wound two years ago. Since then, he has developed bronchitis, but has been kept reasonably well controlled with occasional use of corticosteroids to reduce the inflammation, and a drug to loosen and mobilise the respiratory tract secretions. However, there is a distinct chill in the air these last few days – often a signal for our bronchitic and arthritic patients to take a turn for the worse. Sure enough, the old dog's chest sounds noisy – almost crackly, and I suspect that his emphysema could be worsening. Rupture of some alveoli allows air to collect around the others, causing further resistance to breathing, so more rupture, and the process continues like a vicious circle.

As Don is coughing and wheezing badly, I prescribe a short course of an anti-coughing drug, only a short course, as coughing is basically a helpful mechanism to dislodge secretions and debris from the chest. It is only when the coughing gets out of hand that such a drug can be useful. A few days' respite might allow Don's chest to settle down somewhat. We also increase the steroid dosage – he has only been on a low dose as and when it has been necessary. No walks until he returns next week. I am slightly anxious with his deterioration; although he is getting old, I thought he would be around for quite some time to come.

As usual, the rest of the day is busy. Alice postpones a visiting company representative until tomorrow 'I'm sorry, but she is due in theatre all day today.' This always makes me smile and conjures up a vision of Julie and me clad in Shakespearean attire, delivering flowery speeches to an attentive crowd.

The day's business began at 8 a.m. with the admission of Darth the diabetic cat. Despite over a week of gradually working up his insulin dose, he is still not stable and we are going to take blood samples every two hours to find out exactly what his blood glucose levels are doing. He is a lovely cat whose particular trick is to lie on his back for his tummy to be tickled. We lather on the local anaesthetic cream, only too aware that when serially blood sampling cats, it is not uncommon for more human than feline blood to be spilled. Unfortunately, the usual ear prick technique yields no blood so we use a very fine needle to repeatedly collect a drop of blood from his veins. He takes it all in good part and we soon fall into the routine of application of local followed by sampling followed by several moments of tummy tickling. It seems to work very well. By lunchtime, the blood glucose level is dropping so the insulin which he had this morning is definitely having some effect.

Routine neuterings take up the rest of our time until Sheila appears with a poorly kitten. Apparently Mum and two kittens have been living in a local timber yard, but when the boss appeared for work this morning, he found the mother and one kitten dead, run over on the road. A search was initiated, and our patient was found, huddling under a pile of logs. When brought in the sawmill office, he could hardly walk, falling weakly from side to side. Sheila was summoned and has brought him straight here. The kitten has no obvious illness or injuries, but feels bitterly cold. A check of his temperature shows it to be subnormal. 'Woody' is on the verge of hypothermia. Last night was rather cold for a four-week-old kitten to spend outside on his own. 'He has livened up a bit even during the car ride,' reports Sheila, so I discharge him into her care. Warmly wrapped up next to her Aga, he will be better in next to no time. I warn her not to feed him until he has warmed up – any food given now will not be digested and will do him no good.

Having worked our way through all the neuterings, we adjourn for lunch where we have a treat – toast with plum jam courtesy of Sheila. Less busy after the summer kitten rush, she has been devoting time to making jams and chutneys to sell. Fruit trees and bushes lie bare for a two-mile radius – not locusts, but our friend. Toast made on the Rayburn is wonderful, crisp on the outside but soft inside. The smell in the kitchen is glorious. Inspired, I even work up to stewing some apples for tonight's supper. As Jay and I suspected, the Rayburn is really coming into its own with the advent of the cooler weather.

Refreshed, Julie and I return to 'theatre' to perform *Incisor removal for small rabbit*. This bun has had his front teeth burred every two months, but this time, his owner has opted for the more radical approach. I am glad that we have been fortified as this is not my favourite task. The first challenge is anaesthetising the rabbit deeply enough so that it does not react to painful stimuli. Like icebergs, there is more tooth under the surface than above the gum line so careful dissection is necessary. They are also deeply curved and fragile, liable to break at the drop of a hat. If a tooth does break during removal, then we have to wait until it regrows and try again. This requires more anaesthetic and another extraction procedure, so it is important to try to be successful first time round. It takes almost an hour before the teeth are removed – fortunately intact. The rabbit is bundled up in bubblewrap and tucked in to a heated kennel.

After the operations, the dogs and I set off up the hill in the car to give the metal detector an airing. There is an Iron Age fort not far from here, and I had hoped that some lesser Iron-Agers might have been relegated to our lesser hill top. On the way, we stop off to leave food for the badgers but notice that there are still some peanuts left from earlier in the week. There is probably so much other food around for them just now – the humid weather will encourage worms and other invertebrates; and there are multitudes of brambles and fungi. I thought I had found a skull the other day, but instead it was a large puffball mushroom partially eroded by insects. Apparently they are delicious if you can get them before the insects do.

Unfortunately, metal detecting up the hill is a big disappointment. Initial excitement on hearing a contact soon turns to despondency after digging up yet another piece of chicken wire or .22 slug. The place is like a rubbish tip. We shall confine ourselves to the beach in future.

The day ends as it began – at 10 p.m. with a final blood sample from Darth, fourteen hours after the first. It can be seen from the results that the insulin is having an effect but it is not lasting for the full twenty four hours, so I make my recommendation that we increase Darth's insulin injections to twice daily. This is not an uncommon finding with cat diabetics – they seem to metabolise insulin faster than dogs – but after today's efforts, Darth's diabetes should be better controlled. These serial blood samples are hard going, but definitely worthwhile.

Chapter 38

We are having wonderful sunny days – then incredibly wet stormy nights. This suits most people – but not the farmers, who are becoming increasingly frustrated about the still unharvested grain. It is drying nicely during the day then is soaked again at night. Some are giving up and attempting to gather still wet crops. This is not ideal as wet grain tends to make the combine break down, and when it is eventually in, much expensive fuel has to be used to run the grain dryers. Profits are not going to be good this year.

We have had an advance notice of a power cut at the farm today. Faults are being mended at the neighbouring farm, and we will be off from 8.30 a.m. until 4 p.m. Not inconsiderable contingency plans swing into action – up early to turn up the Rayburn, fill thermoses for tea and turn heating on in the surgery. Luckily, it is a quiet day for Fern surgery – only one consultation is due, Sheila's ops having been diverted until later in the week.

There is good natural lighting in the consulting room and the emergency lighting comes on when the power is off. Being well-insulated, the surgery stays warm for several hours and we have plenty back-up in the shape of torches, hurricane lamps and a bottled gas heater if necessary. In the event of an emergency, the anaesthetic machine requires no power and the pulse oximeter is battery operated; only the x-ray machine, steriliser and clippers are irrevocably lost. There are plenty of instruments and drapes already sterilised, and if necessary an ordinary razor can be used to trim up an op site – although razor rash becomes a likely hazard for any unfortunate patients. Another nuisance is that the answering machine will not be functioning – thank goodness for the call diversion facility. Alice arrives in Clayfern a few minutes early for me to divert the phone to her, then waits there until I arrive back at Fern. For my consultation in the farm surgery, I temporarily divert incoming calls to my mobile phone – as the surgery phone is cordless, it is also afflicted by the power cut.

Overnight it rained incessantly and the wind howled round the house. Jay set off at crack of dawn for an early meeting, and rings to warn me to proceed into Clayfern with caution – there is considerable flooding, and some hefty branches have landed on the road. Proceeding cautiously, I am thankful for the trusty Tundra – it may be a heavy old thing which drinks petrol and doesn't go very fast, but it is as solid as a rock in uncertain driving conditions. With increasing petrol costs, we had considered changing it, but today's hazards remind me how trustworthy it is. The geese are splashing about in Abbeygate's flooded fields when I pass. As the farmer was out muck-spreading in them recently, the birds must now smell atrocious.

The day starts badly with a call from a neighbouring practice. One of my clients has gone there for a second opinion. Although not showing any obvious symptoms when I last saw her, the dog has since developed a symptom which makes diagnosis very easy. 'She was had a follow-up appointment for last week but didn't turn up,' I tell my colleague feeling vaguely aggrieved – not with the colleague but with the owner. As always with only vague symptoms are showing and a specific diagnosis has not been reached, any vet's approach is generally to treat the symptoms and keep monitoring the situation, ready to investigate further if no progress is made. For some reason, my approach did not inspire confidence in this particular owner who evidently decided not to bother returning to any vet. It was only when the dog's condition worsened that she headed for pastures new. Vets are used to the vagaries of client behaviour – only last week I had a client of this vet requesting a second opinion from me. I agreed with everything that the vet had said and done, but the client was reluctant to return, preferring to carry on with this practice. I suppose that you can't please all of the people all of the time, but all the same, the situation rankles, and I will probably spend part of the day brooding on the injustice of it all. I wish I could be the type of person who can just brush such things off, but I never can. I find myself being exceptionally careful with the next customers – repeating instructions and checking to be sure that they have fully understood my plan for their pet.

The surgery also brings in Leo, the Cushing's disease dog. He is doing very well, drinking a mere three pints per day, but, like many others in this horrible weather, he is suffering from a touch of arthritis. Some anti-inflammatory pills should sort him out. His owner looks years younger – getting uninterrupted nights' sleep is obviously doing her good.

Don too has improved following his brief course of anti-coughing drugs. I supply his owner with more steroids and request his presence again in two weeks. He will be maintained on the steroids and come in for regular checks to monitor his condition. He will never be cured, but hopefully we can control him for a good time to come.

Into Stramar after surgery to collect the results of my successful bids at the auction. Some chemists' jars and … the clippers. Sneaking them home, I secrete them in the corner of the museum. Theoretically, my plan is to restore them to working order and sell them, but, as with most of my schemes, this work will not occur now but at some vague time in the future when I suddenly have a surplus of leisure time.

I have planned to spend the rest of the day at home, blitzing the neglected in-tray. The first item is a practice performance survey form. The notional salary for partners is approximately twice my earnings, so my figures have minus signs in front. It will be embarrassing to be compared with my peers, but I think that my lifestyle is infinitely superior. While I am metal-detecting or visiting auctions, they have their noses firmly to the grindstone. This really is the perfect job if not for the nearly continuous time on-call.

One of many phone calls is to order a folding car ramp for Kippen. Leaping in and out of the Tundra has become increasingly hit and miss. Our technique now is to stand prepared as he leaps in, ready to grasp the flagging rear end and propel it carwards. I am convinced that the dog thinks 'Oops, I'm being grabbed – hair away' as his helper inevitably ends up coated in tan fur. This technique does nothing for the descent where all his weight lands on his fore legs (his most painful areas) and we have had the occasional belly-flop which must be painful after which he scrambles up, embarrassed, shrugging off any solicitous attention. Theoretically with the ramp, he should be able to stroll in and out quite the thing. At the price, we could practically buy him his own car *How* much?' I gasp on hearing the price. However, nothing is too expensive for our dog so I order it just the same. The thin white-coated metal used for collapsible clothes maidens looks rather flimsy but I am banking on the assumption that, once extended, the triangular shape lends stability. We shall see.

For a change, this past weekend has largely been devoted to Jay's business. Last night, we hosted an open evening for past customers. This involved much socialising with glasses of wine, and basically showing off all the business has to offer. As is usual with such events, neither of us particularly look forward to them until we are in the thick of it, then we find ourselves quite enjoying it. An adage which I find very helpful is that *Strangers are only friends which you haven't met yet.*

I had a particularly enjoyable conversation with a lady who has been a nurse in intensive care for over fifteen years. She remembered the days before pulse oximeters when artificial respirators were either on or off (no gradually weaning off the respirator on to normal breathing). The staff judged purely by the colour of the patient's mucous membranes whether they were receiving sufficient oxygen. 'From what we know now, some poor souls must have been barely fifty per cent oxygenated,' she commented in amazement (minimum expected nowadays is around ninety per cent). Discussing the ever-increasing complexity of modern equipment, she agreed that intensive care staff these days are a cross between nurse and technician. When an alarm sounds, it may either be due to a problem with the patient –

or with the machine. 'I can remember the old E.C.G. machines,' she said, 'They had to be switched off for ten minutes rest every few hours.' For my part, I reminisced about schoolgirl Saturdays spent with the local vet. We used to anaesthetise patients with an ether-soaked pad of cotton wool in a tin can punctured with holes. Such quaint tales seem incredible in today's high-tech medical atmosphere. All in all, the evening was very successful and Jay gained enough new business to keep us ticking over for some time to come.

When we finally got home, Jay collapsed exhausted into a favourite chair while I did my bag-lady bit up the hill with the dogs. We had our first sighting of Honky for weeks. I threw some apples but he disappeared into the woods. There was a strong smell of stag urine by the fence line. Both Honky and Charlie must be gearing up for the rutting season. Apparently, if you are a stag, weeing into a muddy puddle and anointing yourself liberally with the scented mud is guaranteed to make you irresistible to the ladies. The surrounding green forest is tinged with mustard – the first signs of the autumn splendour to come. As I walked home through the woods, it occurred to me that I can differentiate between fox, badger and deer urine. What a strange skill to possess.

Wednesday rolls round again, thank goodness – just morning surgery to be got through then, emergencies permitting, I am left to my own devices until evening surgery. First in is a kitten with a bald, scaly patch behind its ear. Coming as it has from a rescue centre, ringworm has yet again to be one of the suspects. Closing the shutters still left on the surgery's elegant Victorian windows, I turn off the room light and approach the kitten with the Wood's lamp (which has been switched on for at least five minutes to ensure that it is emitting the correct wavelength of ultra violet light). Probably about half the species of ringworm found in cats fluoresce so a negative finding is not a guarantee that the patient is clear, but there are no doubts about this one – the entire area almost glows. So of course do flecks of dust and my fingers (which have probably collected powder from counting out pills), but the ringworm fluorescence is very distinctive – an apple-green hue; once seen never forgotten. It is good to have a positive diagnosis. 'Have any of you developed any bald patches?' I make conversation while counting out a supply of tablets. Laughter makes me raise my head to see Mrs Owner affectionately patting her husband's exceedingly bald pate.

Both current diabetics are in for progress reports. There is to be a Pet Diabetes Awareness Week in October, and I prevail upon the owners to write a small article on life with a diabetic pet which we can feature in a window display. After years of producing window displays, both Alice and I are flagging a little in thinking up fresh topics. A focus on diabetes will let us off the hook for a couple of weeks.

Once finished, I head again to the auction in Stramar where yet more chemist's paraphenalia is to be sold. There are several sets of the brightly decorated glass jars known as shop rounds, and I put in modest bids for them all in the hope of getting some. It would be rather a financial disaster if I ended up with them all, but I think I will be fairly safe. Julie and I have an antique fair coming up, and the bottles are generally quite popular.

Alternative career as an antiques dealer out of the way for the day, I head home for a dog walk. It has been a wonderful crisp, sunny morning but rain is forecast, and sure enough, a solid band of dark cloud is approaching from the West like a grey eiderdown being drawn across the land. I rush in, grab a bag of windfall apples and dogs, and drive up the hill. Heading towards the deer pen, we pass toadstools growing in profusion – there are yellow crocus-like ones; deep browns; crimson and white spotted *fly agaric*; large meaty ones like Mexican hats and clusters of others resembling parasols on a beach; toasty-browns with golden centres and tiny white chocolate-drop-like miniatures. I make sure the dogs do not linger, especially near the last. On a Christmas walk through the woods, our last dog mistook them for doggy chocolate drops and guzzled some before we could intervene. Panic-stricken, knowing how poisonous many toadstools can be, we tried to rush her back to the car, but she plodded along as usual. After a few minutes, she began gulping and retching, was violently sick and was her usual self from then onwards.

As we approach the deer pen, Honky, Mum and Gray are lurking by the fence. 'Come on,' I holler, bowling apples towards them. The flightier Mum and Gray speed away in an elaborate semi-circle back into the woods, while Honky merely glances in our direction. He is engaged in a staring contest with Charlie, his son, who has remained in the pen. Charlie is concentrating on digging up the ground with his foreleg then anointing his head and other important parts. Honky merely stares. The small herd of hinds stand behind Charlie. The stags are probably weighing each other up as adversaries for the forthcoming breeding season – the rut. Before Honky escaped from the pen, Charlie was no great threat. In the first two years of his life, he was allowed to stay with the hinds during the rut, but the last two years, Honky has increasingly chased him away and he has lead a solitary existence at the opposite end of the pen. I doubt that he is strong enough to seriously challenge his father, although he is heftier than he was. Honky is magnificent – full head of evenly balanced antlers, neck thickened and hairy due to surging hormones. I wouldn't challenge him, but the fence wire between them has given Charlie false bravado.

Heading home, I think I feel rain but it is droplets propelled upward from the stubble. Water collects in the cut straw and scatters when brushed by my wellies. However rain is predicted and coming up the valley is a homogeneous sheet of grey obscuring all features of the landscape. Time to move quicker.

Beating the rain, I start the supper early and set it on the stove to cook slowly before settling to inspect my new toy – the pulse oximeter/carbon dioxide monitor. Yes, I succumbed – at great expense. A recent article in the *Veterinary Record* predicts the future of the veterinary profession as a network of regional hospitals with satellite surgeries like human general practitioners. The GPs will refer all complicated cases to the hospitals. It is bound to come, it is impossible for all surgeries to keep up with the prices of new, increasingly sophisticated equipment – and to gain specialist expertise too. Present day graduates are educated to the peak of expertise with cutting-edge technology, and are often dissatisfied with mundane practice life. After an all-too-short period, they vote with their feet and leave the profession. At a conference recently, one specialist was even quoted as saying that we need to lose our *James Herriot* image. Why? Specialists may be flavour of the month just now, but they are not always needed. A simple GP can alleviate much suffering by curing simple things; and not all clients want or can afford the full monty. I'm sure I am not alone in thinking that the *James Herriot* image is really pretty special.

Anyway, this latest pulse oximeter has come with a vast instruction manual which is heavy going. I make myself comfortable in the rocking chair by the Rayburn to scan the contents. One of the more indigestible passages goes as follows:

If the carbon dioxide sensor is initially connected and operating and then;
the carbon dioxide sensor is unplugged, or
the airway adaptor tube is removed from the carbon dioxide sensor, or
the airway adaptor tube becomes damaged or
the light path is blocked, or
a carbon dioxide sensor failure occurs
then a medium priority (equipment) audible alarm is started (unless the audible alarms are disabled or
unless an audible high priority (animal) alarm is in progress).

Good grief! Taking this in is going to take some time.

I wake somewhat bleary-eyed next morning. While Jay was watching football, I spent all yesterday evening perusing a 1760 and an 1890 map of this area, trying to pin down exactly where the old road might have gone. The new road is in place on the newer map, but there are tracks over the hill which appear to correspond roughly to the original old road seen on the 1760 map. There is not much detail on the older map, and comparison between these maps and the present-day one is not easy as they are all different scales. After much work with a calculator, I have eventually come up with guidelines for further investigation *on site*. There is more afforestation now than in the past, and few obvious features to use as frames of reference, so my instructions seem rather complicated – *Pace out 176 yards up the stream from northwest corner of east woods; double-check by pacing 80 yards due south from the top of Fern Law.* Luckily, there are only two routine operations today, so there may be a chance to put theory to the test this afternoon.

After morning surgery, *another* visit to Jock the electrician's shop. He has still one or two jobs to finish at the farm surgery, and we are still waiting for him to put an electricity supply into the museum. I have been calling in once a week to remind him, but now that the weather is turning cooler, I am intensifying my campaign. The frequency and fervour of my visits will be increased until we finally get some action. 'He's just rushed off his feet with grain dryers breaking down,' explains his long-suffering assistant Bunty, 'If only folk would get them serviced in July before they need them. But I'll see that he comes up at the beginning of next week.' The poor woman does her best, but Jock is a law unto himself. It is just the unfortunate Bunty who takes the flak from disgruntled (indeed desperate) customers. Coming home, the thought strikes me that Jock could have done the work in July when he *wasn't* servicing grain dryers.

Operations finished and safely handed out, it is time to test some theories about the old road. Armed with dogs and compass, I head to the North-east corner of the east woods and follow the stream uphill, counting my carefully regulated and measured paces. Unbelievably, within yards of the measured distance I can see remains of an old bridge across the stream, and a track – which I always thought was a fire break in the trees – heading through the woods. Compass in hand,

I follow the track to the edge of the plantation. Incredibly, pacing due North from here brings us to the top of Fern Law, just as anticipated from studying the old maps. Isn't it wonderful when things work out just as you expect them too.

Feeling elated, I summon the dogs and we retrace the entire route followed by the old road. I am presently reading a book about the old Scottish farmtouns (farming communities) and can vividly imagine who might be travelling on this route, heading past Fern Farm and on to Dhu property: perhaps a merchant selling basic wares, a horseman heading to the smithy near Abbeygate Farm or even an orra loon off to collect flour or oatmeal from the mill at Dhu. From the book, it appears that most farm workers existed virtually on a diet of oatmeal in various guises – not least the porridge poured into a drawer in the unmarried men's bothy so slabs could be cut off to stave off hunger pangs during the long busy day. Our house once consisted of two cottages and an attached bothy – perhaps some of these very men trekked along this very path. The next project is to trace the road in the opposite direction, but that must wait for another day.

This evening we are off for a much-needed weekend off in Pitdreel. Any chance of a long lie in the morning is once again scuppered by dogs desperate for a wee, so, struggling into clothes, we head off to the point. It is a still, misty morning – the tide out and the horizon obscured by haar. The mournful sound of the foghorn blares in the distance. Cormorants dry their wings on the exposed rocks, looking like mini 'flashers' and eiderducks bob in the waves. Some seals have hauled out on the rocks – their heavy expirations and barks quite reminiscent of our rutting stags. First walk of the day over, we return for a leisurely breakfast, the make-up of which can be decided at the last moment – it is such a novelty to be so close to the shops. While Jay nips to the general store for butter, milk and marmalade, I pop next door for some fresh bread and rolls. The beguiling smell of baking bread from the bakers tends to make breakfast a foregone conclusion. Blood up for more medical antiques, the morning is spent in a trawl round the local antique shops, but no luck, just a package of stamps for Alice's collector husband. All we ask is that if there is anything valuable, then we get a cut!

The afternoon sees us metal-detecting on the beach. The dogs are in heaven, charging headlong into the water. Fintry looks scared of the crash of waves on seaweed, but gets over it, while Kippen wades ever deeper and is bowled over by the incoming tide. We are poised to rescue him but he seems to be enjoying the experience. I make a mental note to increase his dose of pills tonight. The detector detects several drinks cans buried in the sand, before a strong signal emanates from deeper underground. Intriguingly, the signal seems to be from something circular. Enthusiastic digging uncovers an old car tyre – obviously a *steel* radial.

The mist returns with the dusk, making our late evening walk spookily atmospheric. Tendrils of mist swirl round the old-fashioned street lights suddenly tugging at childhood memories – as a young child, one of my pastimes was to accompany the local *leerie* (lamplighter) on his route round our small town, carrying a long pole with which to light the gas mantles. 'Can you remember what the leeries actually *did* with their pole?' I ask a bemused Jay. 'I can't help you there – we had electric lights,' is the smug reply. This is not a reflection on our relative ages, I hasten to add, only the difference between a country and a city upbringing in the early sixties; it obviously took longer for electrification to hit small town streets.

The dogs are regular vandals on the evening stroll, straining on their leads to follow up fascinating smells or grab dropped chips from the nearby chippie. Living in a town – albeit a very small one – is obviously a novelty for them as well.

Chapter 39

There is much roaring up the hill this morning as both stags get into the spirit of the rut. The young stag is nearly black after plenty enthusiastic wallowing. Part of the courtship ritual is to urinate in mud then roll in the resulting mire – 'He wouldn't be roaring like that if he was on the same side of the fence as his father,' says Sheila darkly, bringing a sick cat in for examination, 'And God knows what his offspring will be like, his antlers are like corkscrews.' Honky meanwhile is mournfully bellowing through the fence, imitating the creak of an old heavy door.

Sheila's cat is slobbering profusely and shakes his head when I try to look in his mouth, sliming

everywhere within a four-foot radius – 'He's worse than a St Bernard' I exclaim, dodging gobbets of slobber as best I can. When we finally get to see in his mouth, it is clear that his tongue is badly ulcerated at the tip. It looks like he has licked up some corrosive substance – household bleach is a hot favourite. Painkiller and antibiotic cover is called for, together with soft warm food.

It must be cat substance abuse week, as tonight yields another case. A young male cat, Jiff, appeared home last night with a smelly, stained leg. His owner sensibly bathed him but he has been shaking the leg and is quite out of sorts. There is still a faint aroma from the leg, familiar but hard to pinpoint ... oil, diesel, creosote? I explain to the owners that there are several potential hazards once an animal is coated with toxic material – the first is skin damage at the soiled site; then there may be mouth ulceration from licking the substance; there is also the risk of gastrointestinal damage if any is swallowed, and finally organ damage if any is absorbed into the circulation. Jiff's mouth is clear and he has been eating, so intestinal and organ damage are less likely, but the skin of the affected leg is rather inflamed and obviously uncomfortable. It can take three to four days for the full extent of skin damage to appear, and we will occasionally see animals brought into the surgery with large skin sloughs after a history of some spillage or soiling. The owner thinks that the danger is past when no immediate symptoms show up, but the skin cells are already dying off, leading to a disaster in a few days' time. As with Sheila's cat, I administer antibiotic, adding corticosteroid in an attempt to reduce inflammation and pain. The owners were correct in bathing the leg immediately but unfortunately only used water. Tonight they are going to repeat the process using *Swarfega* or washing-up liquid – both good at dislodging oily deposits. They are also going to mount a search round the nearby sheds and garages to try to find the source of the contamination.

The last patient is disappointing – a cat who had a tear on his hip sutured last week. The wound has broken down and is badly infected. Suspicious as to why this has happened, I suggest blood tests to check for any immuno-suppressive viruses, as well as cleansing and re-suturing the wound. The blood is duly taken and Jay will drop it into the lab in the morning on the way to work. Meantime, I administer antibiotics and painkiller (again) and settle Squeak into a kennel for the night.

Nobbled by Sheila earlier in the day, I set off at dusk to put her ducks away. It is nearly dark just after 7 p.m. but while I herd recalcitrant birds into their house, the dull thrum of the combine harvester still reverberates across the field, and the powerful headlights lurch towards me through the dark. Colin and John are obviously going for broke to finish the harvest before the much-forecasted rain. Apparently, this has been the worst harvest since 1985, and there is considerable disgruntlement and depression within the farming community.

First job of the next day is to see to Squeak in his kennel. Unfortunately, his blood results are damning – he is positive for feline immunodeficiency virus, an infection very similar to human immunodeficiency virus. As in humans, the virus lowers the body's defences and leaves them prey to infections which would never usually cause a problem.

I *thought* I smelt a rat with this cat. Unfortunately, the extent of Squeak's problems are underlined by the results of his blood analysis – his white cell count and platelet count are both low. The former are necessary to fight infections, and the latter are important for efficient blood clotting. Cats infected with FIV can live for years and Squeak was so much better after the treatment given on Tuesday night that his owner and I opted to tidy up his wound and see how things go – *Give him enough rope to hang himself* – sounds a bit stark, but is essentially the way of it.

He is very cheerful this morning, yowling for food, nice clean wound. As he is an outdoor cat and pesters his owner unmercifully if kept in the house, we decided that he should stay here for a few days to allow his wound to begin to heal in a clean environment, and to encourage him to rest. At home, he would be following his owner about, but he has little else to do in a kennel but sleep. Certainly he looks the picture of a happy, healthy cat this morning. He was slightly stand-offish when he first came in, but is now pathetically grateful for any attention. This happens a lot with hospitalised patients and must be similar to the bonding that occurs between prisoners and their captives: the Stockholm effect I believe it is called. Certainly having inmates causes a big chunk to be taken out of my day, devoted to feeding, cleaning and just generally talking, cuddling and playing with them. There is an added side-effect in that I get rather more attached to the patient than I would like – if things don't go well, then it is a thoroughly miserable experience for me as well as for the owners.

Thursday is generally Sheila's day for routine operations – although she does tend to spill on to most other days too – and she has been busy trapping ferals so the day is going to be busy. This batch seem to be an accident-prone lot. The first spay has a band of scar tissue completely round her abdomen just in front of her hind legs – she has probably been caught in a snare at some time. It is not pleasant to think of how she must have suffered before she escaped. Luckily, she appears fit enough, but it has left her a little pinch-waisted like a Victorian lady with a corset.

The next cat is worse, he has no back foot, just a tangle of ankle bones embedded in a mass of dark tissue. A car or train probably did the deed, and he has been running about like this for weeks until the neighbours were put in contact with Sheila. Several other charities were contacted, but none turned out. Although I do get annoyed with Sheila sometimes for taking on too much work, I can see how hard it is for her to refuse when everyone else has. Unbelievably, the cat is in good condition and has been eating well (unlike Squeak, he has good body defences), so he gets castrated and the leg amputated. The folk next door to the site where he lives have been feeding him and are prepared to give him a home in their shed. Although they cannot touch him, they have got quite fond of him.

Years ago, in my city practice, we used to get animals in quite regularly with limbs amputated by trains. Trains seem to do quite a good job of it. Possibly they cauterise as they go? In later years, we hardly saw any. I did wonder whether this coincided with the advent of faster trains which took no prisoners. I warn Sheila that the operation is not for the squeamish – the cut muscle tends to twitch in an off-putting fashion, and the sawing through bone has seen off many observers in the past.

'I just shut my eyes at the bad bits,' she says cheerfully. I can't resist replying 'So do I!' In fact, the cat's muscle has wasted considerably in the weeks post-accident so the job is done in double-quick time. Sheila will keep the cat in one of her kennels until he is due his stitches out, then he will return to his new home. Like Squeak, it is quite likely that this period of enforced captivity will tame him up, so on his return he may be friendly enough to ingratiate himself into the good Samaritans' nice warm house.

Despite our non-routine neutering session, there is time before evening surgery for a decent walk. It is a crisp autumn day, mellow sunlight bathing our progress through crunchy tan leaves. Looking down into the farmyard, I can see the combine in the yard, no doubt getting its once-over before its winter hibernation. The sound of the grain dryer drifts upwards in the still air. No time is being wasted, the freshly harvested field is being limed by a farming contractor – to counteract excess acidity in the soil. Round by the thinking stones, John is burning straw lying in the field, too spoilt by the rains to bale. He has lit each end of each furrow and the flames are wicking along , raising multiple plumes of smoke – it could be a volcanic valley. The heat haze distorts the field and forest in the distance. Burnt fragments rise on thermals, dance wildly then, suddenly released, plummet earthwards. The loud crackling of the fire echoes in the wood behind the stones, sending Fintry off at the gallop in search of noisy creatures. The whole scene is very impressive, and I watch the show from my perch before ambling back through the woods.

I have a mission to accomplish here at some time – Jay's mother has a new hobby – folk-painting, where old kitchen and farm utensils are revitalised by being painted with bright colouful roses and daisies. There is an old rubbish tip in the woods where past generations of farm incumbents have dumped their rubbish with a happy disregard for the environment. The diggings of wild creatures have exposed some interesting finds such as my hen pail and an old pitchfork, and I have seen old enamel kettles and tins lying under the ferns. I have volunteered to collect some likely utensils for Mary's forthcoming visit.

'No time like the present,' I grunt, sliding down the steep mossy banking in pursuit of a half-buried kettle. It has no bottom ... but I don't expect that will matter if it is just to be an ornament. Lying in the vacated hole is another interesting find – it is covered in mud and moss, but it does look very much like a miniature enamel bath. Perhaps the lady of the house had a doll's house. Anyway, I throw it in the back of the car intending to give it to whoever of the D*olls' house six* next appears at the surgery.

I have seen Jiff, the oiled cat, on a daily basis since he first came in. He is being a real cliff-hanger – will his skin slough, or will it not? Tonight, he is improved, but his skin is still red and obviously uncomfortable. He walks as if someone has spilt hot water on his trousers. His owner's detective work has paid off, he found a tank of central-heating oil surrounded by a moat of uncovered oil. He has informed the relevant people, and steps have been taken to seal off the oil. At least no other animals will get caught.

By one of life's strange coincidences, Mavis of dolls' house fame drops into the surgery for a repeat prescription and becomes the proud owner of the 'bath'. After thanking me, she has only one thing to say on her way out of the door 'Get digging!'

Jiff and owner are already in the waiting room when I arrive at Clayfern surgery the following morning. My heart does that little dip that it does – *Has the skin begun to fall off?* If the whole area sloughs, then we will have real problems. No need to worry, Jiff is in fact much improved, the only reason for their early appearance is that they have an appointment later this morning, and it seemed sensible to get the trip to the vet's over with early. Advising Jiff's owner to keep an eye on the leg – he knows what to look for now – I sign them off until next week.

It is a light ops day, only two routine neuterings, so there is plenty time to attend to Squeak, who remains very cheerful, and to sort items to sell at tomorrow's antique fair. I stand in the museum surrounded by my collection, trying to decide what to part with. I am still very much in the collecting phase of my interest. In the background, I hear the roaring of the stags. Looking up the hill, I can see Honky camped by the fence like a protester at a military base, roaring balefully to himself. Charlie is still at his digging and anointing. His roaring has an intriguing variation to the usual out-of-tune groaning – he is making *oof-oof-oof* sounds like an outboard motor. Watching and listening to their antics really does add spice to our days.

Before morning surgery on Saturday, Jay and I are unpacking our wares at the Stramar antique fair. There is the usual feeling of happy anticipation, the thrill of the chase. Julie and Bill are also laying out their stock 'Is that Noritake?' I enquire, trying to appear knowledgeable 'No, it's very tacky!' Bill replies, deadpan. 'You can put your glasses on my salver,' I offer, watching Julie unwrapping a set of crystal goblets. Quick as a flash, Bill plonks his spectacles on the silver tray. He is definitely on form today. There is the usual visitation by the other dealers before the hall opens to the public.

My chemist's jars go quickly – probably under priced as they are snatched away with such alacrity. Never mind, we are in profit and feel like real traders. I do my usual disappearing act for morning surgery, then dash back to find we are having a good day. One trader has some wares which might interest me – they do indeed. One is an 1836 graduation certificate from the Dick veterinary school in Edinburgh. The graduate had attended for two years (we do five years now) and was thereby qualified as a vet. The certificate is actually signed by William Dick, the very founder of the veterinary school which only opened its doors in 1823. In the same house clearance were also two old instruments which the dealer assumes are also veterinary tools. I think so too. Even better, he has two delicate blades ensheathed in tortoiseshell cases – these are *lancets*, the human equivalent of the stouter veterinary *fleams*: both instruments were used for blood-letting, a common treatment for all sorts of ailments. At the end of the day, the caterers give us doggy bags of their leftover scones and cakes – apparently we are their best customers.

Flushed from today's successes, we are just settling down for an evening in when the telephone goes. Ferdy the cat has been sick today and now appears collapsed – there goes our cosy evening. When he arrives, the cat looks dreadful. He is lying flat out with dry gums, sunken eyes and cold feet and ears. His temperature is below normal – he is in shock, but why? The only symptom of note apart form the vomiting is that he might have been drinking more than normal, his owner thinks, but it is hard to be certain as he usually drinks from the garden pond.

As I examine him, possibilities run through my head – severe gastroenteritis, tumour, kidney or liver failure, and more. I can feel a large bladder in his abdomen and express its contents into a dish before testing it with a urine dipstick. It is loaded with glucose, ketones and blood. Diabetes moves to the top of the diagnostic table. Although Ferdy has not eaten for twenty four hours, a drop of blood loaded into the glucometer (a device for measuring glucose levels in blood) gives a reading so high that it is off the scale. Ferdy is almost in a *keto-acidotic* coma. As diabetics cannot utilise blood glucose for energy, the body breaks down other body tissues to provide an alternative source. This breakdown produces toxic byproducts (which we measure as ketones) which poison the system.

As he is such an outdoor cat, the owners have missed the most obvious clues – the increased drinking and urinating. The most pressing concerns are to raise Ferdy's temperature and to dilute the toxins in his blood stream. Heaters are cranked up to achieve sauna-like temperatures, bubble-wrap is broken out and, with difficulty, I find and insert a catheter into a vein, running fluid in as rapidly as I dare. After twenty minutes fluid, I inject a small dose of quick-acting insulin. In the normal treatment of diabetics, we use long-acting insulin so that only one or two injections are necessary in a twenty four hour period, but in an emergency, short-acting insulin is used to rapidly bring down the blood glucose levels. The drip is slowed to a maintenance rate, and I take another blood sample in an hour – glucose level still off the scale; body temperature hasn't moved much either, not encouraging. More insulin injected and on we go.

After three hours, it is sadly obvious that we are getting nowhere, the cat is looking worse – if that is possible – he has developed heart irregularities and is more unconscious than conscious. Enough is enough – I telephone his owner and break the sad tidings that we are not winning; with her permission I put him to sleep.

I have no sooner draped myself over the settee in anticipation of one of the caterer's scones and a cup of tea, when the phone goes again. I go to answer it with the usual feeling of incredulity that it should ring again so soon. Illogically one feels that one should somehow be immune to further calls after a busy session. Unbelievably, it is also a diabetic cat, but this one has gone in the opposite direction. She has been on insulin and has no glucose in her blood stream. Like Ferdy, she is collapsed, cold and shocked, but the glucometer measures a resounding zero when her blood sample is inserted. She has either had too much insulin, too much exercise or too little food, and all the glucose has been hauled from her circulation. Her heart is worryingly slow and deliberate, often a prelude to imminent death. There is no fuel to power her brain and she is unconscious. Unfortunately, her owners have just come in and found her like this. If they had been with her, they would have seen the earlier signs of *hypoglycaemia*: slow and tottery at first, degenerating into fits, then finally coma. Her outlook is poor but we have to try.

Poor Jay is once again press-ganged into wrapping the patient in bubblewrap, holding the oxygen mask against her face and attempting to raise non-existent veins for me to canulate. In desperation, I finally hit a vein using a hypodermic needle and slowly inject concentrated glucose solution before connecting to a drip. Not surprisingly in such an extreme case, our resuscitation efforts fail. Not a happy evening, although it somehow seems less traumatic when the patients are virtually unconscious. Wryly, it crosses my mind that we are certainly in practice for diabetic awareness week.

It is still nearly dark at 7 a.m. but the stags are shouting as disharmoniously as ever, accompanied by a pair of owls. A skein of geese go over, also honking off-key. Why is it that all winter creatures vocalise out of tune?

Up the hill for the morning walk with the stags roaring in the background like prehistoric monsters. They keep it up all night, and must be somewhat exhausted by now.. Staring at the east woods from the thinking stones, a movement catches my eye. A fir branch is waving frantically up and down. I can see Honky's white outline in the background – could he have got his antlers entangled? Moving closer, wondering what to do if this is the case, I am relieved to see the stag moving off into the woods. In his wake is a trail of devastation – trunks and branches stripped of bark, and shredded branches holding on by the merest threads of mangled wood. The poor lad must be really frustrated. At this fraught time of year, I think we'll give him a wide berth. 'I don't remember her having a khaki leg,' I think, watching Fintry returning to the car. The little sod has rolled in deer doo-doo. She will need a bath when we get home. As I drive down the hill with the windows open, I admit that it could be worse – fox dirt is truly disgusting whereas deer is really not too bad, just a rather musty agricultural aroma.

Driving to work, I can see hordes of brown and white geese in the fields. They seem uneasy, with odd batches swirling skywards and moving to a safer pitch. There is always one who can't quite keep up and flaps frantically in the others' wake. Squeak is with me today. He has been doing so well that he is going home today, and will be picked up from Clayfern surgery. It is always quite a relief to have an empty surgery again – at least until Sheila appears after morning surgery with her latest batch of neuterings. However, they don't have any hidden extras today so we are finished by lunchtime. This is good news for me, there is time to exercise the dogs, have a bite to eat and manage to attend the art group in Clayfern. This is a loose-knit assembly who meet in the local community centre. We have a teacher but there are no rigid lessons, we paint what we like, while he is on hand to advise and answer queries. The two hours out of the day doing something completely different are very relaxing, and no one takes themselves too seriously. Most of us are probably there for the social crack as much as anything.

Don't ask me how, but in the coffee break, we get on to the subject of my clippers from the auction. One of our number used to have a croft in days gone by and remembers entering a neighbour's byre one day to find one crofter cranking the handle and cutting another's hair. It was harvest time and there was no spare time to visit the barber. There is an amusing postscript to this story – apparently the shorn crofter had an English wife and when he next visited the village barber, the barber cast a disbelieving glance over his crop before carefully enquiring 'And was it an *English* barber that cut your hair last?'

Still reading the farmtoun book, I find that it was the usual practice on the touns for one of the cottars (married farmworkers) to cut all the other farmhands' hair: the cottar's croppin', as it was called.

Squeak is in for a check-up during evening surgery. He is bright enough but his wound is healing more slowly than normal. I think we'll just keep on with the antibiotics as well. The next client brings in her cat, but asks if Alice can hold the animal. 'She's not a bad cat, is she?' I enquire, slightly puzzled. 'Oh no, she's lovely,' her owner replies, 'But I'm being treated for cancer and the drugs have knocked out my immunity.' 'We've just had a cat in with the same problem,' seems the only logical comment.

A rude shock during morning surgery two days later – Squeak has taken a turn for the worse over the last two days. The stitches have broken down and he is pallid and lifeless. There is no other option but to put him to sleep. It seems so unfair when he was doing so well, but, I suppose, thats life. He was a nice little cat – I will miss him. The next patient is also depressing – a small rabbit who was in on Friday with inflamed eyes. I was a little anxious about him at the time as there was a suggestion of thickening about the eyelids, and this can be a symptom of *myxomatosis*, a serious viral disease of rabbits. However, the rabbit was eating and appeared quite bright so I gave him some treatment, explaining my fears to his owner – or rather his owner's mother, often the common situation with children's pets. Poor Mum gets all the dirty work. 'I think you might be right,' she says sadly, lifting the now quiet and miserable bunnie out of his box. He is a lot worse and we decide to call it a day, although I do give Mum the option of continuing with treatment. I have tried treating victims of myxomatosis, but have very seldom been successful. They have an unfortunate habit of showing an initial improvement, then hanging in the balance for a few days before going downhill again, a routine which is hard on everyone's emotions. The lady's mother is terminally ill in hospital, and she feels that the family cannot cope with another long-drawn out trauma, I am inclined to agree. 'The next one will be vaccinated,' she says firmly.

Not the best of days. The cure is a leisurely amble through the east woods gathering some kindling for the fire. At least tomorrow is a day off.

We are indulging ourselves as Jay's mother is visiting and having a day off today. An expedition is planned – to the *Barras*, Glasgow's famous weekend market. Sheila is going to see to the dogs at lunchtime but I am up early to exercise them before we go. I am wakened early anyway by the crowing of Sheila's cockerel – 'Is he not locked in with the others?' I enquire when I speak to her about the dogs. 'Its not mine, he's been abandoned!' she tells me. This is a novelty. Both vets and charities are used to the occasional dog or cat left on their doorstep, but a cockerel …? I shouldn't think Mr Fox will leave him alone if Sheila cannot entice him into a safe haven overnight. The fox comes round even if she is just a little late putting the hens and ducks away.

It is pleasant up the hill this morning – another gorgeous October day. We catch four roe deer unawares in the stubble field and watch them bolt for the woods. Geese honk overhead, their undersides catching the early sun. A pheasant answers their honks with its chattering cry. Honky and Charlie are both lying down, one on each side of the fence. It seems to be something of a stalemate. They are probably both desperate for something to eat but neither likes to make the first move. It would be interesting to watch to see who weakens first but I mustn't lose the advantage of our early start.

The *Barras* are the same as ever, just as in my student days. I became the proud owner of a sit-up-and-beg bicycle then, and commuted happily to and from the vet school for the last two years of the course. I don't think I would like to face the traffic on a bike nowadays. You can find anything at the *Barras*, old and new clothing; old and new furniture; household supplies; food stalls; and our favourites, the bric-a-brac stalls. We are attracted to the anonymous, dusty boxes at the back of the scruffiest stalls – that is where you find the real bargains. Mary is in there like a ferret, rooting for likely objects to be folk-painted. At the end of the day she has collected an old shoe last, a woodworking plane, an old oil lamp and a battered rolling pin. Carrying that lot about is good exercise, and no prizes for guessing what we will be getting for Christmas.

The food stalls are popular too – we start with doughnuts, then after an hour of rummaging, visit the seafood bar in the heart of the market for big steaming bowls of mussels in their barnacled shells, and peeled prawns.

'They have *clabby dooes!*' I exclaim, reading the menu board, and Jay braces for the familiar reminiscence. As a student, I learnt scuba diving, travelling to the west coast of Scotland which boasts excellent diving in the deep sea lochs cutting far inland. Clabby dooes are large mussels, the shells almost the size of my hand. Proudly bearing three home in my diving bag one day, I rang two friends and invited them round for *moules mariniere*. Being Norwegian, my friends were very 'into' fresh produce, and this seemed to be my chance to shine. As they settled round the table, I poured everyone a wine – the remainder of that added to the mussels on the stove – and lifted the lid with a flourish. What a surprise! I had expected the mussels' size to correspond with their shells, but in fact, they were no larger than ordinary mussels. All that shell to house such insignificant wee things. So, instead of a large beefy mussel each, we had a large quantity of wine soup with a solitary mussel nestling in the corner of the bowl, all but obscured by strands of spring onion. That was the last of my efforts at haute cuisine. I confined any future attempts to impress the

Norwegians to the production of guid Scottish fare such as stovies and skirlie. Jay must have heard this tale several times but still laughs loyally whenever it is aired, and the episode certainly amuses Mary.

The day passes quickly: some books and socks for Jay; a jacket for me and an old optician's test kit – a home-made box housing dozens of lenses and the familiar poster with different sized lines. The familiar excuse now is that it has been bought 'to sell on'. We pass on the horse's harness (too mouldy) and fill up on chips and hot dogs before finally hitting the road home. We have only been away for five hours but feel very rested and relaxed. It proves the point that a change is better than a rest.

Chapter 40

The big excitement of the day is the commissioning of our new biochemical analyser. Owning such a machine has been out of the question in the past as they are so expensive, but the company has come up with a scheme for renting them, and, as usual, I have succumbed – for a trial period anyway. We have a good service from the local lab, but the thought of obtaining results within minutes is very attractive. Murphy's Law frequently prevails with the really sick animals turning up on Friday evening or at weekends when the lab is shut. The company representative is here, so are Julie and Alice and the atmosphere is almost festive. I am a great believer in safety in numbers when learning to operate complex machinery, but the device is remarkably simple. The screen 'walks' the operator through the procedure one step at a time.

'I need my glasses to see the screen,' mumbles Julie, beginning again our long-running joke about growing older together in harness. Even nowadays in colder weather, operating sessions are interspersed by trips to the loo and she visualises that in ten years, we will only be able to tackle cat spays or castrations (both quite short procedures) – 'Or get catheters fitted.'

Of course, being semi-geriatric, it has slipped my mind that we need blood to analyse, so while the nurses and rep. sort out the buns for elevenses, I go in search of a victim. It would be interesting to know Kippen's blood situation, I think, luring him to the surgery with a chew. The poor dog is probably thinking 'Oh no, *another* hair cut.' His leg is trimmed up and anointed with local before the blood-letting. The blood is then spun in the centrifuge – this separates the blood cells from the plasma, the clear fluid on which most biochemical tests are done. The machine works by shining light through the test fluid, but unfortunately Kippen's sample produces a very milky plasma. This is because it is *lipaemic* or fatty. This is why blood samples are best carried out on starved patients – the milky colouration may affect the tests. I muse that it might be tricky with Kippen to get six hours without food – it would probably have to be syringes at dawn! We run the tests anyway, following the instructions on the screen. The machine provides a handy countdown *5 minutes to results, 4.50 minutes to results* etc, building tension nicely so by the final entry *Prepare for results* Julie suggests she should bring me a chair and perhaps a double brandy. The results appear both on a little till roll and on a more elaborately printed sheet (to impress the punters). By and large, the old dog's results fall within normal range; two are elevated but this is probably due to the fatty sample. I will probably re-check him at a later date. Anyway, mission accomplished, another arrow added to our diagnostic quiver.

Quite a dramatic emergency tonight – a young cat was attacked by the family dog two hours ago and the owner reports that she has just 'gone quieter.' The understatement of the year. The cat is lying on her chest with her nose touching the floor. Her head is floppy and her eyes are semi-dilated and non-responsive to light. Her circulation and pulse are okay but she is definitely 'out to lunch.' I can feel a depression on the top of her head – indicative of a skull fracture. The damaged bone has been pushed inwards. What to do next? I decide to go with medical treatment initially, with the possibility of surgical intervention if there is no response. The latter course would be a last resort. She would be a tricky anaesthetic and vets are not skilled neurosurgeons. Any surgery would be limited to attempting to move impacted bone out of the brain. I administer steroids to reduce inflammation and pain, antibiotic and a diuretic (drug to induce urination) to drag fluid out of the possibly swollen brain, then institute checks every five minutes, remaining in the surgery with a cup of tea and a magazine. For an hour she remains static, then an improvement is seen – she passes urine and becomes gradually more responsive. After two hours, she is compos mentis again. I ring the owner with the glad tidings. I suspect that human medics would be rather envious of our patients' impressive powers of recovery

By morning, our in-patient is completely back to normal, purring happily and tucking into a large breakfast. She will come into Clayfern surgery to be handed back to her owner. After tidying her up and feeding her, it is time for the morning dog walk. We have only time to walk along the track past the farm. The farmer has begun to provide hay for the cattle in the field, and they are clustered round the circular metal frame which encloses the large bale. There is not much of yesterday's left, and they head rapidly towards the gate when the tractor approaches with this morning's ration.

Morning surgery is busy, and it is a rush to return to the farm surgery in time to admit the morning's operations. We have some charity neuterings and three dentals. That will keep us out of mischief for the day. The puppies for neutering are a cute lot. Despite being from the same litter, there is tremendous variation in their appearance and temperament. First out is Miss Anxious, a white, long-haired female who seems to be carrying all the world's worries on her shoulders. Diligent cuddling on Julie's part does not erase the anxious expression from her face, and a tail wag is out of the question. Just as well we are doing her first or she would no doubt be worrying in the kennel. The next pup is completely the opposite: Mr Cool, a lanky black chap, lies happily on his back while I prepare his anaesthetic injection. Julie tickles his tummy and the pup squirms in delight and tries to nibble her ears. The prick of the needle goes unnoticed as patient and nurse engage in an intimate conversation, tail-batting gives way to a brief yawn then he is suddenly unconscious. Mr Hyperactive, a shrimp of a pup, yells for attention from the kennel thus ensuring that he is done next. Despite his earlier sedative injection, he is a real handful for Julie to restrain, while I go cross-eyed trying to aim for his vein. The little ones are always the worst. Luckily, puppy veins stand out well and in a shake of his tail, he too is unconscious. We both enjoy our puppy days – they are always such happy little people. An hour after the last one is finished, they are playing in their kennel. Even Miss Anxious is persuaded to produce a coy tail wag. Obviously the ordeal was not as horrible as she had feared.

A quick cup of tea, a sandwich and a toffee doughnut and we are ready to face the afternoon. On some Tuesdays, we do not have the luxury of a break, and carry on till after 4 p.m., by which time it hardly seems worth having lunch. Dental work is always left until last as these are messy procedures. The ultrasonic scaler and the drill produce a fine mist which contains bacteria, and it is generally accepted that such a mist can take over an hour to clear from the environment. It is also because of this that I wear a mask while performing dental work. Having said that, Julie reckons that, while waiting for a piece of doughnut, my dogs produce more spray than the dental scaler. The first dog is easy, merely a scale and polish. Even although his mouth is not bad in the scheme of things, it still takes a good thirty five minutes to remove all debris from each tooth, then polish the surface until it is perfectly smooth. Any rough patches provide a focus for plaque and tartar to collect on. Now he has a clean sheet, so to speak, it is important for his owner to carry on with home dental hygiene. A daily brushing with special pet toothpaste is just the very thing. Pet toothpaste is not minty like ours, but has exciting flavours like chicken, malt and beef. This cleverly increases the pets' cooperation, and teeth-cleaning sessions work well when turned into a fun time for the animal.

The second dental is slightly more taxing. This dog has cracked his canine tooth while chewing on a stone. The sensitive dental pulp is exposed, causing discomfort and allowing infection access to the tooth root. There are two treatment options – root canal treatment or tooth removal. The former would require referral to a dental specialist and can be relatively expensive, so the owner has gone for removal. The canine tooth is a big solid tooth with as much root under the surface as there is crown visible.

Dog and cat teeth are much more firmly attached to the jaw than human teeth are, and, without the high-speed drill, we would be in for a miserable half an hour or more attempting to dig out the tooth. As the tooth has not been loosened by infection, I opt for a surgical removal. This involves first freeing the gum tissue on each side of the tooth, then the drill is used to remove the bone covering the root. Finally, a channel is cut on each side of the root and an elevator introduced to break down the remaining attachments. Once the tooth is lifted out, the gum tissue is stitched over the resulting cavity – much easier and more painless (for both patient and surgeon) than physically digging out the tooth.

On to dental number three, this time a cat. The poor chap has a condition peculiar to cats: *feline odontoclastic resorptive lesions*, known colloquially as *neck lesions*. For some unknown reason in some cats, the enamel at the junction of the tooth crown and root is resorbed exposing sensitive tissue. Affected teeth are painful, and if the disease process has been on the go for a while, it is quite common for the crown to break off entirely leaving the root embedded in the jaw. Dentals on such patients can be a nightmare as the teeth become extremely fragile and much time can be spent winkling root fragments out from deep within their sockets. Just a smidgeon too much pressure, and the depressing crack of a shearing crown resounds in our ears. After the neck lesion teeth are finally out, there are still several diseased teeth to be removed. Two teeth have three roots and have been likened to tripods embedded in concrete. The drill is invaluable here too – all I need to do is to section the tooth into three single-rooted parts which are relatively easily extracted. An hour later, the final dental is finished, leaving a mere twenty minutes to whip the dogs round the field before leaving for evening surgery.

Typically, evening surgery is mobbed so it is a shattered vet who finally arrives home after 7 p.m. For a small country practice, we do have our moments. I remember waking up next morning thinking 'Well, my body's wrecked but at least my mind feels fresh.' After this morning's surgery, I feel I have the matching set. Each case has been a challenge – no distinguishing features to make diagnosis easy, like wading through mud. Surgery over-runs by half an hour, followed by a further half an hour's telephoning either to refer cases or to chase lab results and report to anxious owners. Yes, all the symptoms are there – we are going away for a long weekend.

The list of complicated cases to discuss with Emma the locum grows ever longer, as does the list to be ordered from the drug wholesalers. Next week is *Pet diabetes awareness week*, and, as we have several diabetics under treatment, I rashly volunteered to produce the window display – forgetting that Jay and I will be away. Today is the last chance to get it ready for Alice to put it up on Saturday. The computer printer is red-hot as I slave over simple but hopefully informative posters. The locum's bedroom has to be prepared and instructions written to cover her stay in the house, including a blow-by-blow account of how the dogs spend their day. We are going to stay with relatives and they are not coming with us. This is the first time that Emma has had to look after them, and I know that they will be appalled if they do not get their daily ration of chews at the appropriate times. Like all owners, I am convinced that they will fret when Mum is not here.

Emma arrives just after evening surgery so I am technically off-duty from then onwards and theoretically free to go off to paint the town red. However, while Emma prepares to visit friends in the area (staying out till after 1 a.m.), we have our supper, watch television and are in bed by 10.30 p.m. If our teenage selves could see us now, they would doubtless be horrified.

We have had an extremely pleasant weekend visiting Tom's family. Full of pride, he showed us his display of bones, pointing out a new skull. 'That was my friend's hamster,' he explained happily, 'I got him to dig it up for me.' 'I'm really impressed that Tom is keeping up his interest in bones,' I commented to Jay later, 'I'm really impressed with his powers of delegation,' was the dry reply.

The weekend passed in a blur of retail therapy and socialising. Jay comes from a very big family while mine is small. Occasionally, I feel the need for solitude and achieve it by walking Mary's dog. The day of one family gathering, my plan backfired. During a lull in the conversation, I announced that I had better take Titch out for ten minutes; 'I'll come with you, Auntie Kate,' piped up Tom, 'So will I'... 'And me,' from Pete and Jeff, 'Just let us get our shoes on,' from our nieces. Like the Pied Piper, I marched along the road closely followed by five kids and a dog. So much for solitude. Seriously though, it was great to see them all again.

Our shopping expeditions were very successful, yielding such diverse items as fan heaters for the surgery; food and quiet fireworks for our impending bonfire night do; and a three-foot high illuminated reindeer for Christmas. That could really irritate Honky.

After Emma leaves for another locum post, I check on an inmate in the surgery – a cat with a lacerated groin which Emma stitched this morning. This cat provides quite a mystery. He has presented with a similar injury at this time of year for each of the last three years. 'Perhaps with the colder weather he tries to climb into a shed through a broken window,' his owner theorises. He must have a really bad memory, I think. It would be interesting to radio-track him next year to solve the problem.

Before evening surgery, Jay and I take the delighted dogs for a walk up the hill. It is dull and windy, and most of the leaves have now fallen. Honky stares at us through the trees, while Mum glides silently away. Since her escape, she has learned to be stealthy. Only months ago, she could be heard crashing around at quite a distance. A buzzard jumps from a branch and parachutes to the track ahead of us, pantalooned legs extended to make contact with a dead rabbit. Suddenly appreciating our presence, he grabs a piece of rabbit and exits skywards before the dogs realise what is happening.

Leaving Jay to light the woodburner and prepare supper, I drive to evening surgery squinting as the setting sun hits the windscreen.

Coming home again, it is now completely dark, the long summer nights but a distant memory.

Our fourteen year old nieces have joined us for the weekend. This is the first time that they have seen our new house, and this is probably the most beautiful time of year to visit. From their bedroom, the coppice of trees shielding the orchard is seen in its full glory: golds, crimsons, yellow and russet form a breathtaking background for orange and red berries. From the kitchen window, I point out our magnificent white stag. He is still dispiritedly circling around the deer pen, but some of his previous urgency has gone. The deer may all be pregnant to his son by now.

I bring a blood sample home for analysis after morning surgery, and proudly demonstrate the workings of our new biochemistry machine to the girls. I love its muted but high-tech-sounding whirrs and clicks as it goes about its business, and am deeply impressed by the smart print-out clearly labelling any abnormal results. In this case, there is evidence of significant kidney malfunction. I am pleased with how quickly a diagnosis has been reached, as this patient was sampled simply because his owner spotted our diabetes window display and realised that an increase in drinking could indicate a problem. A urine sample suggested a diagnosis and the biochemistry has confirmed it. Such prompt diagnosis allows us to treat the dog appropriately, and hopefully prolong his life. I am well pleased that our window display has improved client awareness, even if it has only helped one dog this time. Early diagnosis and treatment is so much better than dealing with a sicker patient later in the course of the illness.

Returning with the girls from a nearby craft fair, we pass local children on their way to a Halloween party at the community centre. Witches, ghosts and goblins rush across streets battered by high wind and heavy rain. Although the weather has turned nasty and going out is not possible, we are going to try to make it a fun evening as befits Halloween. While Jay whips up a large pan of stovies (our speciality), I raid the museum for some of the more intriguing exhibits. While supper cooks, the girls have to guess what they are. There will be prizes for the one with most correct answers. Aileen wins the first point by identifying the horse tail docker; Carol the second with the dental syringe; neither gets the tooth key (the instrument originally used to extract teeth). To Carol, the brass hernia clamp looks like a device to shut a gossip's mouth (she has been watching too many horror films!), while Aileen thinks it might be a horse's hair piece (what the fashionable horses are wearing!). Both right with the pill moulds, half-right with the tonsillectomy guillotines – they both reckon that *something* is amputated by the vicious blade, but cannot come up with what. They cringe when I tell them, both glad that their operations are well in the past. Carol identifies the electric shock machine as an electrified pestle for grinding powders, and Aileen's final guess has us all laughing, she thinks that the brass pill-making machine – a mahogany strip of wood with u-shaped brass indentations which matches a similar layout on a mahogany board – is a mane crimper for horses. Why does she think that horses are obsessed with hair and beauty? After much debate and awarding of extra points for imagination and originality, we proclaim the match a draw and dole out the prizes, admired objects bought covertly at the craft fair.

Aileen helps me to carry the equipment back to the museum while Carol gives Jay a hand to set the table. 'Oh look!' I exclaim, 'There's our frog.' 'What's his name?' Aileen asks. 'He hasn't got one,' I reply. Carol comes to view our little mascot who stands stock still, trying to blend into the stonework beside the museum. 'Gherkin!' she suddenly shouts, crunching on the very same. That is absolutely spot on – the colour and size of her snack exactly matches the frog. 'I don't know how you can eat that now,' the sensitive Aileen asks, squirming in disgust. 'Easy,' Carol replies, crunching loudly on the last of the frog's namesake.

All dawns peaceful and quiet, the high winds and rain have finally gone, as indeed have our nieces. We appear to have an orange garden – all the leaves have been shaken off by the gale and now paper the grass and flower beds. I risk a trip up the hill. It is off limits during the winds as trees often fall like matchsticks – a branch nearly flattened Kippen one gusty day. Sometimes the track is blocked by fallen trees but it is fine today, just a few branches easily thrown to the side.

Leaves lie inches deep as we trek through the woods. The place is alive with squirrels, they are on the ground either burying or retrieving nuts and give Fintry much sport. She is not too fussed about chasing rabbits or roe deer, but squirrels really seem to rattle her cage. They are up the tree trunks and half the forest away before she reaches their previous position but she obviously lives in hope of surprising a slow or dull-witted one. The forest smell is beguiling this morning, spicey and fruity with the occasional aromatic whiff of fresh cut wood as we pass pine branches ripped off by the wind. The golden leaves and larch needles brighten up the ground and more daylight filters through the denuded trees. Previously secret nests are revealed for all to see. There is a sudden commotion as panic-stricken wood pigeons fight their way skywards (if they just kept a bit quieter, perhaps they would alert less predators), and the raucous alarm call of a jay catches their drift. The whole forest is now on guard. More subtle roe deer glide through the distant tree trunks, completely unobserved by the dogs, and no doubt every squirrel is now aloft.

The sun is setting as I drive to evening surgery, and the western sky is spectacular – pink and aquamarine with delicate brush strokes of snowy white clouds. Against this backdrop, a group of rooks fly in to roost in the tall beech trees, calling tunefully to each other.

It is dark after surgery, a cold clear night with millions of stars. I can see my breath in front of me. I call in for petrol and wait to pay the bill. In front of me are two children stocking up for the evening with sweets. Memories of childhood days spent in the local tuck shop flood back as they carefully choose from the selection of penny sweeties on the shelf. First choices are discarded in favour of more exotic delicacies; then reinstated again. The decisions are obviously agonising and the whole procedure takes a good ten minutes before they depart clutching one of this, two of that and several of the other. The attendant and I reminisce when they have gone 'My favourites were *Lucky Bags*,' she says. Mine were *soor plooms* and *pineapple chunks*. Inspired, I buy two fudges for our after-dinner treat, but for some strange reason, when you are grown-up and have (relatively) lots of money to buy goodies, choosing is somehow not as exciting as it was when you were a child.

Chapter 41

An early trip up the hill to take advantage of a gorgeous November morning. There is no wind and it is a sharp, clear day – the air as refreshing as a plunge into ice cold water. The Laigher is still in shade, but pink tinges the northern hills, milky-white clouds mimicking the snow-capped summits. The sun is just rising above the southern hills as we approach the thinking stones, tinging the dying leaves a vivid gold. A skein of geese passes over one way, cawing rooks the other and a woodpecker flits from pine to pine. A flock of tits also moves between the trees, trackeable by their tinkling calls. It appears that all in the avian kingdom are commuting to work. As we walk back along the track, the sun moves higher in the sky, blanketing one side of the hill in rich autumn hues. Kippen lags behind, bathed in a golden glow and surrounded by misty breath – our golden boy, I think sentimentally, the Littlest Hobo.

Wednesdays are normally a quiet day, but a case requiring prompt attention appears during morning surgery, a male Scottie dog who keeps trying to urinate but manages only a dribble. This is potentially an emergency situation. Voiding urine is the body's way of passing toxins out of the system and if urination ceases then urine builds up in the bladder (which in itself is horribly painful), and toxins dam back into the circulation making the patient feel extremely ill. If the situation is not rectified, the bladder can actually burst resulting in peritonitis, shock and eventual death.

Jake is going to keep us occupied over the next few hours. I try to insert a catheter into the dog's bladder, but it stops dead only inches from the tip of his penis. There is obviously an obstruction; probably a bladder stone which has found its way into the urethra. Like a funnel, the urethra narrows on its way to the external urinary opening

– this is particularly pronounced in male dogs. Jake will need surgery to remove the stone. I buy us some time by carefully introducing a hypodermic needle into the distended bladder through the body wall and using a syringe to draw off nearly a hundred ml. of urine. Then Alice helps me to set up a drip before Jake comes with me to the farm surgery where Julie will be waiting. The sick little dog lies quietly in the back of the car with his bag of fluid tied to the dog guard. It seems a little strange perhaps to be adding fluid to a system which can't get rid of it, but the damming-back of urine causes serious disturbances in the body's normal electrolyte balance; so much so, that anaesthetising the patient before beginning to correct the imbalance can result in a dead patient.

The dependable Julie arrives at the farm surgery before me and has prepared the x-ray machine for action, so we transfer the depressed Jake straight on to the x-ray table and position him on an x-ray plate. Although he has received no sedative, he is unnaturally quiet and stays lying on the plate while we back slowly out of range and press the exposure button. X-rays are potentially dangerous things and we have to take precautions for our own safety. We try to avoid being in the x-ray room when a film is shot. The patient is usually rendered cooperative with sedative or even general anaesthetic, and sandbags and ties are used to position them for the picture. There are lead shutters on the machine which can be used to limit the area exposed – we aim for the smallest area necessary to give a useful result – and lead clads the x-ray table to reduce scatter. Being an extremely dense material, it absorbs x-rays and minimises reflected beams. If we need to be anywhere near the machine during an exposure, then we don lead aprons and gloves. We also wear exposure meters which are sent away to be developed every few months and this reassures us that we are not receiving stray radiation.

The developed radiograph confirms my suspicions – Jake has a urinary stone lodged inches from the tip of his penis. This is a common site for obstruction as the urethra narrows significantly here.

The next step is to anaesthetise Jake and remove the stone. Once the area is prepared, I insert a catheter which again is stopped by the stone. However it gives me a guide as to where to open into the urethra. It does not take long to cut on to the catheter and locate the stone, a solid beige-coloured crystal lodged firmly in the urinary tube. Luckily, it is relatively smooth and has not caused too much damage to the urethral mucosa. Urine flows out of the wound as soon as the stone is removed. The x-ray did not show up any other stones either in the urethra or bladder, so the procedure has been gratifyingly quick.

Some surgeons will close the urethrotomy wound, but others, myself included, prefer to leave it open until it heals by itself. Urine will still appear from the wound for the next few days so we will need to warn the owners that Jake's aim will be hopeless for a while. The stone will be sent for analysis at a commercial laboratory. There are several kinds of stones that can be produced in the urinary tract and treatment varies depending on their make-up. Certain stones can even be slowly dissolved by feeding a special diet. If the stones are in the bladder and not causing acute symptoms, they can be monitored by x-ray while the diet is fed – it is quite impressive to produce a series of x-rays showing the stones receding over a period of time. The patient is then switched on to a diet devised to reduce the chances of stone production.

Later in the day, Jake's owners come to visit him. I want to keep him in overnight to monitor his progress. Also, the first twenty four hours post-op are inclined to be rather messy with urine and blood, so he is best confined in a kennel, not redecorating the family home. I give him a clean Vetbed before the visit. With both blood and urine, a little goes a long way and numerous red patches on the bed tend to upset owners. Jake accords his folks a rapturous welcome and the little family have a happy half an hour together. Jake's 'dad' cringes and visibly pales when I explain the operative technique and lift the dog up to demonstrate the wound. Why is it that males take such things personally? Women don't react this way when ovariohysterectomy or mammary tumour removal is discussed. Jake's owner's response stirs an almost forgotten memory from my time as a city vet.

One day I received an emergency call from the police who were in attendance at an accident. A large dog had attempted to jump the railings out of a park but didn't quite make it and was impaled – directly through the scrotum. The scene when I arrived was quite dramatic – two policewomen were attempting to take the weight of the poor dog while their two male partners lurked a good six feet away, looking visibly queasy. Blessing the new generation of anaesthetic drugs which can produce insensibility and pain relief in one small injection, I swiftly administered a generous dose and waited till it took effect. When the dog was asleep, we simply lifted him up and off the railing. When I say 'we,' it was exclusively a female effort as the two burly policemen felt unable to give assistance. The dog came off the spike with a resounding *schloop* which actually caused one of the coppers to turn a sickly green and the other to be physically sick in the gutter. With the unconscious dog safely stowed in the car, I sped off to the surgery where castration was necessary to repair the damage. The dog made a complete recovery and the policewomen no doubt got considerable mileage taunting their colleagues about their less-than-perfect performance at the scene.

Jake is quite cheery the next morning and the large deposits of blood and urine have reduced to a more acceptable spotting. His owner comes to pick him up before morning surgery and I cram yet another load of stained vetbeds into the washing machine. Let's hope that we don't get any emergency admissions before the backlog is washed and dried. The bedding shelves in the surgery have dwindled to a few threadbare towels.

Three rather special cat neuterings are due in today – the three kittens which we delivered by caesarean section some months ago. Pouncer, Bouncer and Flouncer have all grown into fine figures of cats, even Flouncer who took so long to resuscitate post-caesarian.

Next is a precautionary x-ray on a vomiting dog. 'He never picks up anything he hasn't been given,' asserts his owner firmly. Oh, yes? That's not what the x-ray shows: several stones and two substantial nails reside in the large intestine. Luckily, a gloved, lubricated finger assisted by a gentle milking action through the abdominal wall manages to remove the offending obstacles without recourse to exploratory surgery. It is a good policy to check for oneself if a foreign body seems like a possibility; owners often are blissfully unaware of what their pets get up to. 'He's been in the garden while we've been re-roofing the shed,' his owner belatedly recalls. That explains the nails anyway. I suspect that stone-swallowing is more of a long-term hobby and he has 'got away with it' up till now. 'He does carry stones about when he's excited – but he never swallows them.' This lady is an incurable optimist, but perhaps now this has happened, she may take greater steps to discourage him 'cherry-picking' from the garden path.

Last but not least, a cat with refractory gingivitis. Many treatments have been tried with no great success, so the last option is to remove all her cheek teeth – a prospect which we would have dreaded without our new dental machine. There would have been much cursing and muttering while I attempted to loosen the teeth using only an elevator. As it is, the air-turbine powered drill quickly and cleanly sections the teeth into single-rooted segments which are easily extracted after loosening with an elevator.

Julie transfers the toothless wonder into a warm kennel while I begin the clean-up effort by slopping disinfectant on the table and giving it a hearty swabbing before wandering off to write up clinical record cards. 'There's a puddle on the ops room floor,' the returning Julie reports, scanning the ceiling for any leaks. 'Oh, that was me,' I shout through from the next room, concentrating on the records. 'Your bladder problem must be worse than we thought,' she shoots back, never one to miss a comic opportunity, no matter how tenuous!

Late afternoon sees me and the dogs up the hill. The woods are less dense now as most leaves have fallen. At the thinking stones, the beech tree leaves are brown and a gentle wind crinkles the dry leaves. The sun is hitting the hill at a slant, casting long shadows. It doesn't move far these days, rising and sinking within only a quarter of the sky. A half moon is up already, the short day is nearly over.

An early morning walk round the field before work leaves me frozen to the marrow. No sun reaches this side now, and a bitter wind makes sticking to Kippen's pace excruciatingly cold. In the past, I have always kept toasty warm by brisk walking but the onset of my companion's old age makes this impossible.

Luckily Saturday morning surgery is brisk but finishes on time. I need a clear run today to get ready for our annual bonfire party. There has been some miscalculation this time – Jay has to work today, so I am left with all the preparations. I am quite looking forward to an afternoon in the kitchen, but am anxious that a strategically timed emergency could leave us unprepared for the night's invasion of hungry revellers.

It takes all day to produce the mounds of food to satisfy our friends. After what seems like hours of peeling potatoes, carrots and onions, a large *jeelypan* of stovies and a casserole of bonfire soup (carrot and coconut) simmers on the Rayburn and a baking tray of *wee willie winky* sausages brown in the oven. Bowls of popcorn, crisps and toffee (McGowan's toffee with the Highland cow on the packet) adorn the kitchen counter together with rolls, plates and a basinful of cutlery. The deal is that we provide the nibbles and main course while partygoers will bring sweets and puddings. A selection of cans, bottles and assorted glasses crowd on to the Welsh dresser.

Satisfied that inside is under control, I turn my attention to the yard. A sturdy table holds a mini-terracotta barbecue for roasting chestnuts (a very popular activity at previous does), together with a knife and salt for seasoning; and I artistically (I think) light tiny nightlights on the low wall below the banking. I have even managed to hollow out a turnip lantern to hang at the end of the driveway. I must admit that ordinary parties leave me cold, but special times like Halloween, bonfire night and summer barbecues have great appeal.

No sooner have I finished, and happily surveyed the results of my labours, than Jay arrives home, followed only moments later by the first of our guests. Everyone is heavily wrapped in woollies and fleeces, and all are bearing some addition to the evening's proceedings. There is no need to act as a hostess with this lot; they can all take care of themselves so we can relax and join the fun.

The wind has dropped, leaving a cold, clear night, perfect for being outside. A large bonfire rages in an old oil drum and the kids bravely try to cook sausages on sticks, losing as many as they succeed with ... tottering back, eyes streaming from the smoke. More cautious souls join in by waving sparklers lit from the flames. Cath's husband Chris 'volunteers' to take charge of the fireworks, and does a sterling job, scrambling up the banking to position rockets, sparkling fountains and Catherine wheels, before masterminding their discharge. We have chosen quiet fireworks as much as possible so as not to scare either our animals or those at the farm. Kippen and Fintry have been installed in the upstairs bedroom with the television to drown out any frightening whirrs or crackles. Kippen would not mind, but Fintry is a bit of a wimp. Close friends nip up to see them occasionally, bearing various edible goodies so their evening is pretty successful too.

A gritter goes past as the fireworks blaze, its orange flashing lights adding to the multicoloured scene. Mountains of food disappear – gone are my hopes of meals for tomorrow. Some groups drift in to sit in front of the woodburner while hardy characters linger round the fire, smoking and chatting contentedly. Best of friends roll up sleeves and tackle washing-up despite pleas to leave it till tomorrow. Eventually folks drift homewards, leaving the odd one or two who stay with us laughing and chatting till the early hours. It seems to have been a successful night, and no one has enjoyed it more than Jay and I. Our first bonfire night in the new house, we really feel as if we belong now.

It is peculiar how often the weather is foggy after bonfire night; is this the result of everyone's bonfire smoke or is it just typical weather conditions for this time of year? An early morning walk up the hill brings us above the mist in a world of our own.

Heading towards the deer pen, we spot Honky and Charlie together on either side of the fence. Two hinds approach as if to speak to Honky the outcast, the situation resembling a prison-visiting session. Further along the track comes a raucous squealing – could there be a group of piglets loose in the woods? No, the racket is produced by two jays shouting the odds at each other. As we pause to listen, another sound impinges – a light crashing coming from a stand of larch trees. A small ginger shape can just be discerned hurtling up a trunk and along several branches, followed seconds later by a near-vertical descent to the mossy ground below. This is a red squirrel, but who knows whether it is playing or in some distress ... it doesn't seem to know that we are here so I suspect that it is playing.

Chapter 42

Our pleasant frosty bonfire night is but a distant memory now. High winds and torrential rain are battering the area bringing flooding and fallen trees, and tearing the last of the leaves from the trees still standing. It is suddenly bleak and wintery. Leaving just before me on the way to work, Jay stops a mere hundred yards along the road. Drawing in behind, I see why – a roe deer lies at an awkward angle, felled by a passing car. My services are not required, the body is well-mangled; the car must have been really travelling. There is so much wildlife on the roads (to say nothing of tractors and other farm vehicles) that driving fast is really rather stupid. Judging by the damage done to the poor deer, the car will not have escaped unscathed. Moving the corpse into a more secluded resting place on the verge, we continue sadly on our way.

First case into Clayfern surgery is a guinea pig seen last week with a sizeable wound on his back. 'It just will not heal,' commented his owner, 'Is there anything you can do?'

As a rule, vets are quite spoilt with our patients when it comes to wound healing. Animal skin is more elastic than human tissue and heals faster, so even large defects will generally fill in remarkably quickly. We are seldom faced with the chronic, non-healing lesions which can be so miserable for humans. Only very infrequently does wound healing grind totally to a halt. In these cases, a vet's inclination will often be to anaesthetise the animal, tidy up the wound and possibly attempt to close it using simple plastic surgery techniques – quite a major undertaking. Before reaching this stage, I will sometimes have a go at acupuncture if the case is suitable. This is what was done last week. The technique calls for fine acupuncture needles to be inserted at intervals round the periphery of the wound, and left in place for five to ten minutes, being given the occasional twiddle. This is no mean feat in a guinea pig. They are renowned for shrieking and struggling hysterically when any vet is brave enough to inject them. Some have even been known to faint or worse, die in terror – not a good advert for veterinary intervention. When working up to injecting a guinea pig, I do mention that a slight risk is involved and try to get the procedure over with like greased lightening so it is a fait accompli before the pig knows what is happening.

Me and my mouth, I thought last week while instructing the owner to 'Hold him firmly,' a futile plea if ever there was one. Miraculously, the stars were kind enough to inflict a non-healing wound on what was the most placid of guinea pigs. He tolerated the needles with barely a squeak, only complaining slightly when I tried a quick 'twiddle.' Amazingly, the effect has been wonderful – the wound has virtually closed over. *We must nurture this pig,* I think to myself as patient and satisfied owner depart. The species are not noted either for their tolerance to veterinary handling or exceptional survival, a fact well known by every parent who has ever acquired one for their kids. In fact, most so-called children's pets are the same, noted throughout the profession for their 'Here today, gone tomorrow' characteristics.

Every vet is familiar with the remorseful phone calls from parents who have just found the guinea pig, rabbit, hamster or gerbil dead and torture themselves by agonising over what they have done wrong. No school holiday is complete without the arrival in the waiting room – complete with large cage trailing straw – of the unfortunate stooge who has been 'volunteered' to look after the school pet. It seems to be a matter of honour for said pets to become poorly as soon as possible after they are taken home, just to underline how incompetent their temporary minders are! It may be that the true purpose of 'children's pets' is to introduce the children to the concept of death.

Back to the farm surgery where Kippen is going to be a guinea pig (so to speak), allowing a representative to demonstrate a blood pressure monitor. These devices have been modified for use in animals, and the prices are just beginning to fall into the affordable range. Kippen appears slightly anxious as the blood pressure cuff is attached to his leg – he probably remembers having to give a blood sample to test the biochemistry machine. As is standard practice, the rep takes several readings, allowing Kippen's initial high levels to return to normal. Suddenly, his pressure shoots up – Julie is behind me waving a chew (well, it is chewsday). We decide to leave Fintry out of this. Wimp that she is, she would practically die of fright. We gave her a bath last night and she was virtually catatonic in the tub.

Kippen is dispatched back into the house and we turn our attention to a cat due in for dental work. He tolerates the cuff well and produces several readings in the normal range. However, after five minutes, he begins to growl and bat his tail threateningly so we hastily remove the cuff. When he goes home, his owner is most impressed to be told that his blood pressure is normal.

Just when we think that we are finished, a client turns up with her big butch tomcat sporting an oozing abscess on his head – undoubtedly the result of a cat bite. The skin of his head is quite underrun with pus which seeps out of the bite wound as I examine the area. 'Eugh,' exclaims his owner, 'And just before lunch too.' 'Its like water off a duck's back to us,' I comment airily, 'In fact, it reminds me of the lasagne we're having for lunch.' Leaving the owner squirming, we admit the cat to drain the abscess – and to castrate him at the same time. The latter will hopefully reduce his urge to venture far and wide, getting into cat fights and losing, as he seems to with unnerving frequency – this is not his first visit with the same problem. Other people's sqeamishness when it comes to blood and gore was always a source of much amusement to veterinary students, who would loudly discuss the roundworms they saw that day while guzzling spaghetti, or identify finer points of anatomy in the Sunday roast. There may have been method in our bravado, as the thoroughly sickened non-vets could be relied upon not to return for second helpings.

It is still gorgeous up the hill later. The larches are a riot of flaming gold. I bring the last of the windfall apples to feed to the deer in the pen. Charlie is tremendously possessive with every apple, chasing away any hind unwise enough to head in their direction. So zealous is he that he is hoist by his own petard – as he chases one hind halfway down the field, the others sneak in from behind and grab a bite.

Our old friend Don is in during evening surgery. The months of work on the massive skin defect on his leg will never be forgotten. Even now, the leg is not perfect but his owner has learnt to live with it and Don is a familiar sight around Clayfern sporting his smart collection of socks. The years have passed inexorably like they do, and Don has suddenly become an old dog. Despite his chronic bronchitis and a touch of emphysema, he has remained remarkably steady over the last year. As with all chronic respiratory conditions, he has occasional flare-ups and is coughing badly. He is already on anti-inflammatory drugs, so today I add a course of antibiotics and bronchodilator pills. I remind Don's owner to stick in with extras such as humidifying the air in the house, 'steaming' the patient by letting the kettle boil for ten minutes or taking him into the bathroom while a bath is run, and carrying out *coupage*, the physiotherapy technique where the whole of the chest wall is gently tapped several times to help loosen stubborn secretions. All these techniques do no harm and can be very beneficial as well as medication.

I don't feel hungry when I get home, and, develop unpleasant stomach pains as the evening wears on. Feeling distinctly rough, I set off to bed early, watching TV while hugging a hottie bottle. It's my own fault for that crack about the lasagne. Presently, Murphy's Law swings into action. There is nothing like being off-colour for attracting out-of-hours calls. We can go for days with nothing, but the minute you risk an early night, the phone is sure to ring ... and it does, at 10 p.m. It is Edith, worried about Meeny who is also off-colour and being sick. Knowing that Edith is a worrier, I ask several questions in the futile hope that I might not have to go out. Some chance, the answer to every question is another nail in the coffin. 'Would she take any food?' (a trick question just to see how bad she really is – apart from Labradors, most genuinely ill creatures do not want to eat).

'No, she's not wanted anything since morning.'

'Is she drinking?'

'No.'

'How often has she been sick?'

'Oh, lots of times.'

'When was she last sick?'

'Just before I rang you.'

Okay, okay, I admit defeat. 'I'll be with you in fifteen minutes,' I reply, wearily.

As usual, the patient looks better than described over the phone and does run to greet me, albeit with less verve than usual. Meeny is a devil for eating unpleasant things on walks and I suspect this is the case again. There is much stomach-rumbling from both of us – we could do a duet. An anti-vomiting drug, some electrolyte solution and a promise to visit tomorrow does the trick. Leaving Edith solicitously hugging the stricken Meeny ('There's my poor girl, Mum will just tuck you in on the settee.') I drag myself home to bed again.

After a mercifully quiet morning surgery, along to visit Meeny. As I reverse into Edith's drive, I see all three dachshunds in the mirror. They are standing watching Edith hang out washing – with their bandy wee legs they look like gunfighters at the OK Corral. Meeny has improved. She has finished vomiting but has now started with diarrhoea. As they say, *Rubbish in, rubbish out.* I know how she feels. 'Did you get my message about Eeny's pills?' she asks. Of course I did. Eeny is epileptic but is well controlled on a drug whose trade name is *Epiphen.* Every month, Edith has the pleasure of ringing the surgery for more of 'those effin' tablets.' The old jokes are always the best – Julie and I still smirk with our anaesthesia double act. 'Big breaths,' one of us exhorts the patient, 'Yeth, and I'm only thixteen,' replies the other, quick as a flash.

When Edith first started on the epiphen joke, I told her about my

295

faux pas in front of Jay's entire family 'I really like this Buchan pottery,' I exclaimed, carrying our new plates to the table for Sunday lunch, and wondering why conversation has suddenly ceased. (Say it quickly, and you'll get the drift.)

We seem to have all but lost the sun permanently at the Laigher, and will remain in gloom now until February. The wind has shifted many of the brighter leaves and the forest is a dull patchwork of muted ginger against the blue-green pines. Both stags are head to head on either side of the fence, and I fear an explosive confrontation, but in fact the encounter is more of a damp squib – after several minutes, they both simply lie down. The red-blooded cut and thrust of the rut is evidently over for this year.

Since the clocks changed, the drive from evening surgery has been in the dark. Now it is also virtually dark on the way in, the four or five strands of orange street lighting adorning the hillside like Christmas decorations. It really will not be long until it is *that time* again.

A final visit to Meeny before Saturday morning surgery. Her illness has parallelled mine – bad on Thursday, so-so yesterday then brighter today. The diagnosis has been made in retrospect for Meeny since Edith found the remains of a very dead rabbit in the garden. I think my Thursday lunchtime chicken leg might explain my plight, but as with so many cases of gutrot, we will never really know.

During morning surgery, there is quite an amusing exchange with one of our clients who has recently moved to Stramar but is still travelling to this practice. 'I expect Stramar is a bit more lively in the evenings than Clayfern,' I say to her teenage daughter while weighing the cat. 'Not really,' answers daughter, 'Clayfern was quite active.' 'Mostly outside our house,' adds mother a trifle wearily. Looking at their record card, I notice that they lived opposite one pub and next door to another.

The onset of more wintery weather has whipped Jay into a 'gathering nuts for winter' mentality, so we spend the afternoon chainsawing fallen trees into manageable logs. After one or two token goes with the saw, I get to load the logs into the car. Honky and Gray watch us from a distance, and the dogs potter around desultorily, wishing that we would stop messing about and come for a decent walk. Leaving Jay to cut the last of the logs, I take the dogs with me to lay a trail of peanuts from the badger sett to the stubble field. It is such a pleasant evening that we thought we might try a badger watch later. All peanuts left in the past have disappeared post-haste, but so far, we have not seen the perpetrators in action. After our evening repast, we set off again up the hill. A large red moon looms through the trees but is soon obscured by clouds. I have my early Christmas present with us – a night-vision scope. We creep up the stubble field and park the car a discrete distance from the pile of peanuts, then settle to see what appears. The scope is great, and we watch Mum and Gray crossing the field, appearing an eerie green through the lens. Several rabbits raise our hopes by appearing suddenly at the edge of the woods before hopping off to graze and socialise in the tram lines. But after an hour and a half, still no badgers. I feel our situation is much like the photographer in a current TV advert for *Kitkat* biscuits. After hours of unproductive waiting by the bear enclosure at the zoo, poised with shutter at the ready, the hero turns his back briefly to partake of a *Kitkat*. While his attention is elsewhere, the bear family dance out of their den in perfect step, do some fancy juggling and unicycle riding then disappear into their den as the photographer turns round. I suspect that our badgers do something similar as we head dispiritedly down the hill again. Finding numerous peanut-filled badger latrine pits on our daily walks only serves to taunt us.

Chapter 43

After a hectic ops session on Tuesday, we have a lighter day scheduled today, only two bitch spays. 'Just as well they're small,' Julie grunts, lifting one on to the table, 'My back has been acting up.'

'So has mine, in fact it's really all down my left side, I think it might be sciatica.'

'Mine is down my right side,' she exclaims, and in a flash, it occurs to us that this coincides with how we stand at the ops table. 'We need a right-handed vet back to ring the changes,' she says – 'And maybe a left-handed nurse,' I retaliate.

Recently we both met an osteopath at a party, and she volunteered to do a home visit for three or more clients. Perhaps an osteopathy party is the only alternative to a naughty nightwear party when you progress deeper into middle-age.

After the bitches are awake, we repair to the house for elevens. I bought mince pies (the first sign of impending Christmas) at Jim's shop, and stowed them in the Rayburn after the first bitch. Julie has a few cat kennels at home, and rehomes unwanted cats on a small scale.

Recently she inherited two old cats whose owner had died. Unfortunately, there is little demand for old cats in the homing stakes, so we assumed they would probably live out their lives with Julie. One, a big fat cat, has been drinking like a fish, while the other, a scrawny little thing, eats like a gannet but still loses weight, so they were both here on Tuesday for blood sampling. The big cat is diabetic and the little one has hyperthyroidism. This morning's tea break is to be spent briefing Julie on each cat's medical requirements. The big cat, Roly, will require daily or twice daily injections of insulin, and her food and exercise must be strictly controlled. The little cat, Tinker, needs tablets three times a day. 'We could re-name them Little and

Large,' Julie muses, 'Or Ee and Ig,' I suggest (after my childhood teddies who were – wee and big).

It is quite sociable sitting by the Rayburn, guzzling pies and going over notes, even more so when we are joined by a mutual friend who just happens to be passing. When she hears what we are doing, her response is immediate 'I'll take them,' she declares. Julie and I stop mid-bite and stare at her in disbelief 'You *do* know that they aren't in the best of health,' Julie says diplomatically. 'They perhaps aren't terribly long for this world, Jackie,' I call a spade a spade. 'That suits me fine,' she replies. Jackie has not long since lost her old cat. Near the end, the cat became dirty and Jackie stoically put up with cleaning up after her. Now she seems to want to return to the same routine. She is happy to take on older cats for a short time, but does not want to commit for longer. Recalling those two, I am sure that the commitment can safely be said to be short term. We decide that they should stay at Julie's so that they start treatment in familiar surroundings, then when they are stable, they can go to their new home. What a good result.

With time to spare, I take the dogs out separately. Leaving Kippen in front of the fire with a chew, Fintry and I power-walk round the field. It makes a change to be warm on a walk, and the brisk exercise should be good for both our waistlines. Feeling guilty on our return, I leave Fintry in front of the fire with a chew and take Kippen for an amble in the orchard. The orchard is sheltered from the wind and a colourful carpet of fallen leaves makes easy walking for the old dog. As he snuffles round, I gather windfalls for the deer. Creepers obscure the wall, and skeletal remains of sticky willy drapes small fir trees round the perimeter giving the area a sense of benign decay – rather like Miss Favisham's room in Dickens' novel. It feels like our very own secret garden. Red berries shine on two holly bushes – I hope they last till Christmas.

Home again, both dogs snooze by the fire while I indulge in a cooking session. The fishman comes today, so fish pie is on the menu.

Halfway through, I realise I have forgotten to buy vital ingredients, so call at Sheila's to borrow what is missing. This happens every time I embark on a cooking spree. Luckily, she regularly misjudges her bread and milk requirements so we tend to even out.

All this activity finds me feeling quite tired as evening surgery draws to an uneventful close. Just one more task to complete before getting home to the fish pie and the fire (I won't bother with a chew; a cup of tea and a biscuit will do me). Mrs Cassidy has had a fall and has asked if I could drop off her cat food. On entering the house, my nostrils are immediately assailed with the pungent odour of cat wee. 'I think one of the sods has gone on the stairs, but I can't manage up with this leg,' she laments. 'Well, we must find out where, and give it a right good clean, or the smell will just encourage the others to do the same,' I answer with a heavy heart, just what you don't need at the end of a full day. So it is, at the end of what has been a long day, I find myself poised on one step, sniffing avidly at the upper treads, and I think to myself '*This* is it, what you trained for five years at university for!'

A typical dreich November day dawns. The vivid colours have gone, leaving gloomier russets and browns. Leaves and fallen branches line the roadside, and I watch out for any suitable for woodburner fodder. Almost every Saturday, Clayfern community centre hosts a coffee morning for the legions of societies and groups in the area. Today it is the turn of the Baptist church – well worth a visit for their excellent home-made jams and second-hand books. They obviously read the same material as Jay and I. After a successful trawl, buying a little something at most stalls to avoid offending anyone, I set off into Stramar to meet Jay for lunch. On days like this, it seems that the entire countryside is out and about. At several sites, landrovers and other 4x4 vehicles cram into offroad parking, disgorging their loads of shooters in oiled or tweed coats and enthusiastic Labradors and spaniels. Let's hope none gets shot or wounded on barbed wire as is so often the case – a. call back from Stramar will not be appreciated. A ploughing contest is being held further along. At least ten tractors are at work, ploughing strips of land, watched carefully by figures in overalls and bunnets. Each patch looks the same to me, but obviously I am no expert. On a farm closer to Stramar, a roup (displenishment sale) is in progress. Lines of equipment lie in orderly rows, everything from combine harvesters and tractors to buckets and forks. The same clusters of overalled, bunneted figures tour the aisles, inspecting the stock, deciding what to bid for. Roups always seem sad events, although some must have happy endings with the well remunerated ex-farmer and family heading off to spend the proceeds in the Bahamas before settling to a happy retirement in a pretty country cottage with none of the hassles that farming brings.

Later, a typical autumnal walk with Sheila and the dogs down the stubble field to the river. A smooth dark shape coasts with the tide before submerging and re-appearing further downstream. Is it a seal? It is frustratingly just at the limit of our vision and we really cannot tell for sure. On an even later trip up the hill as dusk falls, a set of eyes are picked out with my torch. Is it a badger? Again, it is not possible to discern a definite shape, but the pattern of movement and behaviour strikes me as very badger-like. Animal sightings today are unfortunately much like the majority of our wildlife photos – distant spots on the horizon.

The week begins with an early call bringing a cat traffic accident. The main damage seems to be to his chest. He can walk around, and his colour and temperature are reasonable, but any exertion makes his chest move in and out alarmingly, and even at rest, his breathing is fast and exaggerated. Through the stethoscope, his chest sounds harsh and squeaky. I think I can hear breath sounds throughout the lung field, but it is hard to totally eliminate the movement of fur against the stethoscope plate. Absence of breath sounds can point to a diaphragmatic hernia, the situation where the diaphragm ruptures and allows abdominal organs to herniate into the chest cavity. An x-ray will help to identify exactly what damage has been done – and whether any surgical intervention is necessary – but a period of stabilisation first seems like a good idea. His oxygen saturation level as measured on the pulse oximeter is eighty eight per cent, poorer than normal (which should be close to a hundred per cent) but not horrendously low. I administer anti-inflammatory drugs and gently fit an oxygen mask – this consists of an Elizabethan collar arrangement with the front end enclosed in clear plastic, and an inlet port at the top through which oxygen is passed. Before reaching the mask, the oxygen is bubbled through a water bottle to humidify it. Quite a cheap piece of equipment in the scheme of things, but very useful and well tolerated by patients. After ten minutes sitting quietly in a cage breathing oxygen, the cat is more relaxed and his oxygen saturation has risen to ninety one per cent. He can stay peacefully like this until morning surgery is finished.

During morning surgery, a phone call from Leo the Cushing's dog's owner – his drinking has increased again, so we increase his mitotane from weekly to daily dosage. 'He's running a bit short of tablets,' Joan mentions. 'I'll order some more,' I say, thinking nothing of it until a call to the suppliers 'The original order specified one hundred tablets,' intones the company contact, 'You'll need another special treatment authorisation.' Arggghh! There goes the day. Fortunately, a call to the Veterinary Medicines Directorate reassures me that we do not have to go through the whole procedure again 'Just alter the original prescription and fax it to us,' is the helpful reply. At the cost of these tablets, you don't order any more than is necessary, and, to be honest, neither I nor Leo's owner expected him to survive for quite as long, but apart from more arthritis and occasional troubles with a bronchitic cough, he is trundling on nicely. Ordering the tablets is probably a risky business – Murphy's Law dictates that the spending of several hundred pounds on drugs is the optimum time for the dog to go rapidly downhill.

Back to Fern to begin the day's operations. The first job is to x-ray Cracker, the RTA cat. A very mild sedative calms him for the procedure, while producing minimal effects in his cardiovascular and respiratory systems. All sedatives have the potential to depress respiratory and cardiovascular function, so it is important to choose with care in a patient whose circulation and lungs may be compromised. It could also be dangerous if he was given nothing, and panicked when we tried to position him for x-ray. As it is, we only move him very slowly and carefully as if, for example, he did have a diaphragmatic hernia, a sharp movement could cause a landslide of abdominal organs into the chest resulting in immediate suffocation. I have seen this happen once, and there was just no time to do anything to save the unfortunate dog involved.

Cracker behaves well, even attempting to purr as Julie gently lies him on his side. It is probably a good sign that he some spare breath to do this. Quickly lining up the x-ray beam, we carefully drape sandbags over his legs to keep him in place. This is a dicey moment, as many animals will attempt to get up at this stage but Cracker thankfully stays put. Whispering sweet nothings to the prone cat, we back speedily out of the door and press the exposure button. A mere tenth of a second later, we whip back table-side to unpack the cat and rescue the x-ray plate. It is then fed into the automatic processor, and one minute later, the developed film appears. I clip it on the light box and examine the picture, while Julie returns the cat to his kennel and re-attaches his oxygen mask. The diaphragmatic line appears intact and Cracker's abdominal organs are where they should be – in the abdomen. There is some diffuse mottled opacity throughout the lung field, but no evidence of either excess fluid or air in the chest cavity. The most likely explanation of the opacity is some haemorrhage into the lung tissue, bruising as a result of the accident. As Cracker seems to be holding his own, there is no need for chest drains or other interference. He will just remain in the kennel under observation for the next day or so, and hopefully the haemorrhage will resolve uneventfully. With the oxygen mask in place, his oxygen concentration is now ninety five per cent, an improvement on this morning.

Onwards then with the remainder of the day's work, mostly routine neuterings. As we work, Julie reports that both Roly and Tinker are doing well. Roly's drinking has reduced by half, and Jackie is going to collect her tonight. Tinker has been offered a home with Julie's neighbour who has been chatting to the little cat over the garden fence, and, as Jackie doesn't mind, she too is off this evening. Jackie will probably have enough on her hands with Roly, and they definitely will not miss each other; in fact, Julie says that they seem to dislike each other intensely and avoid each other whenever possible.

Our final operation is the removal of a sinister-looking lump on a guinea pig. Guinea pigs are not the easiest of creatures to anaesthetise. Several of our multi-drug knockdown combinations – so effective in other small species – have no effect in guinea pigs, and aiming for veins is not really a practical proposition. I opt for a sedative drug followed by masking down with a relatively new gaseous anaesthetic – *Isofluorane.* For small creatures and very frail patients, this drug has several advantages over the routinely used *Halothane.* Its main disadvantage is that is horribly expensive, although the price has been coming down with the advent of more than one manufacturer in the veterinary market – nothing like some healthy competition! This guinea pig is used to being handled, a great advantage in the small furry stakes.

Terrified creatures release massive quantities of the fright-and-flight hormone, adrenaline, into their circulation and can often die at the drop of a hat from a heart attack, one of the main reasons why successful surgery on little beasts was so fraught with risk in the past. Other factors which will also have contributed to the demise of these patients is their increased risk of hypothermia and hypoglycaemia. The operation goes smoothly and the pig is back in his box munching a carrot within the hour. I think that the advances in anaesthesia is one of the biggest changes I have noticed in my quarter of a century of vetting. (Good Grief, is it really that long?) As a young vet, a dog coming in with a cut pad near the end of Saturday morning surgery meant a wait for a sedative to take effect, then a full anaesthetic, then the inevitable two hours waiting for the patient to be compos mentis enough to go home. Many Saturday afternoons and evenings were ruined in that way, whereas nowadays, we use a rapid knockdown agent which can be reversed when the job is done and the dog is on its way, bright as a button, within the hour. There is seldom any need for undignified struggles with stroppy or downright dangerous patients, just a quick jag and they are at our mercy.

The day rushes past, and the poor dogs are only walked at 4 p.m. Light is nearly fading as we wander in the woods, the dogs prospecting while I gather pine cones for a florist friend. My slow progress is ideal for Kippen, and there is the added advantage that we will gain an impressive festive wreath for Christmas. Fintry investigates pheasants chirring in the undergrowth, then scuttles swiftly back to my side when an owl starts to hoot in a tree above her. With ghostly cawing, rooks head in to roost against the sinking sun. It is a good time to be out when the kingdom of the sun surrenders to the kingdom of the moon. I wish we could stay out longer but evening surgery beckons.

During evening consultations, I have occasion to blood sample a little dog to perform a routine blood test. I don't think there is much wrong with the dog but the owner wants me to go ahead. She (the owner) does seem a little anxious tonight. 'Its like getting blood from a stone,' I comment, making conversation as my syringe gradually fills. 'Is that a problem that it should be flowing so slowly,' she jumps on my throw-away line. Reassuring her while I withdraw the needle, I pass a biscuit reward to the dog who has been very good. 'Oh my God, there's something wrong with his mouth, he's having a fit,' she shrieks, totally panicked. 'He's eating a biscuit, Sheena,' I answer wearily, thinking no more ad lib, then seeing her obvious distress 'Are you okay?' It turns out that her husband died suddenly at the weekend, aged forty two. Poor woman, what she really needs is a friendly shoulder to cry on for a few minutes – and a clean bill of health for her dog. We'll run the blood and get her back in a couple of days for a check-up, and probably one or two times after that. I doubt that there is much wrong with the dog, but the contact will do Sheena the power of good. This would be a good lesson for a student – never dismiss an excessively anxious client as a nutter; there may well be a very good reason for their distress.

Another sad ending is in store for Corrie, our thromboembolism cat. Despite being on aspirin, the symptoms have recurred, and, more typically, he is yowling in pain. A quick painless injection puts an end to his career as our only successful saddle thrombus case. Emotionally a little down, I return to Fern and in to see Cracker. He is bright and purrs gently when I remove the oxygen hood. There is no deterioration while I nip into the house to retrieve a plate of chicken saved for his tea, and he scoffs the lot. By bed time, he is behaving almost like a normal cat again. It is definitely all roundabouts and swings in this job.

Chapter 44

After a routine Saturday morning surgery, I am driving home anticipating a leisurely afternoon when the pager shrills. I pull off the road and read the message: *Please telephone Richard, the cat is sitting on the floor.* Richard is Jackie's husband – renowned at being handless with animals. Is Roly running rings around him? I wonder – not greatly worried – reaching for my mobile phone. Not so simple, alas. The message should have read – the cat is *fitting* on the floor. Sounds like she has gone hypoglycaemic. I speed home while the hapless Richard (left alone for the day) attempts to scoop the cat into a box and rushes to meet me.

Low blood sugar seems the most likely diagnosis (not rocket science when the patient is a diabetic), and the first step for the thrashing Roly is to attempt to insert a canula, take a blood sample then connect her to a glucose drip. Thank goodness Jay is at home as Richard looks in danger of collapse himself. 'She didn't eat all her breakfast,' he gasps, shaking her from box on to table.

Between them, he and Jay gently restrain Roly and hold an oxygen mask to her face while I quickly process the blood sample. Her blood glucose levels are in her boots. An anxious few minutes passes before her jerking movements slow and her eyes gradually become focused, losing the awful glazed appearance present only moments before. Soon, she even attempts to sit up.

'She could do with eating something,' I say, disappearing into the kennel room to open a can of cat food and present it to Roly. She sniffs it then ignores it. Jay dashes into the house to unearth some chicken left over from last night – same result. Suddenly, with no warning, Roly begins to fit again and I increase her intravenous glucose. When she stablises again, we collect more tasty morsels and lay them before her – a veritable smorgasbord. Yet again, she sniffs unenthusiastically before embarkings on an even more violent fit, dislodging her intravenous catheter after only a small amount of glucose solution has hit her circulation. It was enough to pull her round from this fit but another must surely be just round the corner if we cannot raise her blood glucose levels. The situation is deteriorating badly. I fail to catheterise her other vein and see failure looming on the horizon. All her veins seem to have gone to ground. Desperate, if unconventional, measures are called for.

'Open a tin of recovery diet,' I instruct Jay: 'Hold her head up,' to Richard, while I grab a nasogastric tube and local anaesthetic solution. A few drops are instilled quickly into her nostril before I slip the tube into her gullet and briskly syringe several loads of the semi-liquid food into her stomach.

'I think she's been through enough,' whispers Richard weakly as we carefully transfer her to a warmed kennel. The poor man looks totally washed out. Ordinarily, I would prefer owners to be out of the way before performing emergency work, but there was no time today and an extra pair of hands was exceedingly valuable. I stay with the patient while Jay takes Richard for a much-needed cup of tea. I don't expect much, and wait in misery for another fit. We have already taken the decision between us that if this happens, we will submit gracefully and put her to sleep.

It is 4 p.m. when Richard eventually departs, leaving Roly with us overnight. It is truly amazing how just one case can screw up the entire day. Time just flies – we have been in and out of the surgery since 12.30 p.m. If you had asked me how long it would take to deal with a hypoglycaemic patient, I would estimate an initial thirty minutes followed by frequent checks. Don't ask me where the time goes – it's like a black hole in that surgery. Then, after the drama, there is still the clearing up. The surgery looks like a bomb has hit it – wrappers from syringes, giving sets and fluid; spent syringes and needles; assorted drug containers on the counter; dirty anaesthetic equipment. The rest of the evening is spent spot-checking Roly; the time intervals between visits lengthening as the night wears on. She has finally eaten so the chances of a further hypoglycaemic episode are thankfully much reduced.

Roly is bright and breezy the following morning but has had spectacular diarrhoea, no doubt as a result of her varied diet yesterday. It is always intriguing how patients manage to get muck on the ceiling of the kennel as well as on the floor, every wall and between the bars of the door. The only untouched area is the litter tray – obviously pelleted sawdust litter is not to her taste. After a quick blood sample to check her blood glucose, she is fed and an insulin dose administered. Richard comes to collect her and the day is ours again – pager permitting – so off we go to do the Christmas shopping which was planned for yesterday. Never mind Roly, I am quite twitchy around the time of yesterday's call and check the pager several times to make sure no messages have sneaked through unannounced.

At last, the shopping expedition is successfully completed, and we store our purchases in the spare bedroom – now nicknamed Santa's Grotto for the duration of the month. It is only as we prepare to take the dogs out that I begin to relax. The shopping has been somewhat nerve-racking as I am in a heightened state of alertness. Jay is a saint to put up with the vagaries of veterinary life, but yet another aborted shopping trip would have gone down like a lead balloon.

Jay checks the chainsaw while I collect a batch of windfalls for the deer. Honky approaches as we cut logs so I stop to hurl the apples. They are getting rather soggy – I hope he doesn't get tipsy. Drunk animals have been an in-topic recently. Sheila's hens were decidedly staggery after she fed them the remains of the berries she used in wine-making, and a friend's dog was found virtually unconscious after pinching sloe gin must destined for the bin. The old soak recovered after a night on a drip, probably with the cracker of a sore head. Even Kippen is partial to a drop of Glayva and has been decidedly wide-eyed after lapping the remains in a glass left by my chair. Jay has been asking what I want for Christmas and these musings give sudden inspiration – I'll have an apple press so that next year we can brew our own cider.

I have been nobbled by the school to give a talk to Primary 3, so any quiet moments during surgery this week have been spent preparing my presentation. With Alice's help, I have decided to use some of our extensive collection of soft toys as props to portray a potted 'Day in the life of a vet.' These unfortunate creatures are always being conscripted for demonstration purposes. *Other* stuffed toys lie on beds or settees; ours suffer the indignity of having their heads stuffed in anaesthetic masks, drips strapped to their legs or, worse, of being stapled or stitched.

Before I begin my spiel, I ask the class of eight-year-olds how many have been to a vet's surgery, and am surprised to see only a quarter put their hands up. Judging from the number of kids accompanying family pets to our surgery, I thought nearly all of them would have had the experience. *Better make this impressive then.*

First up is Fluffy, an attractive black and white stuffed toy who is today masquerading as a new kitten. This is cunningly included to introduce the concept of preventative medicine, and, watched by a sea of impassive faces, I run through vaccination, neutering and worming. The class visibly brighten when I hold up my prized exhibits – a tapeworm and a roundworm preserved in pots of formalin. Protracted theoretical concepts will obviously not do here – what they want is blood and gore. Rootling in my box of tricks, I pull out our next patient, a sad-looking bulldog with a bandaged foot. Red felt-tip blood shows through the bandage. The audience is completely riveted as I explain what Bertie's fate is to be. He has to have his leg stapled – 'And this is how he looks afterwards,' I explain, whipping off the bandage to reveal a neat row of staples. So far so good, I now have their undivided attention. Floppy the rabbit appears next, sporting an impressive set of overgrown incisors – painstakingly stuck on by Alice. A short visit behind the scenes (into the cardboard box) allows the teeth to be added to the growing exhibit pile which is to be examined after my talk.

The piece de resistance is our Grommit pyjama case who has been off his food and vomiting for two days. I adopt a professional solemnity as I palpate Grommit's stomach – 'There is something there! Grommit must be admitted for x-ray.' Another grope in the props box produces an x-ray (of Duke the ball and potato-eater) showing Grommit's foreign body. Another pause for effect before said ball is produced in the flesh. The class are tremendously impressed by this finale although perhaps a little hazy as to how the ball came out of the patient's stomach. We'll leave that till next year.

For the second phase of the visit, they sit round their tables while I dispense the exhibits for their perusal, and make the rounds with our pulse oximeter. They all want a go, getting quite competitive about it ('I've got ninety nine per cent; you've only got ninety seven!') and it crosses my mind that a tidy profit could be made if I charged for a health check. Occasional questions drift across the room as I attach tiny fingers to the machine – 'Can we take the teeth out of the container?' 'Yes.' 'Can we take the worms out?' '*No.*' Meantime, I have hit a snag, one child has no reading on the machine 'Miiisss, Alec isn't registering.' 'That's not unusual,' the teacher remarks wryly. Fortunately, a reading finally shows, but Alec's heart rate is going steadily up … a hundred …a hundred and ten…a hundred and twenty… I disconnect quickly and move smartly on to the next victim before Alec self-combusts.

The final quarter of an hour has been left for questions. Callum goes first 'You were treating my guinea pig but he died.' 'No Callum, that is a *statement*, not a question,' the teacher steps in immediately; my bacon is saved. 'Do have to be clever to be a vet?' and 'Do you make lots of money?' require a little fancy footwork, but even at the top of the hour, questions are still coming thick and fast, and I wonder if I am to be here all day, until the teacher calls a halt, explaining that another guest is expected – a fireman. After a vote of thanks I escape, passing our local fire chief in full regalia. That will make the tiny pyromaniacs' day.

Next day, I am walking briskly up the high street after depositing my car in the garage for its service. 'Hiya, Kate,' 'Hello Kate,' I am greeted by children heading down the road to the school. Once in the surgery, there is a knocking at the window, and I turn to spy several cheeky faces peering in and waving madly. I have had celebrity status since the school talk. Some kids are altogether too familiar, not savvy enough to sense that my easy-going manner in the classroom does not always extend to the surgery, especially when under pressure. Still, fame is transient, and we are off tonight for a few days at Pitdreel to steel ourselves before the Christmas rush. We have had no time off for two months, and I must admit to getting rather twitchy after that length of time without a break. I must work on the time-off situation in the New Year.

Poor Jay is already in the middle of a pre-Christmas rush and will need to leave me and dogs for work on some days, but at least we will have some relaxation and a chance to finish Christmas shopping. The magic of Pitdreel works immediately. We take an evening walk to a vantage point overlooking the harbour and stand in a howling gale while the dogs decide which patch of grass to favour with a wee. A half moon shines across the water, illuminating the bay as do the flashing lighthouses out on the dark expanse of water. A trip to the chippie for fish suppers sets our holiday off to a good start.

Chapter 45

Up early yet again for the dogs – a long lie would be nice but isn't possible while they will not urinate in the concrete yard. However, we have a plan. Careful observation has shown that they enthusiastically water seaweed on the beach, so we return from our walk with a bagful of seaweed to spread on the flagstones. Jay is leaving tonight for an early appointment tomorrow so if I don't fancy a walk, it will be luxury just to let the dogs into the yard before bed.

Unfortunately, things do not go as expected. At 11 p.m., I duly open the back door and the dogs troop out. As they inspect the new surface in the yard, I realise to my horror that a swarm of flies from the seaweed have migrated into the house and are dancing and bobbing round the kitchen light. Swatting proves a mistake, barely denting the dark cloud and leaving black smears on the ceiling. This is like a bad horror movie, there is no way I am going to bed with this lot in the house.

Luckily cold logic eventually supercedes helpless panic. Like Sigourney Weaver in *Alien*, I swing into action. *So they like light, do they?* Extinguishing the kitchen light, I flick on the switch in the hall and wait with bated breath. It works! The buzzing mass transfers its affections to the hall ceiling. Next, porch light on and hall off. Once they are contained in the porch, I shut the hall door, switch off the porch light and, with a flourish, open the outer door on to the street. With me flapping a magazine wildly to persuade them, the invaders give in and make their way gradually to the nearest street light. Having single-handedly cleared our territory of the insect menace, and feeling ridiculously pleased with myself, I switch off all lights and head to bed.

Once dawns breaks, an early mission to surprise any remaining flies – lights off; door swiftly opened and shut, the offending seaweed stuffed back into its bin bag and we head off for our walk. At the point, an orange-pink sky bathes the bay, followed by the appearance of a vast orange sun which lumbers slowly above the horizon. Half an hour later, it is obscured by cloud. One advantage of early rising is that you frequently get the best of the day.

With Jay away, the morning is my own. I plan to spend it indulging in a ceremonial walkabout as practised in Clayfern … and presumably most small villages countrywide. At the surgery in Clayfern, we stock a range of ethical pet food which is available in two, five and ten kilogram bags.

The bigger the bag, the more economical the purchase. The pet food representative cannot understand why we sell more two kilogram bags than any other size, and has no doubt decided that either (a) we do not explain the economics of the situation to our clientele, or (b) our clientele are a bit thick. Not a bit of it. It just happens that the two kilogram bag best fits our customers' requirements. It is compact, easy to carry … and runs out in a reasonable time. This enables the surgery to be on the regular itinerary of the locals. A typical day might go as follows. For someone at the top of the town, they might call in at the baker's, our surgery, the greengrocer's, the post office and the chemist's, pausing for a chat in each thus ending up at the community centre just in time for a mid-morning coffee. This is an incredibly civilised way to spend a morning and is just what I have in mind.

I start off at my favourite shop The Fisherman's Mutual. It sells everything – clothes, kitchen utensils, ironmongery, gifts and fishing gear, the list is endless. Every so often, they must receive a job lot of designer gear as the occasional batch of Calvin Klein T-shirts will be found amongst the yellow waterproof seaman's overalls. I buy gloves for Jay who has given up being a tough guy and has even been squeezing into my fleece jacket against the snell Pitdreel winds; and a hat – or cap really – for myself. It has earflaps which pin above the head when not required. I feel like Deputy Dawg in it (*that* shows my age) and must look a sight, but needs must in sub-arctic temperatures

… oh, and a sieve for the kitchen. Along the waterfront, waves smash on the rocks and my eyes water mercilessly until I turn into a narrow wynd leading to the fish shop. I am going to cook us a special lunch. I enjoy cooking but am not very adventurous while on duty. It can be disastrous to get an emergency call in the middle of a complicated culinary manoeuvre. After the fish shop, the greengrocer, the chemist, the grocer and the novelty shop – the last for gold spray to transform teazel and cow parsley into Christmas decorations.

Back home, I create as the rain pelts down. It is a treat to potter while watching morning television and slurping wine. With perfect timing, a paella finally takes shape just as Jay appears through the door. Oh yes, this is living.

With Jay back, we all head to Elie for our morning walk. Rubies can be found at Ruby bay – Julie (who lived here once) says they are like pieces of red glass. Well, we find plenty pieces of red glass but they are definitely not rubies, they have bits of the manufacturer's name on them. As we head along the cliffs, Fintry is behaving oddly. She walks ahead then suddenly stops and stares into space then continues on her way. We are just getting mildly concerned when we realise what is happening – she is spotting the lighthouse flashing on the point. Funny little dog. She waits until Kippen takes the lead – just in case anything nasty might happen. We hurry to catch up with him as he persists in snuffling on the very edge of sheer drops. His footing is not so sure as in days gone by, so we escort him like agitated sheepdogs, continually chivvying the uncooperative old dog away from the edge. It would be just typical if one of us humans fell over.

After the dogs are fed and watered, Jay and I leave them to head for St Andrews where I have arranged for an eye test with the local optician – or optometrist as they are now called. I have noticed recently an occasional blurring of vision when doing delicate close-up work. At first, this happened mainly during cat dentals, my least favourite procedures, and I wondered briefly if this was a psychological aversion, but it is increasingly clear (or not clear really) that I may be long-sighted. I don't want to end up like my first boss. While stitching up wounds, he would snap frantically with the scissors in the vague direction of the suture ends to be cut, causing much hilarity among his young, able-bodied staff. Despite this quirk, he remained an exceptionally gifted surgeon and faltered at no other stage of the surgery.

I view any medical procedure with deep interest and soon engage the optician/optometrist in a comparison of our patients' retinas (the area at the back of the eye which perceives images and transfers them to the brain). He offers to let me view his own eye with his 'scope. It is really rather boring, containing no tapetum (the reflective layer which gives other species such fantastic colour displays) and consists only of a few blood vessels threading through a dull orange field. I'd rather be a veterinary ophthalmologist.

It is finally established that I do require glasses for close-up work, and I am passed on to an assistant to choose the style. There are various options, but I end up going for the *professional/intelligent* category. After all, who in their right mind would pick any of the others; *sporty, way-out, feminine* (i.e. thick?). Touching on type of material for the lenses, I enquire about cleaning and mention the possibility of occasional blood spatters 'Don't tell me any more,' the assistant cringes, obviously not used to such exacting specifications (or enthusiastic surgeons?).

Wednesday is a half-day in Pitdreel, but the traders are sacrificing their afternoon off to erect the village Christmas tree – freshly cut by the look and smell of it. There is to be a ceremonial switching-on followed by late night shopping on Friday. I must ask Emma if she would mind staying a couple of hours longer so we can participate.

A late walk with the dogs to our beach. The sun has set and the sky is the lemon/aquamarine blend so typical of winter evenings here. The moon appears, bleaching the rolling breakers an improbable white like that in the typical above-fireplace picture of white horses galloping along a beach in moonlight. We disturb a curlew who flies low and swift, his haunting cry raising hairs at the back of my neck.

Out again tonight, in fact back to St Andrew's for a trip to the cinema (we really party when on holiday). The cinema here is reminiscent of the cinemas of our youth. None of your multiplex rubbish or slick ticket counters. At five minutes to six exactly, the ticket-seller appears carrying two wooden boxes and clambers into her booth. Unhurriedly she settles into her chair and arranges the boxes side by side. One contains tickets, little raffle-ticket-like tabs of coloured paper; the other the money. Be there two or two hundred in the queue, this routine never varies. 'Stalls or balcony?' she suddenly asks a bemused Jay who, taken by surprise, opts for stalls – the favoured seats for theatre- goers, but the second class of the cinema world.

The main auditorium is BIG. Murals of local scenes decorate the walls, while in the corner stands a clock with an illuminated face. Not working, in fact hasn't been as long as I can remember. There is a musty aroma, probably emanating from the faded velvet seats. Suddenly there is a brief cry as an unfortunate customer leans too far back in his seat and is deposited in the lap of the person behind. Another broken chair – useful to note their position and sit behind them to ensure an unimpeded view of the screen. I couldn't say what film we saw, but the entire experience was extremely enjoyable. A visit to a modern multi-screen cinema is not a patch on one to this survivor from a time gone by.

The last day of our break dawns. The Christmas-tree lighting will be the finale. As it happens it is almost a damp squib. As a straggly bunch cluster round the tree in the driving rain, an ancient Landrover screams round the corner into the square and screeches to a halt. Santa leaps out, switches the lights on with no preamble and disappears smartly into his grotto in the café. 'You could have got by just booking Emma for an extra half an hour,' Jay whispers as the throng rapidly disperses into the shops to partake of the proffered mince pies and glasses of wine. The shopkeepers have put on a good show and we spend some time circulating and munching the odd pie, but time marches inexorably on: like Cinderella, I have to leave to be home by midnight – or in my case, by 9 p.m.

While Emma briefs me on the significant cases of the week, there is a knock at the door – a deer has been run down just along the road; it is still alive, can we do something? Both vets scramble to assist. The deer – a little roe – looks perfect as we approach, head up, ears revolving, but her rear end is a bloody mess. There is nothing for us to do but put her to sleep. What a contrast from our happy Christmas spirit of only an hour ago. Emma departs shortly afterwards, leaving me sinking in a post-holiday mire, unwilling to be dragged back to the realities of veterinary life. It is hard to be festive when you have just put Bambi to sleep.

Chapter 46

Wet and windy still. Up the hill, the dogs wallow in their own private sea. The standing water comes up to Kippen's elbows. We have only minutes to enjoy this novelty before the first call of the day – to put an old dog to sleep. I fear that this might be the beginning of the Christmas run. Deaths are inevitable at this time of year, but the contrast with festive merry making serves to make them all the more miserable. These owners are all for leaving the dog with Jay and me, but I persuade them to stay. From the dog's point of view, it must be frightening to be suddenly abandoned with strangers. It is best that the owners are there to comfort and calm them. I explain that the procedure is virtually painless, all the patient feels is a pinprick, but even that is minimised with a smear of local anaesthetic.

Luckily Jay is here to hold up a vein for me so all the owners have to do is to concentrate on their pet.

I trim up the foreleg vein and apply local anaesthetic before drawing pentobarbitone into a syringe.

This is an overdose of anaesthetic and the dog will merely go to sleep. Some owners come for this procedure with fear and dread saying 'Oh, he knows.' Gently I counter that he doesn't. All he knows is that his beloved family are upset and that in itself upsets him. Superhuman task that it is, it is best that owners try to keep their emotions reined in and brightly reassure and chat to their pet. The needle slips smoothly into the vein and deep within me, a small knot of tension releases – always a tense moment. Once the syringe is empty, the dog sighs deeply and folds gently on to the table. 'Is that all it is?' is the frequent shocked comment. It is a really peaceful way to go and, in hindsight, owners are pleased they stayed. The reality is so much better than what they might have imagined. Quickly I mention that the dog may gasp or even quiver slightly – both purely reflex actions which occur after death. His eyes stay open unless the lids are manually closed. Surprisingly, this is the relaxed position for eyes – hard to believe when one is fighting to stay awake.

We have planned to put up our Christmas decorations today, and are soon hauling them from the attic. 'Perhaps the illuminated reindeer will annoy Honky and we will end up with an irate stag in the living room,' I laugh. 'There's one here now,' says Jay, launching Kippen into the room wearing flashing antlers bought in a merry moment while on holiday. He quite suits them and plays up to the occasion while Fintry, true to form, decides to be scared, but about-faces smartly when some festive chews appear.

During the course of the day, I end up putting another dog and a cat to sleep. So far, my weekend total is two dogs, a cat and a deer. 'Put Bambi's lights out when you come upstairs,' shouts Jay as we head to bed. 'I'm good at that,' I mutter, giving in to a moment of sarcasm marking the beginning of our annual Christmas 'grim-reaper' phase.

In the newsagent next day, I bump into Primary 3's teacher. 'I've posted their thank-you letters through your door,' she mentions, overheard by a small pupil who pipes up 'I didn't write to you, I wrote to the fireman.' Teacher and I glance at each other and giggle 'That's put you in your place,' she laughs. Certainly has. My celebrity phase must be over.

The letters make enjoyable reading, containing such gems as 'Thanks for bringing the machine to show us we are alive,' and 'I tutched a wurum and I was very happy.'(*strange* child.) It is dry today for a change, but seriously windy. I am a little reluctant to take the car through the trees up the hill in the gale but risk it. All other walks in the fields are completely water logged. I need to stop several times en route to haul branches off the track and can only hope that none fall as we are passing. I did think of getting Jay an off-road driving voucher for Christmas, but slithering and sliding up here will do. At this time of year, the car is a uniform grey-brown. There are several trees down

– we must get up with the chainsaw to chop up some logs. Each type of wood burns differently – pine is good for resuscitating half-dead fires while beech burns for ages. I have carrots for the deer, and both Honky and Charlie come running when they hear 'Cooommme on,' and the rattle of the bag.

I collect more pine cones for the florist, and once home, lay them on a tray by the Rayburn to dry.

Then it is time to stock up the fireside with coal and logs, arrange washing on the pulley and prepare the supper. Chores seem to multiply in winter but at least the garden has stopped growing.

Grim-reaper phase continuing, this week I have put to sleep approximately four times our average number of pets (if there is such a thing as average). Another stressor at this time of year is the distinct impression we have of being manipulated by some clients. They have so much on, that the ill animal is not noticed until after surgery, or at the very last minute. Two extra operations today fall into this category. One is a rabbit whose incisors are vastly overgrown. This has not just happened, but the owner turned up this morning completely out of the blue, and we cannot put it off until the next ops day – it is hardly the rabbit's fault. The next is a dental which was due in yesterday but whose owner simply failed to appear, having had something more exciting to do. Again not the dog's fault so we squeeze him in as well.

Being pushed for time does not make for a relaxing operating session and the situation is made worse by the unexpected deterioration of a dog seen earlier in the week. On Monday, Lilac, a sweet little cross-collie bitch came in for a check-up. Nothing spectacular, just a little quiet and eating less than normal. An examination found no abnormalities. She was cheery enough in the surgery, accepting a few biscuit treats, and, as she had been in season two months earlier, I suspected the beginnings of a false pregnancy and dispensed hormonal drugs. Now she has eaten and drunk nothing for the last two days and is looking decidedly peaky. Still no symptoms to hang one's hat on; what could it be? At this stage, the world is our oyster. She will have to be admitted for fluids and tests.

Our only good luck this morning is that Sheila has come to collect some cat food and mentions she is heading into Stramar. Rapidly, we collect some blood from the miserable Lilac, and Sheila takes a sample to drop off at the lab so that we can get a rapid result on haematology (the relative numbers of various cells in the blood). The biochemistry sample we run ourselves, but again no abnormalities show up. Top contenders in the differential diagnosis list so far are infected womb – less common in younger dogs and usually accompanied by some symptoms, but possible – and foreign body – certainly common in younger dogs, but also generally accompanied by symptoms such as vomiting or tender abdomen. Nothing obvious shows up on x-ray; some gas in the guts but no specific sign of any obstruction. We put her on a drip and await the haematology results which are faxed through later in the day. Surprise, surprise, nothing abnormal. My main interest in the haematology results was to see if the white cell count was increased. This occurs if infection is present, and a large increase would be suggestive of a pyometra (infected womb).

After a day on a drip, Lilac has brightened up a little so I send her home with some recovery diet and an appointment to be seen tomorrow. If there is no improvement, I resolve to open her up just in case there is a foreign body present which is not showing up on x-ray. Having ruled out everything else, an exploratory is our final diagnostic aid. It seems incredible that after batteries of tests and examinations, there are still the odd cases which defy diagnosis. I always feel slightly guilty at this stage, as if it is a personal failing not to have a result, but console myself thinking about the human patients who can spend their life undergoing tests and still not be diagnosed. The possibility of major surgery rather sabotages any plans Julie and I might have for tomorrow. We will be on hold until Lilac reappears in the morning.

The day dawns too soon. Jay and I were at a Christmas party last night, and I could do without the prospect of Lilac hanging over the day. As I feared, she is no better this morning, having eaten and drunk nothing. At least that gives us the green light to go ahead, I think as I install her in a kennel. It would be worse if she had rallied temporarily then gone off again, drawing things out for several days. At least if we find nothing today, then we know she must sink or swim with supportive treatment.

In Clayfern what should come in but *another* rabbit off its food for nearly a week, and yes, his cheek teeth are badly overgrown with sharp spikes growing into his tongue. 'She could have brought him in before now,' I grumble testily to the hapless woman delegated to bring the patient in for her friend, 'We already have one emergency operation and it *is* Saturday. Will you ask her to ring us at 2 p.m. He should be able to go home then.' 'Oh, she's gone shopping and won't be home till teatime – and I've got no transport.' 'Lucky I'm in tonight then,' I grunt, 'Vets do have a life away from the surgery, you know.' I do get ratty at Christmas time, but it isn't this poor woman's fault. She is obviously disgruntled with her friend as well.

The next consultation lightens my mood. An elderly cat with an elderly owner brought in by her son. The cat is losing weight and not eating as well as he used to. His mouth is disgusting. 'I think its probably his teeth but I'll check everything else anyway,' I say, clamping the stethoscope to his chest. Concentrating on my task, I am dimly aware of the old lady speaking incessantly during the entire examination.

'I'm sorry, I couldn't hear you, what were you saying?' 'She thought that,' puts in her son. It reminds me of one of these foreign translation sketches where the foreigner gabbles on for ten minutes only to be translated as 'Yes' or 'No.' Surgery is hectic and I am late returning to Fern. Julie is ready and waiting, and her eyes widen as I carry in the rabbit. 'Sorry, not my fault,' I explain. Luckily, Lilac is already pre-medicated so we can begin immediately. The first finding is food in her stomach; a bit slow in clearing after twelve hours. Following the gut down, the intestine appears rather dark, and not quite its usual pink self. 'It may be just a severe enteritis, but it's a little strange to have no vomiting or diarrhoea,' I muse, finding it harder to follow the path of the intestine. Normally, one goes over it hand after hand, like paying out rope, but this is not happening. Finally, I pull out an entire clump of intestine which seems twisted on its mesentery (the tissue which suspends the abdominal organs) and manually unravel the twist. 'The guts have gone pink!' Julie reports. Well, that's a surprise.

Twisted organs can cause acute life-threatening problems in other species but is seldom seen in dogs or cats (apart from gastric torsions in deep-chested dogs). I would have expected such a case to cause considerable discomfort but Lilac has always been quite relaxed when her abdomen was palpated. Not quite believing it, I check all the other organs, finding nothing untoward. You see something new every day. Lilac is stitched up and returned to her kennel with her drip still running, and we turn our attention to the rabbit.

A spike of tooth is gouging a trench in his tongue and must have been horrendously painful. Lilac awakens while we work, but curls up quietly in the corner of her kennel. At the end of the rabbit's op, Julie hears movement and goes to check. A bizarre sight meets her eyes – Lilac has chewed through the i/v line, and a large puddle of fluid is spreading on the kennel room floor. More seriously, blood is spurting from the end still attached to the dog who is moving round the kennel. It looks like a mad axeman has been at work. The severed line resembles a fire hose, jerking this way and that, spattering walls, floor, ceiling with blood – and Lilac was a white dog. This shows the value of checking recovering animals with great regularity. Lilac has not lost very much blood but a little does go a very long way. It takes a long time to close off the catheter and clear up. We occasionally have dogs pull catheters out, but severing the line is a first.

It is now 3 p.m. and at last we can stop for a lunch of tea and mince pies. Lilac's owner rings and we arrange for her to go home at 4.30 p.m. Julie departs after lunch and I take the despondent dogs out. The weather has gone suddenly colder and there is ice where there has previously been water. It is a pleasure to be on firm ground for a change. Up the hill, the pager goes off – nothing too taxing, just a dog with diarrhoea which I arrange to see after the walk. A few days on a special easily digestible food should do the trick.

In the interval before Lilac's owner is due to arrive, I rush to make something for supper and re-light the woodburner which has gone out due to extreme neglect yesterday. Well, I can't do everything. Donning rubber gloves, I am the midst of dragging charred coals into a large bag when the pager shrills yet again. Muttering some choice Anglo-Saxon words, I scan the digital message *Please telephone Jill as soon as possible.* It is Jill's dog who has the diarrhoea, what on earth can have happened now? He wasn't particularly ill at all. As I dial, I run through the case again – could I have missed something significant? No – when Jill got home with Bruce, she found that her other dog had eaten a packet of rat poison left on the table. 'What is the name of the product?' is my first question, then 'Give him some salty water to make him vomit while I look up the details of the active ingredient, then I'll call you back.'

The bi-monthly Cd-rom on canine medicine is very useful for this sort of scenario as the information it contains is bang up-to-date and can be accessed rapidly. As I feared, Ralph has eaten one of the newer anticoagulant rat poisons. This is unfortunate, as it is particularly efficient (i.e. good at causing internal bleeding leading to death by interfering with normal clotting mechanisms: okay for rodents; not so good for dogs). Treatment is to supply the body with vitamin K. Charcoal is also worthwhile giving if the poison has only recently been taken in. Its purpose is to reduce absorption of the poison out of the gut. A quick check of my supplies shows that although some vitamin K is at this surgery, the bulk of it is in Clayfern. A rapid call to the chemist confirms she has charcoal tablets in stock and although it is nearly closing time, she will wait for me to drive in.

'He has been sick and brought up a heap of stuff' Jill reports when I telephone. Good, as it sounded as if he had eaten a lethal dose. I explain my dash to Clayfern and arrange to meet her back at Fern in twenty minutes. After injecting vitamin K and writing a prescription for a month's supply of the tablet form which she can collect tomorrow in Stramar, we struggle to get some charcoal tablets down the anxious Ralph. Like Lilac, he is also white and, after the messy struggle, the irrelevant thought crosses my mind that we have ended up with both red and white, and black and white dogs today. Ralph will be on vitamin K supplementation for three to four weeks, during and at the end of which we will take blood samples to check clotting times. As he has been sick and brought a fair amount of bait up, it is possible that we are treating unnecessarily, but better to be safe than sorry.

It is now 6.30 p.m. and I have not stopped all day. Typically Jay is due home late and has not been here to help in any way. After two hectic days, I feel absolutely flattened. Events have moved seamlessly up to the time for the rabbit to go home so at last the surgery is finally empty and all kennels clean. Washing my hands yet again, they feel like parched pads of sandpaper or these little wonder sponges which achieve double their size when left in water. They almost visibly swell when lathered with hand cream. Bliss! An hour later, the fire is lit, the tea is cooking in the Rayburn and I try to relax on the settee. Not easy with a tension headache and tons of adrenaline whizzing round the system. The worst possible scenario is to take all evening to wind down – then get another call.

Slept right through until 8 a.m. – must have been tired. I uneasily await the 10 a.m.

consultation with Lilac. If she is not responding I don't know what else to do with her. She turns out to be no worse but not very much better, so I put her on a drip for an hour just to play safe. While we wait for the fluid to run into her circulation, she eats several proffered biscuits so I feel quite optimistic.

Up the hill with the dogs en famille. It is bright and frosty with no wind, a beautiful day to be out and about. Honky comes at the gallop when he is called and gobbles carrots with relish.

Meanwhile, the dogs gobble frozen deer droppings which seem to be particularly desirable. It must be to do with texture as well as taste. The low rays of sunshine illuminate cobwebs shrouding the freshly ploughed field, making them twinkle like natural fairy lights. It reminds us to spray dried teazel and briony with gold paint for Christmas decorations.

Back home, there is a message to call Ralph's owner. He has been sick a couple of times and his owner is panicking. I reassure her that this is probably just the results of his intake of grain, concentrated salt solution and charcoal, and recommend a light diet. The poor woman is going to be on pins for the next few days.

Chapter 47

This morning is blissfully free of our usual routine operations as Sheila is having a day out in Edinburgh. In an attempt to generate some seasonal cheer, I am collecting Edith and bringing her to see the new house. It will be pleasant with mince pies and clotted cream in front of the fire. One snag is that Lilac is due in again – if she is poorly then the cosy plan will have to be abandoned. Luckily, Lilac is doing well and is approaching normal, so I zoom off to pick Edith up like a child let out of school early.

The grand tour of the property ends in the museum where Edith (an ex-nurse) revels in the familiar tools. 'My goodness, they could fairly bleed,' she reminisces, clutching a lethal-looking set of tonsillectomy shears – 'And some patients just had to walk home afterwards.' This makes me very glad that we are living in the twenty first century.

We achieve our coffee and mince pies without interruption, and exchange Christmas presents. I am pleased with one of my offerings – a small *parrot plant* begged as a cutting from my aunt with Edith in mind. The flowers are shaped like a beak; red-edged with a bright yellow interior. I have had the cutting for a while and , as do all house plants in our care, it is beginning to look a little peaky. This is even better from Edith's point of view – a challenge. Her present to me will also be much appreciated – two vouchers for a visit to the theatre.

After this pleasant oasis, clients' strange behaviour resurfaces with a trio of out-of-hours calls.

One dog has been limping for three months; one has been losing weight for a similar period and a cat has had diarrhoea for a week. Perhaps the owners are subconsciously making sure that there are no impediments to an enjoyable Christmas but, at less than a week to the big day, they are not giving us long to sort out the various problems.

I escape up the hill to feed 'my' stag. I can now predict where to find him depending on the weather. It is windy today, blowing from the east so he will probably be in the west side of the woods. He is, lying down in a scraped-out hollow but gets up as I approach and moves towards me showing no fear. He is a magnificent beast, muddy-brown from wallowing, with a fine set of antlers.

I feel so privileged to be so close to him. I throw carrots which he follows and devours, then raises his head enquiringly for more. We must get him a big bag of Tesco's carrots for Christmas. These are his favourites, the large dirty carrots which come in sacks for horses are looked on with disdain. That's all we need, a picky stag.

The shortest day, and it feels it. Not only dark but also misty, the world begins and ends within three hundred yards. On the early dog walk, the sounds of cattle roaring for their breakfast and frustrated hens still locked in their night shed echo eerily through the gloom. We pass the farm muck heap which is covered in a mass of cobwebs, looking as if enclosed in a delicate white net. I hear the odd car going by as we traverse the field but cannot see who it is. This increases the somewhat isolated feeling produced by the mist. We recognise most early commuters as they do us, and it is confirmation that all is well with the world when John, Annie and the old chap in the old Volvo wave as they pass on their way to work.

First into Clayfern surgery this morning is a cat who Emma operated on yesterday to remove her hyperactive thyroid glands. Her owner has been warned about the potential danger of low blood calcium and how this initially makes the patient twitchy. If not treated at this point, the patient can begin to fit and ultimately die. Little Netta has bad ears so her head shakes anyway making diagnosis difficult, but she does seem to be a trifle tottery when she walks so I play safe and administer intravenous calcium slowly and admit her for observation.

Next is an outdoorsie type of client recently moved into this area. 'Do you know anywhere in these parts where I can shoot pigeons over rape?' He enquires. I can be of no help, but consider flippantly that I didn't know pigeons did rape. Are they only shot for that, or for minor dismeanors as well? The unfortunate client looks rather bemused, not used to the warped McKelvie sense of humour.

One of the good things about single-handed practice is that clients tend to come because they like your manner. If they aren't impressed then they go elsewhere. There is none of the 'putting up with one vet while hoping for the one they really like' situation which can occur in multi-person practices. My poor flock are occasionally subjected to my feeble attempts at being humerous but seem to accept it as part of the package and join in with good grace, giving as good as they get.

Last minute blood samples today before the Christmas break. It is so easy to get anxious about losing access to our usual support services over the holidays, but in fact, the gap is only minimal as most of our suppliers are only shut for two days. Unfortunately, as Christmas is on Monday this year, we will have to get through four days without supplies or lab services. I take blood to check Netta's calcium levels, blood from a possible kidney-failure cat and blood from Ralph the rat poison dog to check for anaemia and monitor his clotting times. His blood hardly comes gushing out and it is a struggle to fill the sample tube – no sign of any anticoagulant effect there. He looks very well, this is hopefully a mere formality.

At the end of the morning, Alice and I feel more like vampires than veterinary staff. I will do the first two samples at Fern on our own biochemistry machine and Ralph's owner has volunteered to take his to the lab for specialist procedures so everything is in hand. With a final check to be sure we are not short of vital drugs, I set off for a little rest and recuperation with my old friend Mrs Cross. Eleven o'clock is a good time to visit as the kettle is always on the Rayburn for what Mrs Cross regards as the secret of her longevity – a mug of coffee liberally laced with a generous slug of Drambuie. Well, it is Christmas. A leisurely hour later, laden with another Christmas gift, I return cheerfully home to clean the house and begin to think about catering for our Christmas visitors.

After the usual hectic run up to Christmas, Saturday morning surgery has a quieter feel. Netta the hypocalcaemic cat is still a little twitchy despite lots of oral calcium. She has had so much that we joke she will be going stiff. I stop at the chemists to collect some vitamin D which supposedly helps the absorption of calcium. I must admit to being somewhat anxious about her; she should be doing better by now. There is nothing for it but to continue with what we are doing.

On an expedition to the supermarket in Stramar after surgery, the pager shrills, almost giving us heart attacks. The thought of a dire emergency requiring instant flight while standing in a long checkout queue with a full trolley is a nightmare scenario. Luckily, the caller is quite laid back 'The dog's had diarrhoea since Thursday but we've just missed your surgery. Are you at Fern as I could just pop along now?' 'No, I'm shopping like everyone else,' is my terse reply, before arranging to see the dog later, allowing us time to get home and unpack. I am lurking in the surgery when the car draws up and I have to laugh when a white hanky tied to a stick appears at the window. This sense of humour business works both ways.

The pace of veterinary life finally began to slacken yesterday – Christmas Eve. Netta is improved and has gone home, but is due in later this morning. It is easier to see her – a two minute job with a pleasant cat and owner than risk a relapse later over the holiday period, and a call at an unsocial hour. Yesterday was quiet except for two calls for advice, and one from someone requesting worming tablets which I suspected was a joke (who rings a vet for worming tablets at 8 p.m. on Christmas Eve for heaven's sake?) but turned out to be the real thing. Acertaining that this was merely a precaution as worms had not even been seen, I politely suggested a trip to the surgery when we open again after Boxing Day. 'I can't believe you're so restrained,' Jay said, appalled. 'Well, its easier than getting angry, and I don't want to spoil our evening.' At this time, we were just about to start one of our Christmas traditions – an in-house treasure hunt for small Chrismas-stocking presents. As usual, our clues were excruciating. For example

'*Here is where you get very clean; Look carefully and a clue will be seen*' lead me to the shower, where my prize was an old veterinary dictionary. 'I picked it up in an old book shop for next-to-nothing', Jay explained happily.

The joy of present giving and receiving with loved ones is not the material value of the gift, but the pleasure of knowing that you know and understand each other so well, and go to some trouble to find the very thing that will be just right. Today's unwrapping session goes to prove that. The dogs of course are not left out and excitedly unwrap their (wrapped) squeaky toys. So excited are they that they also attempt to unwrap ours before settling down to play. Typically, Fintry's is de-squeaked in a record ten seconds, and she then tries to get hold of Kippen's. The old chap gives her no quarter; the only ones who can have his toy are Jay and me. Even with his bad legs, he still enjoys a game of 'catch' while lying down. We throw it, he catches it then drops it to start again. They also have new collars – red. Apparently red is a good colour for dogs from the *feng shui* point of view, according to a doggie magazine in the surgery, and, at his age, Kippen needs all the help he can get.

An hour of unrestrained unwrapping later, we recline exhausted on the settee, reviewing our booty. Sheila's offering is a fluffy cat which is activated by pressing his foot. Initial purring is followed by hysterical growling and screaming, a fitting reminder of our feral cat days. The battery is inserted through a velcro-edged flap in its side 'I wish they all had that,' I muse – 'And a switch to turn them off,' Jay adds. Over the years, Julie and Bill, and Jay and I have exchanged cat and badger gifts ad nauseam. We have now moved on – they are concentrating on the nautical theme with items for Pitdreel, while we are retaliating with anything to do with frogs (loosely stemming from Bill's unfortunate encounter with a frog while tiling the yard – another story). My hands and feet are warming up nicely in battery-heated gloves and socks while Jay prepares a cocktail with the new cocktail book and implements.

Before lunch, we all head up the hill to give Honky his festive dinner. Succulent new carrots have been bought especially for the occasion and are much appreciated. I detour into the stubble field to deposit piles of peanuts for the badgers, accompanied by my faithful hounds. Jay is a little hurt that they have both followed me, but soon realises that this is not loyalty but the expectation of a handful of peanuts. Back home to see Netta who is doing well today, and finally, our Christmas dinner. The Rayburn has acquitted itself admirably, which I must admit is something of a relief.

We are just beginng to clear up when the phone goes 'I'm so sorry to disturb you today, but my cat came in half an hour ago and his breathing is really fast and jerky. He was fine earlier this morning.' Down to earth with a bump. While the cat is being brought out, I review the possible causes of such sudden onset symptoms – trauma due to traffic accident, pneumonia, fluid in the chest due to tumour or heart malfunction all spring to mind. All will probably involve considerable time spent in the surgery. Damn and blast! The last thing I could do with after such a mammoth meal. I was thinking more of three hours on the settee.

The cat comes, and looks surprisingly alert. 'He seems to have perked up on the way,' explains the embarrassed owner, a nice lady not given to false alarms. An examination discovers that his temperature is high, his eyes are watery and his lymph glands are enlarged. Close questioning reveals that he has been heard sneezing once or twice recently. Off the hook, thank goodness. The cat looks as if he has a respiratory virus and it turns out that the room that he was in was very warm. His increased breathing was merely him panting to try to cool down. An anti-inflammatory injection and an antibiotic is all that is required. 'I left my husband doing the dishes,' she laughs, relieved. 'So's mine,' I reply, 'Perhaps we should spin this out for a few minutes longer till they're finished.' Every cloud has a silver lining.

Chapter 48

We are gently easing back to work after the Christmas break. Getting up in the dark again is dire. The weather has got colder and colder since Christmas, cars and roofs are covered in layers of frost and the roads are particularly icy since the water draining off the fields has frozen, leaving solid rivers of ice stretching from one side to the other. Jay is helping me with morning surgery as Cath is on holiday.

The frantic feel to the place has gone now, and the surgery remains quiet until moments from closing time when several customers troop in. All been having long lies, no doubt.

Back at the Fern surgery, we have one or two minor procedures to carry out. A kitten x-ray to find out if it has fractured its pelvis – it hasn't; rest and painkillers should do the trick. Then a rabbit with bad teeth who really *should* have joined our pre-Christmas rush. I don't think he will have had much of a feast on Christmas day. On being returned to his cage after his teeth trim, he dives straight into the bowl of food and makes up for lost time. Netta comes in again. She seems alright today, but persists in having the occasional shaky do. She is going to stay at the surgery over New Year as her owner is a nurse and is due to work some very long shifts, leaving the cat on her own. While we pore over her work rota, Netta roams the surgery, inspecting interesting corners before making a bed for herself amongst the stored bedding. 'She really is quite at home here,' her owner laughs. I just wish that she could make some more convincing progress. Despite large quantities of oral calcium, and vitamin D to aid its absorption, her calcium levels remain low. Some species require sunlight for vitamin D synthesis – perhaps we should take Netta up the hill and expose her to the sun like a primitive sacrificial offering.

Without Netta, but with the dogs, we head up the hill after the kitten and rabbit are collected.

There has been some powdery snow, giving a dusting to the fields. If only there were more, it would be ideal for ski-ing or sledging. It is also bitterly cold, probably about six degrees below zero. Jay's present of the heated gloves and socks is proving prophetic. Bundled up like Michelin men, we scrunch satisfyingly through the snow to the woods, Honky's likely haunt in this weather. When I shout, he heads over purposefully. No mistaking his intentions, *he wants carrots*. I feel like Nanook of the North, enclosed in my winter gear amid snow-covered firs, communing with a semi-tame stag. He comes so close that I can hear his crunching and see minute details on his antlers and skin. He holds my gaze with liquid tan eyes. From beside the water trough, Jay laughs and I look up enquiringly to see Charlie, Honky's son who is still in the pen, bobbing his head frantically up and down by the fence, distraught at missing the goodies. While I continue with Honky, Jay takes Junior a handful.

The sky is intriguing as we head for home – broad swathes of purple, blue, cream and pale orange decorate the western sky. Could there be more snow to come? After surgery, we pause in our brisk dash into the house to listen to the blood-curdling screams of a fox looking for a mate. I hope someone picks it to put it out of its misery! Jay has been shopping for essential supplies so tonight we have a treat, the first of – I hope – many cocktails, a Blue Balalaika (vodka, cointreau, blue curacao, lemon juice and ice, as if there wasn't enough around). This hobby is well worth encouraging.

We are still in that strange half-world between work and holiday. The village is dead as I head to the Clayfern surgery; only one or two intrepid souls braving the frost. Other parts of the country have had snow – WHY CAN'T WE? Everyone talks of snow with trepidation, but all my childhood fantasies involved snow, sledges and frozen forests, and I love it. There are several visitors to the surgery, some being the aftermath of our pre-Christmas rush. Stitches out for Lilac, now a hundred per cent, and check-ups for others. After some coaching, Netta's owner is injecting her today and tomorrow morning before leaving for her day shift. I hope all goes well There are more ops today than we've had for a week – two private cat spays and a dental, and the same for Sheila. 'I wish we got more "owned" cat spays,' I think, finishing the second one before Sheila arrives. I can do cat spays in my sleep; they are no trouble and are a welcome financial boost.

As I work through Sheila's (heavily discounted) spays, the snow begins to fall in earnest. Luckily all today's owners have been primed to phone early about their pets so they can go home before the weather closes in. By 2 o'clock they have all gone, and we load the last of Sheila's into her car.

Into the car and up the hill bearing gifts for the livestock. Up here, there is absolute stillness, the only sound the slight hiss of heavily falling snow. Honky spies us from a tangle of felled logs and fairly sprints across. 'Oh, heck!' I think, slightly wary of his uninhibited approach, 'Come *on*, Kippen,' I gesture frantically to the deaf old dog who is snuffling absently on the field, totally unaware of the impending arrival of approximately a hundred and fifty kilograms of speeding stag. Luckily Honky stops about ten feet from us and begins on the carrots that I have thrown. I hope I have not created a monster. If he gallops like that at other people, they will have heart failure – and what happens if they don't have carrots? Even a gentle nudge with that antler-bedecked head would be no joke. On reflection, that is unlikely to happen. He is quite shy when anyone strange comes along with me and keeps well away. I have to leave my companion and walk towards him. Just as well really.

The track down the hill is treacherous. Any braking and the car slides towards the steep drop on one side. I have to engage first gear and crawl down at a snail's pace. The road to Clayfern is slippy too and I arrive late. Luckily the surgery is quiet, but typically, the pager goes off as Jay and I are on our way to friends for dinner. 'The dog seems very stiff and reluctant to get up,' is the information the owner gives me over the phone. 'Has he had much exercise today?' I enquire. 'Just a minute, I'll ask my son.' After a pause, the slightly embarrassed owner reports 'It appears that he was run into by a sledge.' A few more questions to make sure that there are no worrying symptoms then I suggest half an aspirin, and promise to telephone in an hour to check that the dog has settled down. At least, that gives us enough time to eat. Fortunately all is well, and it is not until very much later that we finally do wend our way home.

Netta the hypocalcaemic cat is staying in the surgery while her owner is working away over New Year. She is a bright little button now and definitely regards the surgery as her second home, marching around after me as I potter. She has put on half a kilogram since her operation, a quarter of her bodyweight. Almost rivalling my weight gain over the holidays. After attending to her, we head up the hill with the chainsaw and a bagful of carrots. This time Charlie and the girls enjoy a snack but there is no sign of Honky. All the while that we are cutting logs, we keep looking over our shoulders for him. The theme from *Jaws* springs to mind. I must keep a carrot in my pocket during all walks to keep him at bay if we encounter him unawares.

After the mandatory Netta visit, for which Jay is dragged in to give the cat someone new to talk to, we enjoy a relaxed afternoon watching an old film on the television and sipping a cocktail — a banana daquhiri, our favourite so far. It is pleasant coorying in by the woodburner while snow begins to fall, eddying and swirling past the windows. The view outside is sombre, the river slate-gray and the trees dark and skeletal, but we are warm in our little den.

After the film, we visit Netta with a saucer of milk. Not a long visit, just enough to break the monotony for her while we switch on the lights in the kennel and ops rooms. Rested and relaxed, we are off to sledge on the field, illuminated by the surgery lights. The dogs are very excited, even old Kippen. In his prime, he would accompany the sledger up and down the slope, often grabbing a passing arm or leg in his excitement, causing many a collision. Now he contents himself with barking wildly and lying in wait at the bottom of the hill for prey to come to him. Soon I have to switch off the batteries in my gloves and even lend them to Sheila when she comes to join in the fun.

Thoroughly exhilarated after the first and last sledging of 2000, we have supper then wash and change before setting off to an Old Year's Night ceilidh, picking Sheila up en route. Bill and Julie are already there, saving a table for our gang. People file in bearing baskets and bags of goodies for sustenance. On our table of twelve, we have crisps, dips, sausage rolls, vol-au-vents, shortbread, dumpling and oatcakes and cheese – and we've all had our evening meals. Soon nearly everyone is dancing. It is a particularly good night and later, the crook of my arm starts to ache. For anyone fairly small, when partners link arms to birl round, the upper arm catches it. Most of us will be extremely stiff tomorrow – but it's worth it. As always, all ears are peeled for the pager but it stays quiet. Home later to our animals, and family phone calls before falling into bed.

What a good way to see in the New Year. It should be quiet tomorrow barring emergencies – but you never just know for certain.

Total unpredictability is both the blessing and the curse of this job.